Issues in Complementary Feeding

**Nestlé Nutrition Workshop Series
Pediatric Program, Vol. 60**

Issues in Complementary Feeding

Editors
Carlo Agostoni, Milan, Italy
Oscar Brunser, Santiago, Chile

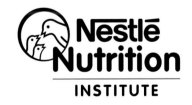

Nestec Ltd., 55 Avenue Nestlé, CH–1800 Vevey (Switzerland)
S. Karger AG, P.O. Box, CH–4009 Basel (Switzerland)   www.karger.com

Printed in Switzerland on acid-free paper by Reinhardt Druck, Basel
ISSN 1661–6677
ISBN: 978–3–8055–8283–4

Library of Congress Cataloging-in-Publication Data

Nestlé Nutrition Workshop (60th : 2006 : Manaus, Brazil)
    Issues in complementary feeding / editors, Carlo Agostoni, Oscar Brunser.
        p. ; cm. – (Nestlé nutrition workshop series pediatric program,
1661-6677 ; v. 60)
    Includes bibliographical references and index.
    ISBN-13: 978-3-8055-8283-4 (hard cover : alk. paper)
    1. Infants–Nutrition–Congresses. 2. Baby foods–Congresses. I.
Agostoni, Carlo. II. Brunser, Oscar. III. Title. IV. Series: Nestlé
Nutrition workshop series. Paediatric programme ; v. 60.
    [DNLM: 1. Infant Nutrition Physiology–Congresses. W1 NE228D v.60 2007/
WS 120 N468i 2007]
    RJ216.N393 2006
    618.92'02–dc22

                                                    2007020744

KARGER   Basel · Freiburg · Paris · London · New York ·
          Bangalore · Bangkok · Singapore · Tokyo · Sydney

Contents

Contents

Preface

Issues in complementary feeding are among the preferred topics of the Nestlé Nutrition Workshops for many reasons:

(1) The dietary requirements of infants in the weaning period and the effects of the different dietary schedules later in life are still poorly explored on a scientific basis, and are mostly the result of family tradition, country socioeconomic background, and common beliefs.

(2) In developing and, to some extent, in transition countries, malnutrition and undernutrition start immediately after the first 6 months of life, that is after the period of exclusive breastfeeding. Therefore, plans to improve the nutritional quality of available solid foods to be introduced, as well as to educate mothers and families to better accustom their children to complementary feeding, have become an issue of considerable importance in public health interventions.

(3) In developed countries and urban areas of transition countries, early forms of qualitative malnutrition, starting in the complementary feeding period, are now becoming more and more common, with unbalanced supplies of both macronutrients and micronutrients.

(4) An increasing demand for food safety and regulatory norms is emerging from the consumers, particularly emphasized for the 'unprotected' and 'weak' segments of the population represented by infants. Both the media and public opinion are quite sensitive to any news raising questions on 'hidden dangers' within the food chain. Food companies, on the other hand, must rely on rapid mechanisms to protect the consumers and themselves from these 'hidden dangers'.

(5) Finally, recent emphasis on the so-called 'bioactive' compounds is stimulating interest on the possibility of improving the quality of the dietary supply with either natural foods rich in bioactive compounds or industrially enriched foods.

Within this context, the contributors of the present workshop have tried to summarize the status of the art in five main areas pertinent to complementary feeding, indicating in parallel the possible emerging areas of interest for both public health and research. These are the breastfed infant as reference, the issues on nutritional quality and safety in complementary feeding, the different roles of cereals on one hand, and meat and dairy products (inclusive of fermented milk products) on the other, and, finally, the different needs and requirements of special groups (e.g., infants with food allergy or celiac disease) have been thoroughly presented and discussed, taking into special consideration the functional value of nutrients and foods in terms of potential positive effects on later growth, development and health.

The different presentations and topics have therefore provided an opportunity to focus on the composite worldwide situation of complementary feeding; the venue in Manaus, in the heart of the Amazon forest, has been to some extent symbolic of a developed area within a developing region.

Speakers and discussants agreed that a 'holistic' approach is definitely necessary for successful complementary feeding. This approach should consider local resources, traditions, nutritional education, issues of hygiene and food safety and, last but not least, the emerging evidence from clinical trials on the different effects of macronutrients and micronutrients in different settings. Hopefully, the papers presented should be of interest for those dealing with infant growth in the various regions of the world and who have to indicate to mothers and families the more appropriate ways of feeding their children.

C. Agostoni and O. Brunser

Foreword

The 60th Nestlé Nutrition Pediatric Workshop entitled 'Issues in Complementary Feeding' was held in Manaus, Brazil, on 22–26 October 2006, and was our third workshop addressing the extremely important subject of complementary feeding and nutrition during the weaning period, since the creation of the Nestlé Nutrition Workshop Pediatric Program in 1981. 'Weaning; Why, What and When' was the topic of the 10th Nestlé Nutrition Workshop in New Delhi in 1984 (eds. *Angel Ballabriga* and *Jean Rey*); the topics dealt with in that workshop are illustrative of the fact that the role of early feeding in later obesity, atherosclerosis and hypertension and the importance of appropriate complementary feeding for intestinal immunity, were already well recognized at that time. Almost 20 years later, the focus of the 54th Nestlé Nutrition Workshop in Sao Paulo in 2003 was 'Micronutrient Deficiencies during the Weaning Period and the First Years of Life' (eds. *John Pettifor* and *Stan Zlotkin*), highlighting the effects of micronutrient malnutrition on behavior and development, on bone growth and mineralization, immune function and infections, and addressed specific strategies to improve micronutrient status, including targeted fortification of complementary foods. Since then, a considerable body of research has accumulated on areas closely related to complementary feeding such as the appropriate time for gluten introduction, allergy prevention, the adverse effects of whole cow's milk during the first year of life and the importance of cereal-based complementary foods. Up-to-date reviews on these and other topics were presented by the invited speakers from five continents, reflecting the global concern for appropriate complementary foods and feeding practices.

We warmly acknowledge the excellent workshop program conceived by the two Chairpersons, Prof. *Oscar Brunser* from Santiago, and Prof. *Carlo Agostoni* from Milan, both of whom are world-renowned experts in the fields of pediatric nutrition and gastroenterology. Many thanks also to Dr. *Marcelo Freire* and his team from Nestlé Nutrition in Brazil for the efficient logistical support and for enabling the workshop participants to enjoy the wonderful Amazonian environment of Manaus.

Prof. Ferdinand Haschke MD, PhD
Chairman
Nestlé Nutrition Institute
Vevey, Switzerland

Dr. Denis Barclay, PhD
Scientific Advisor
Nestlé Nutrition Institute
Vevey, Switzerland

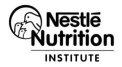

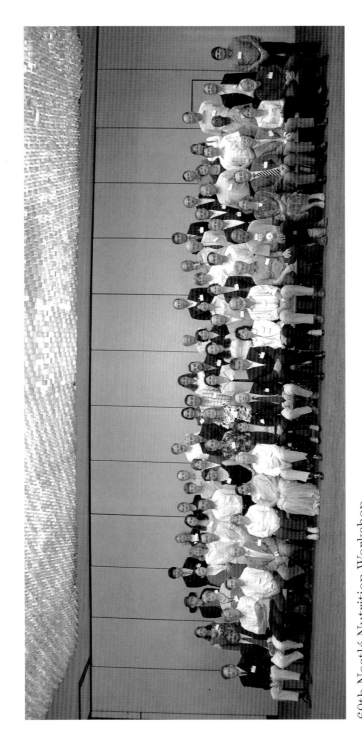

60th Nestlé Nutrition Workshop
Pediatric Program
Manaus, Brazil, October 22–26, 2006

Contributors

Chairpersons & Speakers

Prof. Carlo Agostoni

Department of Pediatrics
University of Milan
San Paolo Hospital
8 Via A di Rudiní
IT–20142 Milan
Italy
E-Mail agostoni@unimi.it

Prof. Kenneth H. Brown

Department of Nutrition and Program
in International and Community
Nutrition
University of California, Davis
One Shields Avenue
Davis, CA 95616
USA
E-Mail khbrown@ucdavis.edu

Prof. Oscar Brunser

Gastroenterology Unit
Institute of Nutrition & Food
Technology (INTA)
University of Chile
Av. El Líbano 5524-Macul
Santiago
Chile
E-Mail obrunser@inta.cl;
brunser@entelchile.net

Dr. Saraswati Bulusu

National Program Manager
The Micronutrient Initiative
11, Zamroodpur Community Center
Kailash Colony Extension
New Delhi 110 048
India
E-Mail sbulusu@micronutrient.org.in

Prof. Magnus Domellöf

Department of Clinical Sciences,
Pediatrics
Umeå University
SE–901 85 Umeå
Sweden
E-Mail magnus.domellof@
pediatri.umu.se

Dr. Elaine L. Ferguson

University of Otago
Department of Human Nutrition
Undergrad Labs, Science 1 Building
700 Cumberland Street
Dunedin 9001
New Zealand
E-Mail elaine.ferguson@
stonebow.otago.ac.nz

Prof. Stefano Guandalini

Section of Pediatric Gastroenterology
Hepatology and Nutrition
University of Chicago
5839 S. Maryland Avenue
Chicago, IL 60637
USA
E-Mail sguandalini@
peds.bsd.uchicago.edu

Prof. Nancy F. Krebs

Department of Pediatrics
University of Colorado
School of Medicine
(UCHSC)
4200 East Ninth Ave-Box C225
Denver, CO 80262
USA
E-Mail nancy.krebs@uchsc.edu

XI

Contributors

Dr. Kirsi Laitinen

Department of Biochemistry and
Food Chemistry &
Functional Foods Forum
University of Turku
Itäinen Pitkäkatu 4A, 5th floor
FI–20014 Turku
Finland
E-Mail kirsi.laitinen@utu.fi

Prof. Kim Fleischer Michaelsen

Department of Human Nutrition
Faculty of Life Sciences
University of Copenhagen
Rolighedsvej 30
DK–1958 Fredriksberg C
Denmark
E-Mail kfm@life.ku.dk

Prof. Lorenzo Morelli

Microbiology Institute
Università Cattolica del Sacro
Cuore (UCSC)
Via Emilia Parmense 84
IT–29100 Piacenza
Italy
E-Mail lorenzo.morelli@unicatt.it

Dr. Francis P. Scanlan

Quality and Safety Department
Nestlé Research Center
PO Box 44
CH–1000 Lausanne 26
Switzerland
E-Mail francis.scanlan@nestle.com

Dr. Atul Singhal

MRC Childhood Nutrition Research
Centre
Institute of Child Health
30 Guildford Street
London WC1N 1EH
UK
E-Mail a.singhal@ich.ucl.ac.uk

Prof. Noel W. Solomons

Center for Studies of Sensory
Impairment
Aging, and Metabolism (CESSIAM)
Avenida 17, 16–89 (interior)
Zona 11 (Anillo Periférico)
Guatemala, 01011, CA
Guatemala
E-Mail cessiam@guate.net.gt

Prof. Dominique Turck

Lille University Children's Hospital
Department of Pediatrics
Clinique de Pédiatrie
Hôpital Jeanne de Flandre
2, avenue Oscar Lambret
FR–59037 Lille
France
E-Mail dturck@chru-lille.fr

Prof. Ekhard E. Ziegler

Department of Pediatrics
University Hospital
200 Hawkins Drive
Iowa City, IA 52242-1083
USA
E-Mail ekhard-ziegler@uiowa.edu

Moderators

Prof. Antonio Celso Calçado

IPPMG
Avenida Brigadeiro Trompowsky
S/N – Ilha do Fundão
21941-590 – Rio de Janeiro-RJ
Brazil
E-Mail acalcado@superig.com.br

Prof. Arthur Delgado

Faculdade de Medicina da
Universidade de São Paulo
Avenida Jacutinga, 352 Ap 81
04515-000 – Moema – São Paulo
Brazil
E-Mail arturfd@uol.com.br

Prof. Clea Rodrigues Leone

Faculdade de Medicina da
Universidade de São Paulo
Alameda Itu, 433 Ap 42 – Jardins
01421-000 – São Paulo
Brazil
E-Mail clealeone@uol.com.br

Prof. Hugo da Costa Ribeiro Júnior

Unidade Metabólica Fima Lifshitz
Federal University of Bahia
Rua Padre Feijó, 29
40110-170 – Salvador, BA
Brazil
E-Mail hugocrj@ufba.br

Prof. Mario Vieira

Center for Pediatric
Gastroenterology and Nutrition
Hospital Pequeno Príncipe
Rua Desembargador Motta, 1070
80250-060 – Curitiba-PR
Brazil
E-Mail gastroped@hpp.org.br

Invited attendees

Mónica Edith Del Compare/Argentina
Gisélia Alves/Brazil
Silvana Benzecry/Brazil
Vera Bezerra/Brazil
Luiza Amélia Cabus/Brazil
Maria do Carmo Melo/Brazil
Ary Cardoso/Brazil
Fernanda Luisa Ceragioli Oliveira/
 Brazil
Mauro Fisberg/Brazil
Rosa Gusmão/Brazil
Christiane Leite/Brazil
Hélcio Maranhão/Brazil
Elza Mello/Brazil
Roberto Nogueira/Brazil
Carlos Alberto Nogueira de Almeida/
 Brazil
Themis Reverbel da Silveira/Brazil
Hélio Rocha/Brazil
Cristina Targa Ferreira/Brazil
Virgínia Weffort/Brazil

Ernest Seidman/Canada
Francisco Moraga/Chile
Enrique Boloña/Ecuador
Monica Reyes/Ecuador
Ollil Simell/Finland
Tuula Simell/Finland
Sayyed Morteza Safavi/Iran
Giacomo Biasucci/Italy
Mario De Curtis/Italy
Marcello Giovannini/Italy
Marco Sala/Italy
Mary Fewtrell/UK
Bede Ibe/Nigeria
Mary Jean Guno/Philippines
John Uy/Philippines
Ricardo Ferreira/Portugal
Salome Kruger/South Africa
Sungkom Jongpiputvanich/
 Thailand
Isdore-Evans Pazvakavambwa/
 Zimbabwe

Nestlé participants

Dr. Marcelo Freire/Brazil
Mr. Rubens Magno/Brazil
Mrs. Marília Rosado/Brazil
Mr. Roberto Sato/Brazil
Louis Dominique Van Egroo/France
Dr. Annette Järvi/Sweden
Dr. Denis Barclay/Switzerland

Dr. Kay Dowling/Switzerland
Dr. Marie-Odile Gailing/Switzerland
Prof. Ferdinand Haschke/Switzerland
Mr. Stefan Kubacsek/Switzerland
Dr. Yasaman Shahkhalili/Switzerland
Dr. Simona Stan/Switzerland
Ms. Deepali Darira/UK

Agostoni C, Brunser O (eds): Issues in Complementary Feeding.
Nestlé Nutr Workshop Ser Pediatr Program, vol 60, pp 1–13,
Nestec Ltd., Vevey/S. Karger AG, Basel, © 2007.

Breastfeeding and Complementary Feeding of Children up to 2 Years of Age

Kenneth H. Brown

Department of Nutrition and Program in International and Community Nutrition,
University of California, Davis, CA, USA

Abstract

Appropriate breastfeeding and complementary feeding practices are fundamental
to children's nutrition, health, and survival during the first 2 years of life. The World
Health Organization recommends exclusive breastfeeding until 6 months of age and
continued breastfeeding for at least 2 years, along with the timely introduction of adequate amounts of complementary foods of suitable nutritional and microbiological
quality. The amounts of energy and micronutrients required from complementary
foods have been estimated as the difference between the total physiological requirements of these food components and the amounts transferred to the child in breast
milk. Recommendations for the energy density of complementary foods and their frequency of feeding have also been proposed. Intakes of several micronutrients, including iron, zinc, calcium, selected B vitamins and (in some settings) vitamin A, remain
problematic because commonly available, low-cost foods contain inadequate amounts
of these nutrients to provide the shortfall in breast milk. Alternative strategies to provide these nutrients include adding animal source foods to the diet, providing fortified,
processed complementary foods, administering micronutrient supplements, or offering some combination of these approaches. Advantages, disadvantages, and possible
risks of these different strategies are discussed.

Introduction

The first 2 years of life represent an especially challenging period for children's nutrition and health because their relatively high metabolic rates and
rapid rates of growth during this period impose proportionately greater nutrient requirements. Moreover, the immaturity of young children's gastrointestinal tract, neuromuscular coordination, and immunological function limits the
types of foods that they are able to consume and exposes them to an elevated

risk of food-borne infections and food allergies. For these reasons, recommendations on optimal child feeding must take into consideration the children's age-specific physiological requirements for essential nutrients, the appropriate food (or other) sources of these nutrients, and proper methods for preparing and feeding these foods. The World Health Organization (WHO) currently recommends that, '…infants should be exclusively breastfed during the first six months of life. Thereafter they should receive nutritionally adequate and safe complementary foods while breastfeeding continues up to two years of age and beyond' [1]. The evidence base for these recommendations will be discussed briefly below.

For this review, the definitions of infant feeding practices proposed by the WHO will be applied [2]. In particular, 'exclusive breastfeeding' is defined as the consumption of no other food or liquids except breast milk and small amounts of medicines or vitamin-mineral supplements for at least 4 and if possible the first 6 months of life. The term 'predominant breastfeeding' is applied when the infant's major source of nourishment is breast milk, but water and water-based drinks, such as flavored water, teas, and herbal infusions, or fruit juices are also consumed. Complementary feeding refers to the consumption of both breast milk and other foods, usually during the period from 6 to ~24 months of age, until the child ceases to nurse at the breast and is able to consume the same foods as the rest of the family.

The physiological requirements for nutrients do not differ for children in lower income countries and economically more developed ones. Thus, recommendations for infant and young child feeding should be similar in each setting. Nevertheless, proper feeding of infants in resource-poor settings is often more challenging because of limited access to high-quality, nutrient-rich foods, inadequate environmental sanitation, and lack of clean sources of water and proper facilities for food preparation and storage. Thus, recommendations for appropriate breastfeeding practices assume even greater importance for infants raised in these circumstances. Although the appearance of HIV infection in some of these same countries has complicated infant feeding recommendations, standard guidelines still apply for the vast majority of infants worldwide, so these general recommendations will be the focus of the present paper.

A complete discussion of all aspects of breastfeeding and complementary feeding is beyond the scope of this review. Several excellent general texts are available on breastfeeding [3] and complementary feeding [4]. Thus, this presentation will focus on just a few of the most salient issues regarding feeding recommendations, with a primary focus on infants and young children in lower income settings. In particular, information will be presented on: (1) the optimal duration of exclusive breastfeeding, (2) energy and nutrient requirements from complementary foods, and (3) available strategies for satisfying the micronutrient needs of young children during the vulnerable period of complementary feeding.

Appropriate Duration of Exclusive Breastfeeding

Exclusive breastfeeding during the first months of life is associated with reduced rates of diarrhea and other infections [5, 6], and a multicenter study by WHO in Brazil, Pakistan and the Philippines indicated that both exclusive and predominant breastfeeding are associated with reduced infant mortality [7]. The pooled odds ratios of mortality associated with nonbreastfeeding declined progressively with increasing infant age, ranging from 5.8 (95% CI 3.4–9.8) during the first 2 months of life and 4.1 (2.7–6.4) for 2- to 3-month-olds to 1.4 (0.8–2.6) for 9- to 11-month-olds.

Current recommendations for the duration of exclusive breastfeeding are based on a systematic review of intervention trials and observational studies carried out in both lower income and more affluent countries, which assessed the rates of growth of infants who were breastfed exclusively for 6 months versus those who were partially breastfed or nonbreastfed, as well as their respective rates of infections [8]. Two of the three available controlled intervention trials were conducted in a lower income country, Honduras. In the first of these studies, infants were randomly assigned to one of three feeding regimens: (1) exclusive breastfeeding until 6 months of age, (2) exclusive breastfeeding until 4 months of age at which time high-quality, packaged complementary foods were started and breastfeeding was continued ad libitum, or (3) exclusive breastfeeding until 4 months at which time complementary feeding was initiated as above along with explicit encouragement to maintain breastfeeding frequency [9]. There were no significant differences in the children's total energy intakes despite the additional energy provided by complementary foods, and there were no differences in their growth velocities from 4 to 6 months. The authors concluded that there was no advantage of introducing complementary foods before 6 months, whereas there may be considerable risks of inadequate nutrient intakes and food-borne infections if the nutritional and hygienic quality of the foods cannot be assured. The second Honduras study yielded similar conclusions, even though all infants enrolled weighed less than 2,500 g at birth [10].

In another large trial conducted in Belarus, more than 17,000 newborns were randomly assigned by clinic to receive an intervention designed to promote appropriate breastfeeding practices. Infants in the intervention group were significantly more likely to be breastfed exclusively at 3 months of age (43.3 vs. 6.4%), and they had a significantly lower occurrence of one or more episodes of diarrhea (9.1 vs. 13.2%) and atopic eczema (3.3 vs. 6.3%) [11]. Based on these intervention trials and other published observational studies, the aforementioned WHO review concluded that, 'the available evidence demonstrates no apparent risk in recommending, as public health policy, exclusive breastfeeding in both developing and developed country settings' [8].

Energy and Nutrient Requirements from Complementary Foods

Estimates of the amounts of energy and nutrients required from complementary foods have been derived by subtracting the mean amounts provided by breast milk to children of different ages from their estimated total requirements [4]. These estimates were recently revised [12], using updated information on infant energy requirements obtained from direct measures of energy expenditure and physical growth, including body composition [13]. According to these updated estimates, the average amounts of energy required from complementary foods are approximately 200, 300 and 550 kcal/day for infants 6–8, 9–11, and 12–23 months of age, respectively.

Similar calculations of the amounts of specific nutrients required from complementary foods is complicated by the fact that existing sets of estimates of nutrient requirements are not always consistent. Moreover, in many cases these estimates are simply extrapolated from older age groups or derived from observations of presumably adequate intakes by apparently healthy children rather than from direct measurements of physiological requirements [12]. These issues have been described elsewhere in more detail, along with their implications for estimating the nutrient requirements from complementary foods [12]. Focused research on the nutrient requirements of young children remains a pressing need.

Energy Density and Frequency of Feeding Complementary Foods

To formulate adequate complementary feeding regimens to satisfy young children's total energy requirements, both the frequency of feeding and the energy density of complementary foods must be taken into consideration. When more meals are provided each day, the complementary foods can be prepared with lower energy density and vice versa. Empirical data from several studies indicate that both factors contribute independently to total daily energy intakes, as illustrated in figure 1 [14]. Using these empirical data, the minimum adequate energy density has been estimated for children of several age groups considering different possible levels of feeding frequency (table 1), using assumptions described previously in more detail [4, 12]. It should be noted, however, that most of the available information on young children's food intakes used for these estimates was collected from nonbreastfed children, so additional data are still needed from those who are continuing to nurse at the breast.

It is conceivable, for example, that overzealous feeding (i.e., excessive feeding frequency or energy density of complementary foods) may inadvertently displace breast milk or contribute to undesirably high energy intakes.

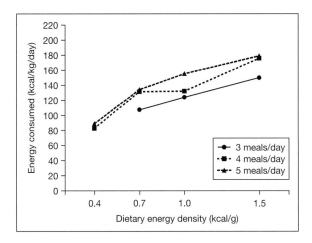

Fig. 1. Effects of dietary energy density and frequency of feeding on total daily energy intakes by young children recovering from severe malnutrition [reprinted from 14 with permission from the *American Journal of Clinical Nutrition*].

Table 1. Revised estimates of the minimum energy density of complementary foods (kcal/g prepared foods) that is necessary to ensure adequate energy intakes from complementary foods by children of different age groups according to the number of meals served per day

Number of meals/day	Age group		
	6–8 months	9–11 months	12–23 months
2	0.71	0.84	1.12
3	0.48	0.56	0.75
4	0.36	0.42	0.56
5	0.29	0.34	0.45

Analysis assumes average level of breast milk intake and total energy requirements as estimated by FAO, 2004 [34]. Assumed functional gastric capacity (30 g/kg reference body weight) is 249 g/meal at 6–8 months, 285 g/meal at 9–11 months, and 345 g/meal at 12–23 months [see 3, 11 for more details].

Indeed, several recent studies have found that increasing the energy density of complementary foods had a negative impact on breast milk intake, although the effects on total daily energy intakes were inconsistent [15, 16]. In one study, total energy intake was increased when the density of complementary foods was raised from 0.5 to 1.5 kcal/g [15], despite minor reductions in breast milk intake. However, no such effect on total energy intake was noted in another study when energy density was boosted by from 0.20 to 0.55 kcal/g by adding oil to a cereal-legume mixture [16]. The different outcomes of these two studies may be due to the distinct ranges of energy density that were used or the fact that the latter study provided each diet for 1 day only, so it is possible that the children had not yet reached a constant level of intake. Additional studies with a greater number of permutations of energy density and feeding frequency are currently in progress to address these issues.

Problem Micronutrients and Strategies to Provide Adequate Micronutrients

As indicated above, the nutrient requirements from complementary foods can be estimated as the difference between the total theoretical nutrient requirements and the amounts of these nutrients transferred in breast milk. Despite the difficulties imposed by the lack of harmonization of current estimates of young children's nutrient requirements, as published by different international groups of experts, we have attempted to identify specific 'problem nutrients' by comparing the observed nutrient intakes from complementary foods in different low-income settings with the range of currently estimated requirements [12, 17]. We defined 'problem nutrients' as those for which there is the greatest discrepancy between their content in complementary foods and the estimated requirements for young children. These analyses indicate that iron, zinc, calcium, selected B vitamins and occasionally vitamin A are often present in limited amounts in home-available complementary foods relative to the requirements for these nutrients. Other investigators have arrived at similar conclusions, using somewhat different approaches to estimate current dietary intakes [18].

Available strategies to supply these problem nutrients include promotion of greater consumption of animal source foods or other nutrient-rich food sources of these nutrients, provision of fortified complementary foods, or delivery of additional nutrients through home-based fortification or micronutrient supplementation. An analytic approach for identifying local foods that can be used to fulfill the nutrient shortfalls has been described recently [19]. This method utilizes information on dietary intake and local food prices to model potential nutrient intakes at particular costs, using linear programming.

Incorporating animal source foods, such as animal flesh and organs, eggs, fish, and dairy products, is often the only way to supply the aforementioned problem nutrients through local foods. However, these foods may be available in very limited amounts in the poorest countries [17], and their relatively high cost frequently makes them inaccessible to poorer households. Moreover, religious proscriptions or cultural taboos may further restrict their use in some societies. On the other hand, a recent study in the US demonstrated the feasibility of including meat in the feeding regimens of young infants [20], and another study carried out in slum communities in Peru found that, following an intensive educational campaign, poor households were able to increase children's consumption of animal source foods. Moreover, the linear growth of children in the intervention communities in Peru was significantly greater than in the control areas, reducing rates of stunting by two thirds at 12 months [21]. Thus, it may be possible to increase children's consumption of these foods in some settings, by using appropriately targeted educational interventions.

Distribution of processed, fortified complementary foods, either through public sector programs or commercial channels, offers an alternative food-based approach to supply problem nutrients [22]. Although such foods can successfully cover current nutrient shortfalls of the home diet, the rapid changes in young children's nutrient requirements during the period of complementary feeding make it difficult to design a single product that meets the nutrient needs of all children in this age range without imposing the risk of excessive intakes by some children [23]. Moreover, the impact of these foods on children's growth has been inconsistent, possibly related to the timing, amount, and composition of these foods, as well as the underlying nutritional status of the study populations [24–26]. Despite the inconsistent growth responses observed in these earlier studies, several recent studies have found positive effects on iron status and/or developmental milestones among children who received these products [27–29].

Addition of micronutrients to current feeding regimens, either through home-based fortification or direct child supplementation, offers a lower-cost strategy than providing a processed, nutritionally complete complementary food. Home-based fortification involves the addition of a prepackaged micronutrient supplement to the child's food once daily at the time of serving. One such formulation, 'Sprinkles', which contains iron as microencapsulated ferrous fumarate (to avoid adverse organoleptic effects of iron on the food), and vitamins A and D, folic acid, ascorbic acid, and zinc, has been shown to reduce rates anemia among consumers, although evidence of its positive impact on other indicators of micronutrient status and growth is still lacking [30].

Micronutrient supplements may be supplied as liquid formulations; chewable, crushable, or dispersible tablets [31], or fat-based food pastes [32]. A complete review of these products and related issues is beyond the scope of the present publication. Nevertheless, each of these formulations has been found to yield positive impacts on selected indicators of micronutrient status, depending on the specific formulation, the preexisting nutritional status of the target population and the presence of conditions that may interfere with nutrient absorption or utilization, but there is only limited evidence of any positive effects of these products on child growth. A recent study compared the effects of Sprinkles, 'Nutritabs' (crushable multiple micronutrient tablets), and 'Nutributter' (a micronutrient-enriched peanut butter mixture) in Ghanaian children [33]. Each type of the supplements was well accepted,

7

and there were no differences in adherence to treatment by intervention group. After 6 months of study, children in the three supplementation groups had greater concentrations of serum ferritin and lower concentrations of transferrin receptors than those in the nonintervention group. Children who received Nutributter had greater final weight-for-age and length-for-age Z scores compared with the other two intervention groups and the control group. Thus, all three products enhanced iron status, but only Nutributter increased the infants' growth. Additional research is still required to define optimal dosing regimens of multiple micronutrient formulations added to complementary foods, interactions among nutrients in the various preparations, and any possible adverse effects on child growth and other health outcomes in particular settings.

Conclusions

Important advances in knowledge have been achieved in recent years with regard to the multiple advantages of exclusive breastfeeding during the early months of life, the optimal timing of introduction of complementary foods, and the appropriate energy density, feeding frequency and micronutrient composition of these foods. However, adequate understanding of the effects of different complementary feeding regimens on breast milk intakes and the ultimate duration of breastfeeding is still lacking. Likewise, more information is needed on the ideal micronutrient composition of fortified complementary foods and the impact of alternative micronutrient delivery systems on young children's nutritional status, physical growth, and neurobehavioral development.

References

1 World Health Organization and UNICEF: Global Strategy for Infant and Young Child Feeding. Geneva, World Health Organization, 2003.
2 World Health Organization: Indicators for Assessing Breast Feeding Practices. Geneva, World Health Organization, 1991.
3 Lawrence RA, Lawrence RM: Breastfeeding: A Guide for the Medical Profession, ed 5. St Louis, Mosby, 2005.
4 Brown KH, Dewey KG, Allen LH: Complementary Feeding of Young Children in Developing Countries: A Review of Current Scientific Knowledge. Geneva, World Health Organization (WHO/NUT/98.1), 1998.
5 Brown KH, Black RE, Lopez de Romana G, Kanashiro HC: Infant-feeding practices and their relationship with diarrheal and other diseases in Huascar (Lima), Peru. Pediatrics 1989;83: 31–40.
6 Popkin BM, Adair L, Akin JS, et al: Breast-feeding and diarrheal morbidity. Pediatrics 1990;86: 874–882.
7 WHO Collaborative Study Team on the Role of Breastfeeding on the Prevention of Infant Mortality: Effect of breastfeeding on infant and child mortality due to infectious diseases in less developed countries: a pooled analysis. Lancet 2000;355:451–455.

8 Kramer MS, Kakuma R: The Optimal Duration of Exclusive Breast Feeding: A Systematic Review. Geneva, World Health Organization, 2002.

9 Cohen RJ, Brown KH, Canahuati J, et al: Effects of age of introduction of complementary foods on infant breast milk intake, total energy intake, and growth: a randomized intervention study in Honduras. Lancet 1994;343:288–293.

10 Dewey KG, Cohen RJ, Brown KH, Rivera LL: Age of introduction of complementary foods and growth of term, low-birth-weight, breast-fed infants: a randomized intervention study in Honduras. Am J Clin Nutr 1999;69:679–686.

11 Kramer MS, Chalmers B, Hodnett ED, et al; PROBIT Study Group (Promotion of Breastfeeding Intervention Trial): Promotion of Breastfeeding Intervention Trial (PROBIT): a randomized trial in the Republic of Belarus. JAMA 2001;285:413–420.

12 Dewey KG, Brown KH: Update on technical issues concerning complementary feeding of young children in developing countries and implications for intervention programs. Food Nutr Bull 2003;24:5–28.

13 Butte NF, Wong WW, Hopkinson JM, et al: Energy requirements derived from total energy expenditure and energy deposition during the first 2 years of life. Am J Clin Nutr 2000;72: 1558–1569.

14 Brown KH, Sanchez-Grinan M, Perez F, et al: Effects of dietary energy density and feeding frequency on total daily energy intakes by recovering malnourished children. Am J Clin Nutr 1995;62:13–18.

15 Islam MM, Peerson JM, Ahmed T, et al: Effects of varied energy density of complementary foods on breast-milk intakes and total energy consumption by healthy, breastfed Bangladeshi children. Am J Clin Nutr 2006;83:851–858.

16 Bajaj M, Dubey AP, Nagpal J, et al: Short-term effect of oil supplementation of complementary food on total ad libitum consumption in 6- to 10-month-old breastfed Indian infants. J Pediatr Gastroenterol Nutr 2005;41:61–65.

17 Brown KH, Peerson JM, Kimmons JE, Hotz C: Options for achieving adequate intake from home-prepared complementary food in low income countries; in Black RE, Michaelsen KF (eds): Public Health Issues in Infant and Child Nutrition. Philadelphia, Lippincott Williams & Wilkins, 2002, pp 239–256.

18 Gibson RS, Ferguson EL, Lehrfeld J: Complementary foods for infant feeding in developing countries: their nutrient adequacy and improvement. Eur J Clin Nutr 1998;52:764–770.

19 Ferguson EL, Darmin N, Fahmida U, et al: Design of optimal food-based complementary feeding recommendations and identification of key 'problem nutrients' using goal programming. J Nutr 2006;136:2399–2404.

20 Krebs NF, Westcott JE, Butler N, et al: Meat as a first complementary food for breastfed infants: feasibility and impact on zinc intake and status. J Pediatr Gastroenterol Nutr 2006;42: 207–214.

21 Penny ME, Creed-Kanashiro HM, Robert RC, et al: Effectiveness of an educational intervention delivered through the health services to improve nutrition in young children: a cluster-randomised controlled trial. Lancet 2005;365:1863–1872.

22 Brown KH, Lutter CK: Potential role of processed complementary foods in the improvement of early childhood nutrition in Latin America. Food Nutr Bull 2000;21:5–11.

23 Dewey KG: Nutrient composition of fortified complementary foods: should age-specific micronutrient content and ration sizes be recommended. J Nutr 2003;133:2950S–2952S.

24 Simondon KB, Gartner A, Berger J, et al: Effect of early, short-term supplementation on weight and linear growth of 4–7 month-old infants in developing countries: a four-country randomized trial. Am J Clin Nutr 1996;64:537–545.

25 Caulfield LE, Huffman SL, Piwoz EG: Interventions to improve intake of complementary foods by infants 6 to 12 months of age in developing countries: impact on growth and on the prevalence of malnutrition and potential contribution to child survival. Food Nutr Bull 1999;20:183–200.

26 Dewey KG: Success of intervention programs to promote complementary feeding; in Black RE, Michaelsen KF (eds): Public Health Issues in Infant and Child Nutrition. Philadelphia, Lippincott Williams & Wilkins, 2002, pp 199–216.

27 Lartey A, Manu A, Brown KH, et al: A randomized, community-based trial of the effects of improved, centrally processed complementary foods on growth and micronutrient status of Ghanaian infants from 6 to 12 mo of age. Am J Clin Nutr 1999;70:391–404.

28 Rivera JA, Sotres-Alvarez D, Habicht JP, et al: Impact of the Mexican Program for Education, Health and Nutrition (Prograsa) on rates of growth and anemia in infants and young children. JAMA 2004;291:2563–2570.

29 Faber M, Kvalsvig JD, Lombard CJ, Benade AJS: Effect of a fortified maize-meal porridge on anemia, micronutrient status, and motor development of infants. Am J Clin Nutr 2005;82:1032–1039.

30 Zlotkin SH, Christofides AL, Hyder SM, et al: Controlling iron deficiency anemia through the use of home-fortified complementary foods. Indian J Pediatr 2004;71:1015–1019.

31 Smuts CM, Lombard CJ, Benade AJ, et al; International Research on Infant Supplementation (IRIS) Study Group: Efficacy of a foodlet-based multiple micronutrient supplement for preventing growth faltering, anemia, and micronutrient deficiency of infants: the four country IRIS trial pooled data analysis. J Nutr 2005;135:631S–638S.

32 Lopriore C, Guidom Y, Briend A, Branca F: Spread fortified with vitamins and minerals induces catch-up growth and eradicates severe anemia in stunted refugee children aged 3–6 y. Am J Clin Nutr 2004;80:973–981.

33 Adu-Afarwuah S, Lartey A, Brown KH, et al: Randomized comparison of 3 types of micronutrient supplements for home fortification of complementary foods in Ghana: Effects on growth and motor development. Am J Clin Nutr, in press.

34 Food and Agriculture Organization: Human Energy Requirements: Report of a Joint FAO/WHO/UNU Expert Consultation. FAO Food and Nutrition Technical Report Series 1, Rome, 2004.

Discussion

Dr. Haschke: With regard to energy density, where you showed that it is of importance in terms of changing the amount of breast milk which is consumed. Can we now move to a recommendation or is it too early? How can it be started at 6 months, at which energy density, and then how can the energy density be increased? Secondly, with regard to your studies in Peru and Guatemala, you said that the amount of cereals consumed was very low; it was higher in the intervention studies than in the two studies. But isn't that also an effect of just being observational and not interventional. Did these infants grow normally or did they show growth faltering?

Dr. Brown: Munirul Islam, a who is based at the ICDDRD, the International Center for Diarrheal Disease Research in Bangladesh, is the person who actually carried out the pilot study. He has just finished a follow-on study which has a number of different permutations of feeding frequency, (3, 4 or 5 servings/day) and energy density (0.5 to 1.5 kcal/g). I don't think we have enough information yet to make formal recommendations. I just showed this information to alert us that we can go too far by promoting either overly dense complementary food or feeding more frequently than desirable, which might have adverse effects on breast milk intake. In terms of the age specificity question, there is no information that I am aware of. In the Bangladesh study the children were 8–12 months of age, but they weren't stratified so as to have a sufficient sample to look at whether there are differences in the different age groups. The second question with regard to what would happen if these children actually received food either through a government program or some sort of subsidy. Would they consume more of these cereal-based fortified foods? Undoubtedly, yes, because that is what we saw. We could double the level of energy intake from cereal-based complementary food by providing these foods free to each household. We provided a plastic sac, 250 g dry weight, once a week, which translates to just a little over 30 g dry weight/day. Based on earlier studies we did, we assumed that children would actually consume about 20 g/day; in fact they actually consumed about 23 g/day. So either they can't consume more or the food is being used for other purposes. I can't tell you exactly why, but we couldn't boost the intake beyond that, even though we were giving more than what was actually consumed. I am sure that it is very culture specific, depending on what the usual feeding practices are. In Peru, for example, mothers are giving milk in addition to breast milk, so that is another source of energy. Other milks are probably the largest non-breast milk source of energy. They often start complementary foods with soups and may pick out certain items from the soup and make a dish specifically for the child. So, even when we give fortified complementary foods to the households, the mothers are still feeding all these other things.

Dr. Haschke: And their growth?

Dr. Brown: These children remained stunted; the final prevalence of stunting was 18%. These were children who were initially selected for being at risk of stunting. Their initial Z score at 6 months of age was less than -0.5; so it was a selected group. But we did not see any impact of the zinc intervention. I can't say whether or not porridge had an impact because all the groups were given porridge, although it was fortified in different ways in the different groups.

Dr. Giovannini: I perfectly agree that the problem of nutritional tradition is very important for complementary food but I have some concerns about the use of chicken livers. We are involved in a nutritional study in Cambodia, and I don't think it is good practice to suggest liver in child nutrition, especially in this country where hygienic conditions are bad. Moreover, in Western countries the use of liver is no longer allowed following the BSE outbreak, and chicken, as we know, is full of salmonella and bacteria.

Dr. Brown: Those are very important considerations. In Peru, chicken liver is surprisingly commonly fed to young children. At least in the communities where I worked in Peru, it is generally viewed as a good thing to feed the children. We found in earlier studies that the use of chicken liver, and controlling for other components in the diet, was associated with increased growth of the children. So at least from a nutritional perspective it seems like a good thing to do. From a microbiologic perspective there is much less concern because it is always boiled in soup, so I don't think we have a problem here. My major concern would be more from a toxicological perspective, and unfortunately I have no information to present. In Peru there is a very well-developed poultry industry, so the chickens are generally raised in closed conditions, at least along the coast of Peru, and marketed through formal markets. But this doesn't really answer your question. I don't know that anybody has done a formal study on possible heavy metal contamination of chicken liver, and this would be worth knowing. It is something that is being used locally and is appreciated by mothers as a valuable component to diet. The only reason it is not used more widely is because not everybody can afford it.

Dr. Fisberg: Sometimes it is very easy to obtain zinc and iron levels over the upper limits, especially in fortified food. In spite of that how do they behave in clinical data? How do they behave when reaching low zinc plasma levels or low anemia or lowering anemia?

Dr. Brown: This is a very important question. I should reemphasize that these results that I presented are all simulations; we have no evidence of any true adverse effect of delivering nutrients at levels greater than the upper level. So we are simply bound by what the current published recommended intakes are. As I said we rely mostly on the dietary reference intakes (DRI) for the upper level that I referred to. There are several caveats; for most minerals the US DRI don't take bioavailability into consideration. I think we could probably go much higher, safely. But I can't ignore the DRI, so we do the analysis using the existing recommendations. The second issue is that in many cases the upper levels are simply extrapolated from adults, there is no empirical information from children to establish the upper levels correctly. The third thing, at least in the case of zinc which I have looked at much more closely, the upper level is just too low for children. Over months we have continuously supplemented children at levels 50% greater than the upper limit without any evidence of adverse effects. We are presently trying to put the literature together to try to make the case that, at least for zinc, the upper level for young children is probably set too low, Dr. Krebs, would you like to comment on that?

Dr. Krebs: There is a general agreement that the upper limit is too low for young children. In fact the procedure that was to be used to establish these limits was not actually followed to completion for the young children. Once they had come up with this proposed level, they did not go back to compare the actual and common intakes, and had they done that they would have seen that there are many children with much higher intakes with no apparent problems.

Dr. Brown: Let me just mention that we have looked at the US data published by the US Department of Agriculture, a continuing survey of food intake by individuals. We found that in the US more than 90% of infants consume more than the upper level for zinc although that percent decreases with age. But even among older children, 30–40% are still consuming usual zinc intakes greater than the upper level.

Dr. Solomons: I would like to return to the Shrimpton slide. How can we use it to frame the entire discussion for the week? That is to say, is the notion that all regions of the world actually assume the zero, because in fact after they get to 15 months they run parallel to that. So does this period represent some sort of adaptation or is it desirable that all the world be on the NCHS curve channels forever? I would also ask, is it complementary feeding alone or are other environmental-related issues important to correct the abnormality that Dr. Shrimpton showed on the slide?

Dr. Brown: For the first question let me refer to what was recently published by the WHO as a new international reference database for assessing growth. This growth chart was put together using what they called prescriptive selection of children, that is children were enrolled in the study because they were adhering to recommended infant feeding practices. They were predominantly breastfed at least until 4 months of age and continued breastfeeding until 12 months of age. They were all selected from communities in which their environmental circumstances, should not have limited their growth, and they were selected to represent all of the world's population, so 6 geographically distinct countries were included. These statistics are published on the internet. Although some of the distributions of the new WHO growth standards differ from those for the earlier CDC WHO reference data, the median values of the new standards are generally similar to those of the prior CDC/WHO data. So at least among individuals who were adhering to the recommended feeding practices, this is the expected growth pattern. Now could you do better in terms of certain functional outcomes by adhering to some other growth pattern? I don't know the answer to that. I think the other aspect that you are probably implying is the issue of to what extent does intrauterine nutrition, or perhaps genetic factors, also program postnatal growth. I imagine that it is something that we will get to later in this conference.

Dr. Solomons: So wherever we put the new zero line projected by the WHO, I assume it is your notion that the world as a whole, by region, should mimic it.

Dr. Brown: My notion is that if children adhere to recommended feeding practices and don't have the environmental circumstances that we think of as being adverse, i.e. contaminated environment, infections, they will follow that zero line.

Dr. Simell: Two questions related to the simulation models which were highly interesting. The first one concerns the assumption that the distribution is normal in the consumption of these nutrients. Do you have any evidence that this is true, especially when we are talking about energy intake for instance? The second question is related to how you handle the child who is expected to be a passive recipient of a nutrient, but factors like satiety and differences in intake affect this. Have you taken this into consideration here? The child is not just a passive recipient of nutrients, the satiety feeling is an important factor in the amount of nutrients consumed.

Dr. Brown: I could talk for another hour just on how the simulations were done. The issue of distribution of intakes depends on the nutrients. In many cases these are nonsymmetrical distributions, and to do the simulations, transformation is needed to try to adjust for that, and we've taken that into account. It is actually even more complicated because what you would like to model is the usual intake of a nutrient and the usual intake of the food that you are trying to fortify, and these are two independent distributions. It simply cannot be done. What we have done is to look at the distribution intakes on given days rather than usual intakes. Then those graphs are superimposed and we find that for most nutrients the 2.5 percentile of usual intake crosses about the 10 to 15th percentile of intake on a given day. I always used the 10th percentile for my cutoffs in establishing inadequate intake relative to the estimated average requirement and excessive intake relative to the upper limit. This work can certainly be refined; this was something we did fairly quickly because we wanted to be able to talk about these points in this setting. The critical take away message here is that it is very difficult to decide what the right level to fortify these foods is, and it may well be age-specific and it may well be country-specific. It is a difficult problem to solve. The second question: children determine what they are eating and we are very much aware of that. In the studies that I described with regard to energy density, the protocol is one that we worked on over years and it has certain aspects which I think are very important. One, we always try to mask the diets so that if you look at them physically, smell them, even taste them, for the most part they can't be distinguished. We add flavoring and ingredients to all of them so that they are masked, and we try to make them as similar to adult test panels without adding anything that we think might independently affect consumption. The second is that we have a very rigorous feeding protocol in which a nursing aide does the feeding. She would get a coded bowl for the child with an amount of food that was far in excess of what the child could possibly eat. The instructions were to fill the spoon, put the fluid in the child's mouth, let the child swallow that, and when the child has swallowed, repeat the process and offer it again until the child shows some indication of not wanting anymore. At that point they wait 60 s and then start again: they offer another spoon, and continue the feeding until the child refuses again, then they wait another 60 s, try a third time, and after that third attempt and third refusal, the meal is considered completed. So all these studies are done using this very standardized feeding protocol to try to control for all those child-specific factors. There are some fascinating things that we have never published in terms of the duration of meals. The children seem to have a certain duration regarding how long they want to eat. When you change the energy density of the food the children eat more rapidly. They swallow the food and are ready for a new spoon faster, but the total duration of a meal doesn't change. So what changes with lowering density is eating velocity, not how long the meal lasts. We also found that if we control for a nursing aide that explains a small but significant part of the variability; some aides feed more rapidly or more than others. So there are a lot of factors that need to be controlled in doing these kinds of studies.

Dr. Leone: You showed the evolution of weight for age Z scores and length for age. Do you have data about the evolution of the body mass index in the complementary feeding groups?

Dr. Brown: We have some data, but I don't have the information with me.

Agostoni C, Brunser O (eds): Issues in Complementary Feeding.
Nestlé Nutr Workshop Ser Pediatr Program, vol 60, pp 15–29,
Nestec Ltd., Vevey/S. Karger AG, Basel, © 2007.

Does Breastfeeding Protect from Growth Acceleration and Later Obesity?

Atul Singhal

The MRC Childhood Nutrition Research Centre, Institute of Child Health, London, UK

Abstract

Nutrition in infancy has been suggested to have a major influence or program the long-term tendency to obesity. Breastfeeding, in particular, appears to protect against the development of later obesity, a conclusion supported by data from four systematic reviews and evidence that a longer duration of breastfeeding has greater protective effects. The size of the effect (up to a 20% reduction in obesity risk) although modest has important implications for public health. The mechanisms involved, although poorly understood, probably include the benefits of relative undernutrition and slower growth associated with breast rather than formula feeding – the growth acceleration hypothesis. This hypothesis is now supported by data from animal studies and two recent systematic reviews, which suggest an association between faster growth in infancy and later obesity in both richer and low-income countries and for both faster weight and length gain. The present review considers the evidence for a role of early growth and breastfeeding in the programming of obesity and the underlying mechanisms involved.

Introduction

The WHO has described the recent dramatic increase in obesity as the most important public health issue facing both industrialized and developing countries. Globally more than 1 billion adults are already classified as overweight and at least 300 million of them as clinically obese. The rise in obesity has been particularly steep in children. In the USA, for instance, the number of overweight children has doubled since the 1980s, a trend that has immense implications for the prevalence of obesity-related chronic disease and future health care costs.

Ultimately, obesity is a result of a cumulative increase in energy intake above energy expenditure. While genetic factors determine a person's susceptibility to weight gain, increased consumption of energy-dense foods (with high proportion of fats and sugars) and declining levels of physical activity have been suggested to be the main causes for the rise in obesity prevalence. However, this simple paradigm of an interaction between lifestyle and a genetically determined susceptibility has been challenged by recent research which suggests that factors in fetal and early postnatal life may also have a profound impact on long-term health. By raising the possibility of interventions in early life, this 'developmental origins' hypothesis has major implications for primary prevention of noncommunicable chronic disease and hence public health worldwide. The present review considers the evidence for the developmental origins of obesity with particular reference to a possible protective role for breastfeeding.

Nutritional Programming of Obesity

The hypothesis that breastfeeding protects against the development of later obesity originates from the more general biological phenomenon of 'programming', the influence of a factor or stimulus acting during an early critical window on long-term structure or function of an organism. The specific importance of nutrition in programming first emerged in the 1960s with the pioneering work of McCance [1]. He showed that rats raised in small litters, and therefore overfed in the suckling period, were larger as adults irrespective of nutrient intake after weaning. In contrast, manipulating nutrient intake after weaning produced little effect on final adult size, suggesting that nutrition acted during a critical, early postnatal window to program later body size. Similar effects of early overnutrition were seen in baboons. Lewis et al. [2] found that overfeeding in infancy programmed greater fat mass but not total body weight in adulthood. The effect size was substantial (baboons overfed in infancy had up to 4× greater omental and perirenal fat as adults). The effect also emerged only after adolescence, demonstrating the late manifestation of some programming phenomena [2].

Since these early observations, early postnatal overnutrition has been shown to program adiposity in many animal models. For instance, Ozanne and Hales [3] showed that mice given a higher protein diet during the suckling period (that allowed catch-up growth) were more obese and had a lower lifespan than those given a lower protein diet. Importantly, the adverse effects of higher protein intake postnatally were most marked in rats fed a 'cafeteria' or obesity-inducing diet from weaning compared to those given standard laboratory chow [3]. This observation suggested an interaction between nutritional programming and later environment, whereby the adverse effects of a higher nutrient intake prior to weaning were greatest in those given a highly palatable, energy-dense diet after weaning.

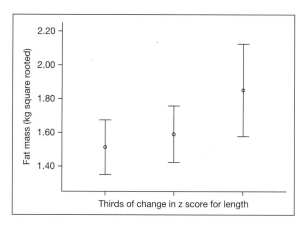

Fig. 1. Fat mass determined by bioelectric impedance at age 6–8 years according to thirds of z score change for length between birth and age 9 months (from lowest to highest) (p = 0.02).

In humans, the concept that early nutrition may influence long-term adiposity has focused mainly on the possible protective role of breastfeeding. However, while there is little doubt that breast milk is the best source of nutrition for the newborn, whether breastfeeding has long-term health benefits remains controversial.

Does Breastfeeding Protect against Later Obesity?

A case-control study by Kramer [4] was one of the first reports to suggest a protective effect of breastfeeding on later obesity. Since then many, but not all, population-based studies have confirmed an association between breastfeeding and lower risk of later adiposity, as summarized recently in four systematic reviews [5–8].

The first review by Arenz et al. [5] confirmed a protective effect of breastfeeding against later obesity (adjusted odds ratio 0.78, 95% CI 0.71–0.85) (table 1). Obesity was defined as a BMI above the 90th, 95th or 97th percentile and the analysis was confined to studies that had adjusted for a least three of several confounding or interacting factors (birth weight, parental overweight, parental smoking, dietary factors, physical activity and socioeconomic status). Age, definition of breastfeeding, or the number of confounding factors adjusted for did not affect these findings and there was no evidence of publication bias. However, there was evidence from four studies of an inverse and dose-dependent effect of duration of breastfeeding on later obesity prevalence.

Table 1. Meta-analyses of effects of breastfeeding on later body fatness

Review	Studies n	Effect size[1] (95% CI)	Duration of breastfeeding effect	Publication bias
Arenz et al., 2004 [5]				
Adjusted[2]	9	0.78 (0.71, 0.85)	yes	no
Owen et al., 2005 [6]				
Overall estimate	28	0.87 (0.85, 0.89)	yes	yes
Adjusted	6	0.93 (0.88, 0.99)		
Study size				
Small (n < 500)	11	0.43 (0.33, 0.55)		
Intermediate (n = 500–2,500)	7	0.78 (0.69, 0.89)		
Large (n > 2,500)	10	0.88 (0.86, 0.90)		
Exclusively breastfed	4	0.76 (0.70, 0.83)		
Owen et al., 2005 [7]				
Overall estimate	36	−0.04 (−0.05, −0.02)	yes	yes
Adjusted	11	−0.10 (−0.14, −0.06)		
Study size				
Small (n < 500)	10	−0.12 (−0.29, 0.04)		
Intermediate (n = 500–2,500)	13	−0.15 (−0.21, −0.08)		
Large (n > 2,500)	13	−0.03 (−0.04, −0.01)		
Harder et al., 2005 [8]				
Overall estimate[3]	17	0.96 (0.94, 0.98)	yes	no
<1 month breastfeeding	5	1.0 (0.65, 1.55)		
1–3 months	14	0.81 (0.74, 0.88)		
4–6 months	15	0.76 (0.67, 0.86)		
7–9 months	11	0.67 (0.55, 0.82)		
>9 months	7	0.68 (0.50, 0.91)		

[1]Data are odds ratios (95% CI) for risk of obesity/overweight comparing breastfed versus formula-fed infants except Owen et al. [7] who show mean difference in BMI (95% CI).
[2]Adjusted for potential confounding factors.
[3]Analysis of effects of breastfeeding duration per month.

The second report by Owen et al. [6] also defined obesity on the basis of BMI percentiles and again found a protective effect of breastfeeding on later obesity risk (table 1). Interestingly, the effect size in four studies that compared exclusive breastfeeding with exclusive formula feeding was similar to that shown by Arenz et al. [5]. However, the inverse association between breastfeeding and later obesity was stronger in smaller than larger studies raising the possibility of publication bias. The effect was also reduced markedly in six studies that adjusted for three potential confounding factors (parental obesity, maternal smoking and social class), with a fall in odds ratio from 0.86 (95% CI 0.81, 0.91) to 0.93 (95% CI 0.88, 0.99). Again, as in the review by Arenz et al. [5], the effect of breastfeeding was not altered by age at outcome and was stronger amongst prolonged breastfeeders.

The third review examined the evidence that breastfeeding reduced average levels of adiposity (i.e. mean values for BMI) rather than obesity per se [7]. This analysis, based on the possibility that breastfeeding moved the upper tail of the BMI distribution to the left but did not shift the whole distribution, found that breastfed infants had a slightly lower mean BMI than those formula-fed (table 1). As with their data on obesity [6], the authors found greater effects of breastfeeding on mean BMI in smaller studies than larger studies. The effects of breastfeeding were also markedly attenuated by adjustment for confounding factors (socioeconomic status, maternal BMI and maternal smoking during pregnancy) [unadjusted mean difference in BMI: -0.10 (95% CI -0.14, -0.06) kg/m^2 compared to adjusted mean difference: -0.01 (95% CI -0.05, 0.03) kg/m^2]. The authors concluded, therefore, that any effect of breastfeeding on later BMI was likely to be influenced by publication bias and confounding factors.

The most recent meta-analysis summarized the evidence that duration of breastfeeding programmed obesity risk [8]. Consistent with previous reviews [5–7], this analysis confirmed that prolonged breastfeeding reduced the tendency to obesity (each month of breastfeeding was associated with a 4% reduction in risk of obesity, 95% CI -6%, -2%), independent of the definition of obesity or age at measurement.

Clearly, the above systematic reviews were based on observational studies, and because of marked differences in demographic and socioeconomic characteristics between breast- and formula-fed infants cannot establish causation. Randomized studies comparing breast and formula feeding are unethical, although data from cluster randomized studies of breastfeeding promotion by Kramer et al. [9] could be informative. Nonetheless, although residual confounding by sociodemographic differences between breast- and formula-fed infants could be influential, adjustment for these factors did not reduce the benefit of breastfeeding on obesity risk to zero. Methodological issues such as differences in age at outcome, definition of obesity, and publication bias also did not explain the protective effect of breastfeeding. The definition of breastfeeding, however, could be relevant to interpretation of published data. In reviews by Arenz et al. [5] and Owen et al. [6], for instance, confining the meta-analysis to studies comparing exclusive breastfeeding with exclusive formula feeding found remarkably similar reduction of obesity risk by breastfeeding (odds ratio of approximately 0.77). Exclusivity of breastfeeding may therefore be central to the mechanism by which breastfeeding protects against later obesity.

Overall, therefore, there appears to be some evidence that breastfeeding protects against the development of obesity, a conclusion supported by data from several systematic reviews which showed that a longer duration of breastfeeding had a greater beneficial effect [5–8]. The size of the effect (up to 20% reduction, table 1) has major implications for the health of populations.

Mechanisms

The potential mechanisms by which breastfeeding protects against later obesity have been extensively reviewed elsewhere [10], and so will be considered here briefly. These mechanisms can be broadly categorized as those that influence behavior or those related to the unique nutritional composition of human milk.

The most common explanation for the beneficial effect of breastfeeding on later markers of health is residual confounding by unmeasured attributes of the family and parents. Because parents who choose to breastfeed may have a healthier lifestyle (especially those who breastfeed for longer) cumulative differences in dietary habits and physical activity over many years could affect obesity risk despite statistical adjustment for these factors at a single time point in some studies [11]. Another behavioral explanation is that because breastfed babies control the amount of milk consumed they may learn to better self-regulate their energy intake, although whether this difference persists into adult life is unknown.

Mechanisms for programming of obesity related to the nutritional composition of breast milk include a number of bioactive nutrients in human milk, which are absent from some formulas (e.g. long-chain polyunsaturated fatty acids [12]). Lower protein and energy content in human milk compared to formula could also affect later body composition. For instance, protein intake in infancy (up to 70% greater in formula-fed than breastfed infants [13]) has been associated with adiposity in childhood [14] possibly by mechanisms that involve an earlier age of adiposity rebound [15], a hypothesis now being tested in European clinical trials. A higher protein intake could also promote obesity by stimulation of insulin release. Consistent with this thesis, formula-fed infants were shown to have higher plasma insulin concentrations than those breastfed from as early as 6 days of age [16].

Finally and most recently, we have suggested that the benefits of breastfeeding for long-term obesity and cardiovascular disease may be due to slower growth in breastfed compared to formula-fed infants – the growth acceleration hypothesis [17].

The Growth Acceleration Hypothesis

The growth acceleration hypothesis suggests that faster postnatal growth (upward centile crossing – particularly in infancy) programs the major components of the metabolic syndrome [17]. Consistent with this thesis, faster neonatal weight gain was shown to program insulin resistance in preterm infants randomly assigned to a nutrient-enriched diet (preterm formula) that promoted faster growth compared to the standard diet (banked breast milk or term formula). Faster postnatal weight gain also explained the associations between breastfeeding and lower later insulin resistance, and between low birth weight for gestation and greater insulin resistance later in life [17]. Furthermore, early acceleration in weight programmed higher LDL cholesterol concentration and explained the benefits of breast milk feeding on later cholesterol concentration [17]. Similarly, acceleration in both weight and length in the first 2 weeks of life was associated with later endothelial dysfunction, a measure of the earliest physiological changes associated with the development of atherosclerosis [17].

The effect of early growth on later cardiovascular outcomes was substantial and greater than the adverse effects of both formula feeding or of being born small for gestation [17]. For instance, adolescents with the greatest weight gain in the first 2 weeks had 4% lower flow-mediated dilation of the brachial artery (a measure of endothelial function) than those with the lowest weight gain, an effect similar to that of insulin-dependent diabetes mellitus (4%) and smoking (6%) in adults [17]. Similarly, for cholesterol concentration, slower neonatal weight gain was associated with 20% lower cholesterol concentration compared to 10% lowering of cholesterol concentration associated with breast rather than formula feeding [17].

Programming by postnatal growth acceleration is potentially a unifying hypothesis which can explain, in part, adverse programming effects seen in infants born small for gestation (who show 'catch-up' growth immediately after birth) and the long-term cardiovascular advantages of breastfed babies (who are relatively undernourished and have slower growth compared to those given formula). This concept is now extensively supported by studies in infants born at term. For instance, upward centile crossing for weight in infancy is associated with higher later blood pressure independent of birth weight [18]. In fact, the adverse long-term effect of faster early growth appears to be a fundamental biological phenomenon seen across animal species as diverse as insects, fish and mammals [19]. Faster growth as a consequence of a higher nutrient intake prior to weaning appears to be particularly important and, in animal models, has been shown to program the metabolic syndrome, obesity and even reduced lifespan [1–3].

Growth Acceleration and Later Obesity

The growth acceleration concept may be particularly important for programming of obesity as shown in two recent systematic reviews [20, 21]. Monteiro and Victora [20] showed that upward centile crossing for weight and length in infancy was associated with later obesity in 13 studies, while Baird et al. [21] found similar findings in 10 studies (odds ratios for obesity risk ranging from 1.2 to 5.7 in infants with rapid growth).

Although these systematic reviews were based on observational studies and so cannot establish causality, they provide compelling evidence for an effect of faster growth in infancy on later adiposity. This effect has been seen for both faster weight and length gain (Singhal, unpubl. data, fig. 1), irrespective of the definition of faster growth, in both high and low income countries, and over time (i.e. for people born between 1927 and 1994) [21, 22]. The effect has also been seen in healthy term infants with normal birth weight and is not confined to infants born small [17, 18, 20, 21] who often show 'catch-up' growth. Catch-up growth, defined as the nutritional recovery and acceleration in growth seen after a restriction to growth is removed, is common in infants born small for gestation as a consequence of intrauterine growth retardation. Catch-up growth is widely associated with cardiovascular disease and obesity later in life. However, randomized intervention studies have shown that growth acceleration as a consequence of a high postnatal nutrient intake has programming effects independent of birth weight for gestation [17], which suggests that rapid growth, and not the closely related phenomenon of 'catch-up growth', is central to underlying mechanisms.

The effects of growth acceleration on later obesity are also not confined to infants fed formula. For instance, breastfed infants with a vigorous feeding style at age 2 and 4 weeks, suggestive of a greater breast milk intake, had greater adiposity at age 3 years [22] and upward centile crossing for length and weight has been associated with later adiposity in breastfed infants with birth weight <10th centile (Singhal, unpubl. data). Similarly, faster weight gain in the first 2 months was associated with higher BMI at 10 years in a large, prospectively followed, and predominantly breastfed cohort from the UK (The Avon Longitudinal Study of Pregnancy and Childhood) [mean, SD BMI of lowest compared to highest quartile of weight change in the first 2 months: 18.1, 0.1 versus 18.6, 0.2 kg/m^2; p = 0.01; Charakida, pers. commun.]. Programming effects of faster early growth therefore appear to be applicable to diverse populations.

The size of the effect of early growth rate on later obesity is substantial. For instance, Stettler estimated that 20% of the risk of obesity at age 7 years is attributed to having a rate of weight gain in the highest quintile in the first 4 months of life [23], an effect size important for public health. However, the relative contribution of different growth periods to programming of adiposity is uncertain. Growth is fastest in the first few weeks after birth, which may therefore be a key window for adverse programming. Consistent with this hypothesis, greater weight gain in the first week of life was shown to program obesity in adulthood [24], a finding analogous to programming of insulin resistance and endothelial function by faster early growth in preterm infants [17]. Again the size of the effect was substantial; each 100-gram increase in absolute weight gain during this period was associated with a 28% increase in the risk of becoming overweight (95% CI 8%, 52%) [24]. Emerging evidence therefore supports the first few postnatal weeks as a critical window for programming long-term health in both humans and animals.

The growth acceleration hypothesis could also explain programming of obesity by other factors in infancy. For instance, an earlier age of adiposity rebound, suggested to be a key risk factor for later adiposity [15], may simply identify children whose BMI centile is high and/or crossing upwards (i.e. children with a faster growth rate) [25]. Similarly, previous associations between an earlier age at weaning (complementary feeding) and a greater risk of later obesity [26] may reflect the influence of greater nutrient (and particularly protein) intake with weaning, on growth rate in infancy. Nevertheless, in both humans and animals, it is not possible to separate programming effects of nutrition from growth, as clearly, these factors are interdependent.

Mechanisms

Animal studies have helped shed light on the mechanisms that link early growth and nutrition with long-term obesity. Of particular interest is the role of the appetite-regulating hormone, leptin, which in the first few days after birth programs hypothalamic neuronal projections related to long-term regulation of appetite and energy expenditure [27]. For instance, rats overfed before weaning have been shown to be overweight, hyperleptinemic, and show hypothalamic leptin resistance later in life [28]. Similar mechanisms may apply in humans in whom leptin resistance in early infancy could be advantageous by allowing infants born small for gestation to increase their appetite and so facilitate catch-up growth. However this programmed increase in appetite could contribute to long-term obesity. In support of this hypothesis, breast milk feeding has been associated with lower leptin resistance in adolescents [29] raising the possibility that relative undernutrition and slower growth associated with breastfeeding in the first few weeks permanently programs a lower appetite. In contrast, formula-fed infants may have upregulated appetite leading to obesity when faced with a highly palatable, energy-dense western diet (analogous to greater obesity in rats growing fast before weaning and fed a highly palatable 'cafeteria' diet after weaning [3]).

Does Breastfeeding Protect against Growth Acceleration?

Central to the hypothesis that relative undernutrition associated with breastfeeding protects against later obesity is evidence that breastfed infants grow more slowly than those formula-fed [9]. Over the first 3 months, however, the rate of weight gain in breastfed infants may be *greater* than those formula-fed as suggested by the new WHO breastfed reference charts [30]. However, these charts were based on data from highly selected populations from six centers worldwide (Brazil, Ghana, India, United States, Norway, Oman) with those from poorer countries represented by subjects from affluent communities [30]. Faster growth in breastfed infants may therefore reflect postnatal catch-up growth following a period of in utero restraint,

Singhal

an effect that is most marked in affluent communities (both in richer and developing countries) where parents from a higher socioeconomic group tend to both breastfeed and be taller. In contrast, data from large epidemiological studies have confirmed the growth-accelerating effects of formula throughout infancy [9]. In fact differences in growth rate between breast- and formula-fed infants may be greatest in the first few postnatal weeks, a time when breastfed infants often lose weight, while those formula-fed tend to put on weight. As suggested by studies in animals [1–3] and humans [17, 24] this difference may be critical for programming of obesity.

Conclusion

There is now strong evidence to support a benefit of breastfeeding for long-term risk of obesity, an effect possibly related to the slower growth and relative undernutrition associated with breast compared to formula feeding. Breastfeeding is therefore a preventative strategy, which is both evidence based and has large potential benefits for public health.

References

1 McCance RA: Food, growth and time. Lancet 1962;2:671–676.
2 Lewis DS, Bertrand HA, McMahan CA, et al: Preweaning food intake influences the adiposity of young adult baboons. J Clin Invest 1986;78:899–905.
3 Ozanne SE, Hales CN: Catch-up growth and obesity in male mice. Nature 2004;427:411–412.
4 Kramer MS: Do breast-feeding and delayed introduction of solid foods protect against subsequent obesity? J Pediatr 1981;98:883–887.
5 Arenz S, Ruckerl R, Koletzko B, Von Kries R: Breast-feeding and childhood obesity – a systematic review. Int J Obes 2004;28:1247–1256.
6 Owen CG, Martin RM, Whincup PH, et al: Effect of infant feeding on the risk of obesity across the life course: a quantitative review of published evidence. Pediatrics 2005;115:1367–1377.
7 Owen CG, Martin RM, Whincup PH, et al: The effect of breast-feeding on mean body mass index throughout life: a quantitative review of published and unpublished observational evidence. Am J Clin Nutr 2005;82:1298–1307.
8 Harder T, Bergmann R, Kallischnigg G, Plagemann A: Duration of breast-feeding and risk of overweight: a meta-analysis. Am J Epidemiol 2005;162:397–403.
9 Kramer MS, Guo T, Platt RW, et al: Feeding effects on growth during infancy. J Pediatr 2004;145:600–605.
10 Dewey KG: Is breastfeeding protective against child obesity? J Hum Lact 2003;19:9–18.
11 Gillman MW, Rifas-Shiman SL, Camargo CA, et al: Risk of overweight among adolescents who were breastfed as infants. JAMA 2001;285:2461–2467.
12 Groh-Wargo S, Jacobs J, Auestad N, et al: Body composition in preterm infants who are fed long-chain polyunsaturated fatty acids: a prospective, randomized, controlled trial. Pediatr Res 2005;57:712–718.
13 Heinig MJ, Nommsen LA, Peerson JM, et al: Energy and protein intakes of breast-fed and formula-fed infants during the first year of life and their association with growth velocity: the DARLING study. Am J Clin Nutr 1993;58:152–161.
14 Scaglioni S, Agostoni C, De Notaris R, et al: Early macronutrient intake and overweight at 5 years of age. Int J Obes 2000;24:777–781.

15 Taylor RW, Grant AM, Goulding A, Williams SM: Early adiposity rebound: review of papers linking this to subsequent obesity in children and adults. Curr Opin Nutr Metab Care 2005;8:607–612.
16 Lucas A, Boyes S, Bloom SR, Aynsley-Green A: Metabolic and endocrine responses to a milk feed in six day old term infants: differences between breast and cow's milk formula feeding. Acta Paediatr Scand 1981;70:195–200.
17 Singhal A, Lucas A: Early origins of cardiovascular disease. Is there a unifying hypothesis? Lancet 2004;363:1642–1645.
18 Hemachandra AH, Howards PP, Schisterman EF, Klebanoff MA: Interaction between birth weight and postnatal growth does not increase risk for high blood pressure at age 7 years: results from the United States Collaborative Perinatal Project (abstract). Pediatr Res 2005;58:1102.
19 Metcalfe NB, Monaghan P: Compensation for a bad start: grow now, pay later? Trends Ecol Evol 2001;16:254–260.
20 Monteiro POA, Victora CG: Rapid growth in infancy and childhood and obesity in later life – a systematic review. Obes Rev 2005;6:143–154.
21 Baird J, Fisher D, Lucas P, et al: Being big or growing fast: systematic review of size and growth in infancy and later obesity. BMJ 2005;331:929–931.
22 Agras WS, Kraemer HC, Berkowitz RI, Hammer LD: Influence of early feeding style on adiposity at 6 years of age. J Pediatr 1990;116:805–809.
23 Stettler N, Zemel BS, Kumanyika S, Stallings VA: Infant weight gain and childhood overweight status in a multicenter, cohort study. Pediatrics 2002;109:194–199.
24 Stettler N, Stallings VA, Troxel AB, et al: Weight gain in the first week of life and overweight in adulthood; a cohort study of European American subjects fed infant formula. Circulation 2005;111:1897–1903.
25 Cole TJ: Children grow and horses race: is the adiposity rebound a critical period for later obesity? BMC Pediatr 2004;4:6–13.
26 Wilson AC, Forsyth JS, Greene SA, et al: Relation of infant diet to childhood health: seven year follow up of cohort of children in Dundee infant feeding study. BMJ 1998;316:21–25.
27 Bouret SG, Draper SJ, Simerly RB: Trophic action of leptin on hypothalamic neurons that regulate feeding. Science 2004;304:108–110.
28 Plagemann A, Harder T, Rake A, et al: Perinatal elevation of hypothalalmic insulin, acquired malformations of hypothalamic galaninergic neurons, and syndrome X-like alterations in adulthood of neonatally overfed rats. Brain Res 1999;836:146–155.
29 Singhal A, Sadaf Farooqi I, O'Rahilly S, et al: Early nutrition and leptin concentrations in later life. Am J Clin Nutr 2002;75:993–999.
30 Garza C: New growth standards for the 21st century: a prescriptive approach. Nutr Rev 2006;64:S55–S59.

Discussion

Dr. De Curtis: In preterm infants, especially in very low birth weight infants, it is suggested that aggressive nutrition should be started as soon as possible in order to avoid catabolism, allow rapid growth and obtain catch-up growth. What is your opinion on the catch-up growth of preterm infants? A lot of people don't think that the Barker hypothesis is true. Do you think that sometimes there is no correspondence between the statistical evidence and clinical importance, especially when the effect is seen in a large population?

Dr. Singhal: I couldn't agree with that more. There is a big difference between epidemiology and clinical care. As a neonatologist I would try to make any preterm infant grow because the most important thing is survival. Most preterm infants fall off their weight centile despite us trying to give them a high nutrient intake. So in preterm infants the situation is incredibly simple, promote growth to help them get off the ventilator and make them anabolic. We know that this will also benefit their long-term cognitive function and possibly their bone health.

Dr. Pazvakavambwa: In terms of your theories on insulin, what is the risk for the infant of a diabetic mother, and what is the outcome in terms of cardiovascular risk compared to the normal infant?

Dr. Singhal: This is a very active area of research. I don't know about cardiovascular risk, but the infants of diabetic mothers are at higher risk of later obesity, although the mechanisms involved are uncertain [1].

Dr. Fisberg: Could you possibly comment more on the influence of birth weight on the further development of obesity? In our experience we have seen that the odds ratio for low birth weight is exactly the same for children with a birth weight of over 4 kg.

Dr. Singhal: The association between birth weight and later obesity is complex because most studies don't separate fat and lean mass. There is an association between birth weight and later BMI, but for lean rather than fat mass [2]. There is also evidence of increased risk of obesity in babies with a high birth weight but there are few studies that use two-component models of body composition to show that this is fat and not lean tissue. There is also evidence that low birth weight increases abdominal fat mass later in life [3].

Dr. Ziegler: Thank you for this very comprehensive review of the existing information and the association between breastfeeding and later adiposity. You probably know that I am a skeptic. The simple fact that the obesity epidemic among children has coincided with a sharp increase in breastfeeding in the United States makes me wonder whether I should believe in causality, that is, breastfeeding causes children to be less obese. So could you please review for us the arguments in favor of causality?

Dr. Singhal: I think that researchers in the developmental origins field must not overplay their hand. The developmental origins hypothesis gives you a tendency, but does not directly lead to obesity. Even if you are programmed to eat more, or programmed for an increased risk of obesity, by far the strongest influence on obesity is your environment later in life, and you will never become fat unless you have a positive energy balance, despite your programming. I completely agree that the environment is the main reason that the obesity epidemic in children has occurred, but that is not to say that programming factors are not important. They are important given the current lifetime environment. In fact there may be an interaction between programming and environment probably mediated via appetite regulation.

Dr. Giovannini: I would like to ask about protein intake. The first point is not only the low protein but also the quality of amino acids. The second point is the quality of intrauterine development and complementary feeding.

Dr. Singhal: There are a lot of issues here. We don't even know what total protein intake does for later obesity. To my knowledge, the trial of Koletzko et al. [4] is the only randomized trial looking at the effects of differences in protein intake on obesity later in life. When you know that protein intake matters in an intervention study, only then can you investigate particular amino acids. It is early days in terms of identifying the nutritional window that influences long-term outcome, but we can see evidence of that process both in animals and humans. There is no doubt that there is an association between birth weight and long-term obesity risk. The question is how much of that is antenatal nutrition, how much due to genetic factors, such as imprinted genetic factors, and how much is due to postnatal growth. I think with the current level of knowledge, all we can say is that there is an association – at least until the results of intervention studies now taking place (e.g. in India) are available.

Dr. Cardoso: Why didn't you put discipline in the list of mechanisms to control obesity? I think that it is very important that the medical team make some comments about discipline during routine examinations for every child. Many things about behavior in their homes, in school and with friends contribute a lot to the weight of the child.

Dr. Singhal: I think that is the next stage. At the moment in the UK there is no such thing as an 'overgrowing' baby for mothers or pediatricians. If a baby is growing fast everybody is happy. We still have the attitude that fatter is better. One of the commonest things I see is a breastfed baby who has been supplemented with formula (often by health professionals) to make him grow faster. The baby was born on the 10th centile, is growing on the 10th centile, but nobody is happy because he is not on the 50th centile.

Dr. Cabus: In clinical practice we have seen children who are exclusively breastfed and they are too fat. Are there any studies that have investigated this kind of growth in normal children who were exclusively breastfed as babies?

Dr. Singhal: The data show that the mechanism is more fundamental than breastfeeding versus bottle feeding. The mechanism for early growth having adverse long-term effects occurs in yeast [5] and may not have anything to do with the type of feeding. A breastfed baby is less likely to accelerate centile upwards than a formula-fed baby, but there are a lot of data to show that the same phenomena occur in breastfed babies [6, 7]. There is no public health message for breastfed babies, suffice it to say that breastfed babies shouldn't be supplemented with formula just to make them grow faster.

Dr. Jongpiputvanich: You mentioned the critical window period of nutrition. But there are two hypotheses: one by Dr. Barker in the prenatal period, and you and Dr. Lucas mentioned the postnatal period. Could you comment further about this?

Dr. Singhal: I think at the end of the day there are going to be different critical windows for different outcomes. Dr. Barker and his team are quite rightly very interested in the antenatal period. Our team believe that postnatal factors are more important because you can more easily intervene postnatally and the effect sizes for postnatal growth (in our own work and that of others) appear to be much larger than the effects of birth weight, e.g. blood pressure. I don't think you can say that this is an antenatal or a postnatal hypothesis. I think that we should be focusing on what interventions we need, what public health policy is needed and what experiments we need to test the hypothesis, rather than saying it is all postnatal or antenatal.

Dr. Haschke: The question regarding the critical prenatal or postnatal window might not be an either/or, it could also be an and. I refer to the study recently presented by Dr. Bergmann in which they looked at two cohorts of mothers with breastfed infants in Germany; one cohort was supplemented with DHA from 32 weeks of gestation onwards and during the lactation period, and the offspring were followed until 21 months of age, and both cohorts were fully breastfed until 6 months of age. At 21 months of age the cohort whose mothers had received DHA had a lower body mass index, the difference being highly significant. So there are mechanisms which we still don't understand and the critical window for programming, whatever it is, might be before and after birth.

Dr. Singhal: I completely agree. In fact at a recent meeting in Sweden we agreed that programming is a life course event. The biology has to be continuous from antenatal to postnatal. That is not the same thing as saying that there cannot exclusively be a postnatal effect. The analogy I would make here is with an antihypertensive drug which has an effect by reducing your blood pressure but doesn't tell you anything about the biology of the high blood pressure in the first place. So breastfeeding can have an effect postnatally but the critical window for biology has to be continuous. So we don't need to make the dichotomy between antenatal and postnatal windows.

Dr. Brunser: We had a peculiar experience in Chile because at one time there was a very high incidence of infant malnutrition. To solve this situation these severely malnourished children, between 3 and 6 months of age, were placed in special centers where they were intensively fed to regain weight. Most of them were subsequently lost from control, but about 30 have been followed now for close to 30 years and they tend to be obese, they are short and tend to have lower intellectual development. So probably, as some people think, there is a window in which, if you increase the growth rate very rapidly, obesity tends to occur. The dilemma is that at that time, 30 years ago, we had to decide whether to run the risk of either the children dying of malnutrition or becoming obese 30 years later, and we decided then that it was probably better to be obese later in life than dead at an early age.

Dr. Agostoni: My question concerns your randomized trial on term SGA infants, there was also a nonrandomized control group taking human milk in this trial. Was the unfavorable association between early weight gain and later blood pressure still working in this group?

Dr. Singhal: Infants who showed upward centile crossing for weight between birth and age 8 months had a higher blood pressure [7] and body fat mass [Singhal, unpublished] whether they were breastfed or formula fed.

Dr. Agostoni: So in this case you take human milk, but it does not protect you?

Dr. Singhal: No, the mechanism is more fundamental than formula versus breast milk [5].

Dr. Agostoni: And with breastfed babies, those who have a rapid growth?

Dr. Singhal: They seem to be showing the same effect.

Dr. Solomons: 30 years ago when I went to work in Guatemala, we had the notion that developing an appropriate weight was important to develop optimal height. I am wondering if your epidemiological and clinical experience in Europe now suggests any kind of causal or dependency relationship between gaining weight and gaining height? This, because for Europeans, height seems to be an important thing. Is there any kind of a floor issue where this could explain why people grow in weight as best as they can as a mechanism to protect their height? Thereafter, they can lose the additional weight, but in the meanwhile one will have achieved the correct height. What is the science relating to this kind of reasoning?

Dr. Singhal: I can only speak about our two intervention studies. In preterm babies, who are incredibly malnourished, infants who received a low nutrient formula showed no differences in long-term height compared to babies who received the high nutrient formula [8], despite big differences in nutrient intake and short-term growth. Similarly, in our trial of infants born small for gestational age, there were no long-term differences in height between groups randomized to different nutrition in infancy [7]. So I don't know if there is any evidence from randomized studies that early nutrition makes any difference to final height.

Dr. Leone: Don't you think that preterm babies depend on the level of immaturity at birth, and is there a causality or a relationship between these? Is there bigger or lesser sensitivity to these factors?

Dr. Singhal: There may be other factors that affect growth. I have focused on nutritional intervention, but obviously morbidity, prematurity, maternal size, genetic, many other factors may contribute to growth.

References

1 Plagemann A, Harder T, Franke K, Kohlhoff R: Long-term impact of neonatal breast-feeding on body weight and glucose tolerance in children of diabetic mothers. Diabetes Care 2002;25: 16–22.
2 Singhal A, Wells J, Cole TJ, et al: Programming of lean body mass: a link between birth weight, obesity, and cardiovascular disease? Am J Clin Nutr 2003;77:726–770.
3 Garnett SP, Cowell CT, Baur LA, et al: Abdominal fat and birth size in healthy prepubertal children. Int J Obes Relat Metab Disord 2001;25:1667–1673.

4   Koletzko B, Broekaert I, Demmelmair H, et al: Protein intake in the first year of life: a risk fac-
    tor for later obesity? The EU childhood obesity project. Adv Exp Med Biol 2005;569:69–79.
5   Longo VD, Finch CE: Evolutionary medicine: from dwarf model systems to healthy centenar-
    ians? Science 2003;299:1342–1346.
6   Agras WS, Kraemer HC, Berkowitz RI, Hammer LD: Influence of early feeding style on adi-
    posity at 6 years of age. J Pediatr 1990;116:805–809.
7   Singhal A, Cole TJ, Fewtrell M, et al: Promotion of faster weight gain in infants born small for
    gestational age: is there an adverse effect on later blood pressure? Circulation 2007;115:
    213–220.
8   Morley R, Lucas A: Randomized diet in the neonatal period and growth performance until
    7.5–8y of age in preterm children. Am J Clin Nutr 2000;71:822–828.

Agostoni C, Brunser O (eds): Issues in Complementary Feeding.
Nestlé Nutr Workshop Ser Pediatr Program, vol 60, pp 31–42,
Nestec Ltd., Vevey/S. Karger AG, Basel, © 2007.

Later Effects of Breastfeeding Practice: The Evidence

Dominique Turck

Division of Gastroenterology, Hepatology and Nutrition, Department of Pediatrics,
Lille University Children's Hospital and Faculty of Medicine, Lille, France

Abstract

Breastfeeding plays a key role in the programming process during early life but, due to confounding factors, it is difficult to draw conclusions on long-term health benefits. The magnitude of the beneficial effect of breastfeeding on blood pressure ($-2\,\mathrm{mm\,Hg}$) and total cholesterol ($-0.2\,\mathrm{mmol/l}$) is likely to have public health implications. However, it is unknot known whether breastfeeding reduces the risk of cardiovascular mortality. Breastfeeding may protect against the development of celiac disease. The protective role of breastfeeding against type 1 diabetes seems likely, but the mechanisms involved are still under discussion. There is no convincing evidence that breastfeeding reduces the risk of leukemia and cancer. Breastfeeding is associated with a better cognitive development ($+3$ points) that is present as early as at 6 months of age and sustained throughout childhood and adolescence. The benefits of breast milk may be related to its high content in docosahexaenoic acid which plays an important role in brain development. Increasing the duration of breastfeeding is correlated with an increase in cognitive development.

Introduction

'Programming' describes the finding that, during critical windows in early life, hormones, metabolites and neurotransmitters are able to have a long-term influence on health. Breastfeeding plays a key role in the programming process during early life.

It is difficult to draw firm conclusions on the causal relationship between breastfeeding and long-term health benefits [1]. For obvious reasons, it is unethical to perform randomized experimental studies involving breastfeeding. Available information is limited to observational studies, and confounding is therefore a concern: educational, socioeconomic, and lifestyle factors associated

31

with the mother's decision to breastfeed; recall bias on the nature and duration of breastfeeding, etc. Even in studies controlling for known confounding variables, residual confounding is still an issue.

The aim of the present article is to review the long-term consequences of breastfeeding on health, with the exception of allergy and obesity.

Effects of Early Growth

Singhal [2] has proposed the postnatal growth acceleration hypothesis, suggesting that faster growth (upward centile crossing), particularly in infancy, adversely programs the metabolic syndrome. Faster neonatal weight gain was shown to program insulin resistance in preterm infants randomly assigned to a nutrient-enriched diet (preterm formula) that promoted faster growth compared with the standard diet (banked breast milk or preterm formula). Several studies have found that breastfed infants are shorter at the age of 12 months compared with formula-fed infants. Investigators recently found in the Avon cohort that children presented at age 7–8 years with a trend toward higher serum insulin-like growth factor-1 (IGF-1) in exclusively breastfed infants as compared with partially breastfed infants and never breastfed infants. The IGF-1 axis would be programmed during infancy, with low IGF-1 values during breastfeeding, and higher IGF-1 levels and, as a consequence, higher growth velocity later in childhood [3].

Cardiovascular Health

Blood Pressure
In the early 1980s a randomized trial comparing the use of banked human milk with preterm formula for feeding premature infants gave the opportunity to measure blood pressure at age 13–16 years [4]. The mean diastolic blood pressure was higher when assigned preterm formula than banked human milk: 65.0 vs. 61.9 mm Hg (95% CI for difference −5.8 to −0.6; p = 0.016). No difference was found for systolic blood pressure.

A first meta-analysis was aimed at determining whether breastfeeding in infancy was associated with lower blood pressure at later age [5]. The pooled mean difference in systolic blood pressure was −1.10 mm Hg in participants breastfed as infants. No difference was found for diastolic blood pressure. Another meta-analysis, including an extra ~10,000 subjects from 3 studies with more than 1,500 participants each, showed that breastfeeding was associated with a 1.4 and 0.5 mm Hg reduction in systolic and diastolic blood pressure, respectively [6]. In these 2 publications, the difference was independent of age at measurement of blood pressure and year of birth, and was reduced in large studies (n ≥ 1,000) compared with smaller ones.

Table 1. Blood pressure (mm Hg) at age 6 years in children who as infants had been randomized to be fed with formula supplemented with long-chain polyunsaturated fatty acids or with formula without supplementation

Blood pressure	Supplemented formula (n = 65)	Formula without supplementation (n = 71)	Mean difference (95% CI)	p
Mean	74.8	77.8	−3.0 (−5.4 to −0.5)	0.02
Diastolic	57.3	60.9	−3.6 (−6.5 to −0.6)	0.018
Systolic	92.4	94.7	−2.3 (5.3 to 0.7)	0.132

From Forsyth et al. [8].

The magnitude of the effect of breastfeeding on blood pressure is similar to the effect of salt restriction (−1.3 mm Hg) and weight loss (−2.8 mm Hg) in normotensive subjects, and is likely to have substantial public health implications [7]. A lowering of population-wide diastolic blood pressure by only 2 mm Hg would reduce the prevalence of hypertension by 17%, and the risk of coronary heart disease and that of stroke and transient ischemic attacks by 6 and 15%, respectively.

The lower sodium content of breast milk may play a role in the reduction of blood pressure, as well as the high content of LCPUFA in breast milk, which are incorporated into cell membranes of the vascular endothelium. A randomized controlled trial showed that dietary supplementation with LCPUFA in infant formula from birth to 6 months was associated with a significant reduction in mean and diastolic blood pressure at 6 years of age [8] (table 1).

Lipid Metabolism

The randomized trial on premature infants previously described [4] made it possible to study lipoprotein profile in 13- to 16-year-old adolescents born preterm [9]. Adolescents fed human milk at birth had a lower LDL to HDL ratio than those given preterm formula. There was a dose-response effect supporting a causal link between breast milk feeding and the lipoprotein profile in later life. A meta-analysis of 37 studies showed that blood total cholesterol (TC) differed with age. TC levels were higher in breastfed than in formula-fed infants (<1 year), due to the very high content of cholesterol in breast milk and to the absence or very low content of cholesterol in most infant formulae (mean TC difference 0.64; 95% CI 0.50 to 0.79 mmol/l) [10]. The mean TC in childhood or adolescence (1–16 years) was not related to feeding patterns in infancy. A recent study from Brazil also showed no influence of breastfeeding on TC among male adolescents [11]. However, the meta-analysis showed that TC in adults was lower among those breastfed in infancy (mean TC difference −0.18; 95% CI −0.30 to −0.06 mmol/l). Patterns for LDL cholesterol were similar to those for TC throughout. Whatever the underlying programming stimulus, long-term modifications in cholesterol metabolism are likely to occur, either by regulation of HMG-CoA reductase activity or LDL-receptor activity. Even if the difference in adult TC of 0.2 mmol/l is modest, a reduction in mean TC of this magnitude in adult life would be associated with a reduction in coronary heart disease incidence of approximately 10%.

Cardiovascular Disease

An important question is to determine whether the effects of breastfeeding in infancy on lipid metabolism and blood pressure lead to a reduction in cardiovascular risk in adulthood. The potentially beneficial effects on lipid metabolism and blood pressure could be reduced by a negative effect on arterial function. Two studies showed that arterial distensibility in 10-year-old children and in adults was related to the duration of breastfeeding [12, 13]. A longer duration of breastfeeding was associated with stiffer arteries. However, the study performed in adults showed no difference in distensibility between participants who had been bottle fed and those breastfed for less than 4 months. Further studies are necessary before drawing any conclusions.

The British Boyd-Orr cohort consists of subjects who were originally surveyed in 1937–1939, when they were 0–19 years of age. The follow-up of this cohort made it possible to show in 63- to 82-year-old participants that breastfeeding was inversely associated with ultrasound measured intima-media thickness of the common carotid and bifurcation as well as carotid and femoral plaques, compared with bottle feeding [14]. These results may suggest a beneficial effect of breastfeeding on atherosclerosis. However, there was no clear evidence of a duration-response relationship between breastfeeding and intima-media thickness. The study of the same cohort based on a larger number of subjects and a systematic review with meta-analysis of 4 studies failed to show any beneficial effect of breastfeeding on cardiovascular disease mortality [15]. The study of the cohort of Caerphilly, Wales, surprisingly showed a positive association between breastfeeding and coronary heart disease mortality. There was however no duration-response effect, which might be expected if an adverse effect of breastfeeding was causal [16]. In contrast, the study of the participants of the Nurses' Health Study showed an 8% reduced risk of coronary heart disease [17].

There is still no convincing evidence that breastfeeding reduces the risk of cardiovascular mortality.

Disorders of the Immune System

Celiac Disease

A recent review of 6 observational studies suggested that breastfeeding may protect against the development of celiac disease (CD) [18]. With the exception of a small study, an association was found between an increasing duration of breastfeeding and reduced risk of developing CD. The meta-analysis showed that the risk of CD was markedly reduced in infants who were breastfeeding at the time of gluten introduction as compared with non-breastfed infants (OR 0.48, 95% CI 0.40 to 0.59). However, breastfeeding may not provide permanent protection against CD but only delay the onset of symptoms.

Inflammatory Bowel Disease

Perinatal events may play a role in the etiology of inflammatory bowel disease (IBD). A meta-analysis from 2004 showed a protective effect of breastfeeding on the risk of IBD: the risk of Crohn's disease (CD) and ulcerative colitis (UC) decreased by 33 and 23%, respectively [19]. However, of a total of 17 studies, only 4 studies of Crohn's disease and 4 studies of UC were of high methodological quality. A pediatric, population-based, case-control study was recently performed in northern France to examine the environmental risk factors associated with IBD [20]. In a multivariate model adjusted for the mother's education level, breastfeeding (partial or exclusive) was a risk factor for Crohn's disease (odds ratio 2.1; 95% CI 1.3 to 3.4; p = 0.003), but not for UC. Children with Crohn's disease were breastfed (exclusively or not) for an average of 2 weeks more than the controls, but the difference was not significant. Further studies are needed to fully understand the relation between breastfeeding and IBD.

Diabetes Mellitus

The protective role of breastfeeding against type 1 diabetes seems likely even if the mechanisms involved are still under discussion. A European multicenter study showed that breastfeeding of any duration was associated with a 25% reduction in risk of type 1 diabetes [21]. The early introduction of cow's milk may in fact be the main contributory factor [1]. It has been suggested that immunization against cow's milk proteins would trigger an autoimmune reaction against pancreatic β cells due to a structural similarity between one or several cow's milk proteins and antigens located on β cells. This hypothesis is further supported by experimental studies in animals showing that feeding with hydrolyzed cow's milk proteins is associated with a lower risk of diabetes. More information will come from the TRIGR study in Finland, randomizing high-risk infants to different supplemental formulae, either a hydrolyzed formula or a regular cow's milk-based formula, after breastfeeding for 6–8 months of life.

Malignant Disease

Breast milk may play a role in the prevention of childhood leukemia and cancer by stimulating or modulating the immune response and promoting its development in early life. Only 2 of the 4 studies considered to be of good methodological quality in the recent review by Guise et al. [22] found a risk reduction of acute lymphocytic leukemia (odds ratios 0.80 and 0.67) associated with breastfeeding. A meta-analysis of 26 studies on breastfeeding and childhood cancer showed that having ever been breastfed was associated with a lower risk of 9% for acute lymphocytic leukemia, 24% for Hodgkin's disease, and 41% for neuroblastoma [23]. However, methodological limitations were pointed out.

In the British Boyd-Orr cohort, as compared with never having breastfed, ever having breastfed was not associated with the incidence of all cancers or of any individual cancer type. However, a meta-analysis of 11 studies, including that of the Boyd-Orr cohort, showed that breastfed women had a slightly reduced risk of premenopausal breast cancer (RR = 0.88; 95% CI 0.79 to 0.98) but not of postmenopausal breast cancer [24].

Cognitive Development

Most studies have shown that breastfeeding is associated with enhanced neurodevelopment. The meta-analysis of Anderson et al. [25] showed an increment in cognitive function of 3.14 points for breastfed infants compared with formula-fed infants. Better cognitive development was present as early as 6 months of age and was sustained throughout childhood and adolescence. Low birth weight infants derived larger benefits (5.18 points) than did normal weight infants (2.66 points). an increasing duration of breastfeeding was accompanied by an increase in cognitive development. A specific role of breast milk is suggested by the randomized controlled trial of Lucas et al. [26], who demonstrated a higher IQ in 7.5- to 8-year-old children born preterm who had received breast milk via a nasogastric tube. The benefits of breast milk may be related to its high content in docosahexaenoic acid (DHA, 22:6(n-3)) that plays an important role in brain development. Breastfed infants undergoing postmortem examination because of sudden death had a greater proportion of DHA in their brain cortex relative to those fed formula (fig. 1) [27]. The role of DHA is further suggested by the fact that DHA supplementation of breastfeeding mothers for 4 months after delivery resulted in a higher Bayley psychomotor development index in infants at 30 months of age [28].

The most important residual confounding factor is the influence of maternal socioeconomic status on the child's cognitive development. A study from the Philippines evaluated the relation between breastfeeding and cognitive development in a population in which breastfeeding was inversely correlated with socioeconomic advantages, as opposed to industrialized countries [29]. Scores at 8.5 and 11.5 years were higher for infants breastfed longer (1.6 and 9.8 points higher among normal birth weight and low birth weight infants, respectively; infants breastfed for 12–18 vs. <6 months).

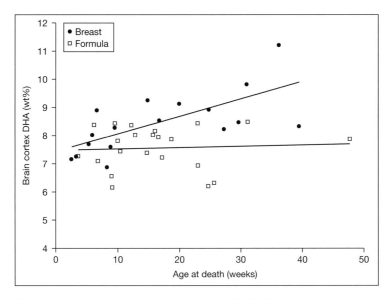

Fig. 1. Brain cortex docosahexaenoic acid (DHA) plotted against age at death in infants undergoing postmortem examinations as a result of sudden death. Results from samples from breastfed infants ($r^2 = 0.72$, $p < 0.01$, n = 15) and formula-fed infants ($r^2 = 0.02$, NS, n = 20) are shown. From Makrides et al. [27].

Little is known about the effects of breastfeeding in adulthood. A positive association between the duration of breastfeeding and cognitive function was observed in 2 samples of young Danish adults, assessed with 2 different IQ tests [30]. In men aged 60–74 years from the Caerphilly cohort, having been artificially fed was associated with a lower cognitive function only in those with a birth weight below the median [31].

A very recent study involving >5,000 US children used sibling comparison analysis. Any confounding factor that is the same for both members of a pair of siblings was automatically controlled for [32]. Breastfeeding was associated with an increase of around 4 points that was mostly accounted for by maternal intelligence. When fully adjusted for confounding factors, the benefit in breastfed infants was small and not significant (0.52; CI −0.19 to 1.23).

Conclusion

Breastfeeding is an unequalled way of providing ideal food for the healthy growth and development of infants. The main advantages on later health associated with breastfeeding are an enhanced cognitive development, as well as lower blood pressure and plasma total cholesterol, although no effect could be demonstrated on the cardiovascular risk.

References

1 Schack-Nielsen L, Michaelsen KF: Breast feeding and future health. Curr Opin Clin Nutr Metab Care 2006;9:289–296.
2 Singhal A: Early nutrition and long-term cardiovascular health. Nutr Rev 2006;64:S44–S49.
3 Martin RM, Holly JM, Davey Smith G, et al: Could associations between breastfeeding and insulin-like growth factors underlie associations of breastfeeding with adult chronic disease? The Avon Longitudinal Study of Parents and Children. Clin Endocrinol 2005;62:728–737.
4 Singhal A, Cole TJ, Lucas A: Early nutrition in preterm infants and later blood pressure: two cohorts after randomised trials. Lancet 2001;357:413–419.
5 Owen CG, Whincup PH, Gilg JA, Cook DG: Effect of breast feeding in infancy on blood pressure in later life: systematic review and meta-analysis. BMJ 2003;327:1189–1195.
6 Martin RM, Gunnell D, Davey Smith G: Breastfeeding in infancy and blood pressure in later life: systematic review and meta-analysis. Am J Epidemiol 2005;161:15–26.
7 Ebrahim S, Davey Smith G: Lowering blood pressure: a systematic review of sustained effects of non-pharmacological interventions. J Public Health Med 1998;20:441–448.
8 Forsyth JS, Willatts P, Agostoni C, et al: Long chain polyunsaturated fatty acid supplementation in infant formula and blood pressure in later childhood: follow-up of a randomised controlled trial. BMJ 2003;326:953–959.
9 Singhal A, Cole TJ, Fewtrell M, Lucas A: Breastmilk feeding and lipoprotein profile in adolescents born preterm: follow-up of a prospective randomised study. Lancet 2004;363: 1571–1578.
10 Owen CG, Whincup PH, Odoki K, et al: Infant feeding and blood cholesterol: a study in adolescents and a systematic review. Pediatrics 2002;110:597–608.
11 Victora CG, Horta BL, Post P, et al: Breast feeding and blood lipid concentrations in male Brazilian adolescents. J Epidemiol Community Health 2006;60:621–625.
12 Leeson CPM, Kattenhorn M, Deanfield JE, Lucas A: Duration of breastfeeding and arterial distensibility in early adult life: population based study. BMJ 2001;322:643–647.
13 Schack-Nielsen L, Molgaard C, Larsen D, et al: Arterial stiffness in 10-year-old children: current and early determinants. Br J Nutr 2005;94:1004–1011.
14 Martin RM, Ebrahim S, Griffin M, et al: Breastfeeding and atherosclerosis. Intima-media thickness and plaques at 65-year follow-up of the Boyd-Orr cohort. Arterioscler Thromb Vasc Biol 2005;25:1482–1488.
15 Martin RM, Davey Smith G, Mangtani P, et al: Breastfeeding and cardiovascular mortality: the Boyd-Orr cohort and a systematic review with meta-analysis. Eur Heart J 2004;25:778–786.
16 Martin RM, Ben-Shlomo Y, Gunnell D, et al: Breast feeding and cardiovascular disease risk factors, incidence, and mortality: the Caerphilly study. J Epidemiol Community Health 2005;59: 121–129.
17 Rich-Edwards JW, Stampfer MJ, Mason JE, et al: Breastfeeding during infancy and the risk of cardiovascular disease in adulthood. Epidemiology 2004;15:550–556.
18 Akobeng AK, Ramanan AV, Buchan I, Heller RF: Effect of breast feeding on risk of coeliac disease: a systematic review and meta-analysis of observational studies. Arch Dis Child 2006;91: 39–45.
19 Klement E, Cohen RV, Bosman J, et al: Breastfeeding and risk of inflammatory bowel disease: a systematic review with meta-analysis. Am J Clin Nutr 2004;80:1342–1352.
20 Baron S, Turck D, Leplat C, et al: Environmental risk factors in paediatric inflammatory bowel diseases: a population based case control study. Gut 2005;54:357–363.
21 The Eurodiab Substudy 2 Study Group: Rapid early growth is associated with increased risk of childhood type 1 diabetes in various European populations. Diabetes Care 2002;25: 1755–1760.
22 Guise JM, Austin D, Morris CD: Review of case-control studies related to breastfeeding and reduced risk of childhood leukemia. Pediatrics 2005;116:e724–e731.
23 Martin RM, Gunnell D, Owen CG, Davey Smith G: Breast-feeding and childhood cancer: a systematic review with metaanalysis. Int J Cancer 2005;117:1020–1031.
24 Martin RM, Middleton N, Gunnell D, et al: Breast-feeding and cancer: the Boyd-Orr cohort and a systematic review with meta-analysis. J Natl Cancer Inst 2005;97:1446–1457.
25 Anderson JW, Johnstone BM, Remley DT: Breast-feeding and cognitive development: a meta-analysis. Am J Clin Nutr 1999;70:525–535.

26 Lucas A, Morley R, Cole TJ, et al: Breast milk and subsequent intelligence quotient in children born preterm. Lancet 1992;339:261–264.
27 Makrides M, Neumann MA, Byard RW, et al: Fatty acid composition of brain, retina, and erythrocytes in breast- and formula-fed infants. Am J Clin Nutr 1994;60:189–194.
28 Jensen CL, Voigt RG, Prager TC, et al: Effects of maternal docosahexaenoic acid intake on visual function and neurodevelopment in breastfed term infants. Am J Clin Nutr 2005;82:125–132.
29 Daniels MC, Adair LS: Breastfeeding influences cognitive development in Filipino children. J Nutr 2005;135:2589–2595.
30 Mortensen EL, Michaelsen KF, Sanders SA, Reinisch JM: The association of breastfeeding and adult intelligence. JAMA 2002;287:2365–2371.
31 Elwood PC, Pickering J, Gallacher JE, et al: Long term effect of breastfeeding: cognitive function in the Caerphilly cohort. J Epidemiol Community Health 2005;59:130–133.
32 Der G, Batty GD, Deary IJ: Effect of breast feeding on intelligence in children: prospective study, sibling pairs analysis, and meta-analysis. BMJ 2006;333:929–930.

Discussion

Dr. Giovannini: A very interesting lecture and I perfectly agree with every point. Breastfeeding is much better in the dietary treatment of inborn metabolic disorders. In the *Journal of Pediatrics* we published a paper regarding the best behavior in phenylketonuria children breastfed for at least the first months of life [1]. This is very important because human milk is lower in phenylalanine and rich in DHA. The second very important point, in *Acta Paediatrica* [2] we showed that women who had been breastfed were breastfeeding more easily. I greatly appreciate the problem of cholesterol; it is an economical and social problem, because breastfed adults have 6.9 mg/dl lower cholesterol than non-breastfed adults.

Dr. Turck: I could not more agree with you. I have to apologize for forgetting to say that breastfeeding can be used in metabolic disorders. In fact in my unit, where we also deal with metabolic disorders, it was after your publication that we started to think about using breastfeeding more than we used to. It is obviously a question of social interaction. In my country the situation of breastfeeding is not very good, with 60% of children being breastfed after leaving the maternity ward. Even if the situation is getting better, the duration of breastfeeding is very low. I think that, from the individual point of view, all the aspects that I showed you are not very interesting, but from a public health perspective, if we want to have some interest from the politicians, points such as cholesterolemia and perhaps cardiovascular risk are important to raise.

Dr. Agostoni: If I can add just a few words regarding amino acid disorders. Two months ago there was a publication showing the positive effects of human milk in children suffering from propionic acidemia and other amino acid disorders [3]. In your review did you have the opportunity to look at the results? It seems to me that the clearest advantage of breastfeeding was shown in children with mental handicaps or at risk of mental handicaps.

Dr. Turck: There was a paper related to the British millennium cohort where previously breastfed children had fewer handicaps than previously non-breastfed children.

Dr. Ziegler: In one of the studies you mentioned you showed that there was no association between breastfeeding and dyslipidemia in 60- to 82-year-olds. There is a similar study showing a lack of association between breastfeeding and, in this case, obesity when the subjects were older. I wish to point out that there is a fundamental difference in breastfeeding as practiced today and probably for the last 50 years where the mother and perhaps the father make the decision to breastfeed, which is influenced by their health beliefs. In contrast, 80 years ago breastfeeding was more or less universally practiced and formula was fed only when there were certain circumstances that necessitated it. The formulas used then were fundamentally different from the formulas that were developed later. So breastfeeding meant something different 80 years ago compared to today.

Dr. Turck: Again it is a combination of an effect on development and also of environment, but of course the formulas in the 1930s have nothing to do with what they are now.

Dr. Seidman: I was intrigued with your data regarding the increased risk of Crohn's disease in children in France. We carried out a very similar case-control study in Montreal. As you know most French Canadian families have a founder effect with genetic origins from the north of France but living in a different environment in Quebec. We studied close to 200 cases of pediatric-onset Crohn's disease and 200 controls who were pair-matched for timing of diagnosis and area of residence [4]. We didn't find that a history of breastfeeding in the first 6 months of life affected risk. I would appreciate your comments. I should emphasize that the rate of breastfeeding in Quebec is extremely low amongst the developed countries of the world, and that might be one consideration. If a family has a history of Crohn's disease, which is by far the leading risk factor for developing Crohn's disease with an odds ratio of 4.6 in our study, it may be that the parents would try breastfeeding more often than the control family with the idea that it would be protective.

Dr. Turck: The results came from a multivariate analysis and we controlled for family history which is, I completely agree with you, by far the most important risk factor for inflammatory bowel disease (IBD) in children.

Dr. Guandalini: My question is actually speculative about the protective role of breastfeeding on IBD. I am sure you have given some thought to why this may be. Has it to do with the microflora that is different between breastfed and formula-fed infants; has it to do with the lower antigenic load from other solids that are taken, or has it to do with the later introduction of complementary feeding?

Dr. Turck: One explanation, which is just speculation, is that because of breastfeeding the infections happen later in life in breastfed children, so there might be a window during which any infection might have some deleterious effect on the immune system, but it is really just speculation. We are more interested by the pollution story because the region is very highly polluted and high particle levels have been found in breast milk and also in tissues from patients with IBD. So we are trying to find out if this could be an explanation. But if the risk is doubled, Crohn's disease is still a rare disease. Even if its incidence is increasing, I think this should not lead us to modify our policy which, of course, is pushing breastfeeding in industrialized countries.

Dr. Barclay: Concerning cognitive development, in the review by Der et al. [5] I think their own study was the only one that had controlled for maternal IQ. In the other studies, maternal IQ was not taken into account. So is it correct that if you control for maternal IQ, the effect of breastfeeding on cognitive development disappears?

Dr. Turck: Other studies controlled for maternal education but this study controlled especially for maternal IQ. I think using the siblings allows you to take into account most confounding factors. In their discussion Der et al. speak of another study with siblings giving the same results, i.e. there is no benefit from breastfeeding. I think that it is a very difficult issue and even if there is an effect, it is really a small one.

Dr. Ziegler: There is one other study by Jacobson et al. [6] where the mother's IQ was actually measured, and when the child's IQ was corrected for the mother's IQ there was no significant effect of breastfeeding on the child's IQ.

Dr. Brunser: I think your observations on Crohn's disease are very interesting. There is work by Hollander [7] who measured intestinal permeability in the relatives of patients with Crohn's disease, and he demonstrated that the parents of children who have Crohn's disease also have disturbances in intestinal permeability. So he thought that if you develop Crohn's disease because your family is prone to Crohn's disease, there must be some kind of disturbance in intestinal permeability.

Dr. Turck: But the risk of Crohn's disease in our study was 5 times higher in cases with a family history of IBD, which was the strongest risk factor.

Dr. Ferreira: I am a pediatric gastroenterologist, not an investigator, so I don't know all the studies as you do. I am wondering if we are not trying to compare something that is not comparable, because even with the power of meta-analysis we cannot reach a conclusion. Is there a study comparing siblings? Sometimes a mother can breastfeed one infant and cannot breastfeed another. Is there a study comparing the two?

Dr. Turck: That was the case in the study by Der et al. [5]. They had 334 pairs of siblings who were breastfed and perhaps 450 pairs with one breastfed and the other not. They could not find any difference in cognitive development between these two.

Dr. Ferreira: And cardiovascular disease in adult life?

Dr. Turck: I have to say that I don't remember. I don't think so, but I am not 100% sure.

Dr. Ferreira: I have another question. Is it possible to think about the gut, not about food but about the gut, because we also see obesity in breastfed infants. Is it possible that babies have a more absorptive gut capacity which in infancy gives them a higher rate of growth and later in life they are more prone to absorb more cholesterol and lipid substances, and more prone to cardiovascular disease, metabolic syndrome and truncal obesity? Is it possible that the problem is in the gut and not in the feeding?

Dr. Turck: I don't think there is a clear answer to your question. At least I can't answer it. To me the main reason for promoting breastfeeding is the pleasure of the child and the pleasure of the mother while she is breastfeeding. This is a scientific issue and a health policy issue, so I can't answer the question.

Dr. Ferreira: All the pediatricians agree that breastfeeding is better but we must try to prove that advantage.

Dr. Turck: There are obviously limits to the meta-analyses and all the studies that have been published.

Dr. Michaelsen: I agree with your conclusion on the studies on IQ. It has remained quite consistent up to the last BMJ study [5] which showed a small (half an IQ point) but non-significant effect. Another US sibling study showed a significant effect of breastfeeding. There are two other pieces of information. One is that there is a DHA mechanism that could explain this and is supported by the results of preterm infants. The other piece of information is the PROBIT study from Belarus by Kramer et al. [8]. I have been at two meetings where some new results from the 6-year follow-up were given. It was a randomized study, where they randomized hospitals to promote breastfeeding or not. So apart from the randomized studies by Lucas and Singhal, this is another kind of randomized study. They underlined that they saw an effect on IQ in that study, not on obesity and allergies. This is some information that might again support that there is a small effect in IQ, which is consistent in many studies.

Dr. Turck: Thank you, this is an important point.

Dr. Solomons: You showed a picture of Dr. Burrill Crohn, and my question has to do with Crohn's disease. How could someone in the 1930s discover a 'new' disease? Where was Crohn's disease before Dr. Crohn discovered it? Was it in fact a new disease of the 20th century or a missed diagnosed disease of antiquity? Dr. Ziegler pointed out the difference between the formulas – then and now. Are there any studies that detail whether the complementary feeding patterns of breastfeeding mothers and artificial-feeding mothers are different? I wonder if anyone knows of any studies on complementary feeding patterns or differential early feeding patterns?

Dr. Turck: To answer your first question, it seems that in the old British medical literature descriptions of what we now call Crohn's disease were made at the end of the 18th century, so that may be part of the answer. The increase in incidence, of course, might be due to a better recognition of the disease. In our region we have a registry that started in 1988 with a system of interviews that allows us to be sure that we haven't missed a diagnosis from 1988 on. In this period we observed a 25% increase in Crohn's disease but at the same time a 25% decrease in ulcerative colitis. I have no answer to your second question.

Dr. Haschke: A very short and nonscientific comment on your historical persons, as to whether they were breastfed or not. There is a comprehensive review on the history of breastfeeding by Fomon published in 1983 and it is clear that animal milk started to be extensively used not earlier than in the mid 19th century, so all your historical persons can be considered to have been breastfed.

Dr. Turck: I am not very anxious about that.

Dr. Agostoni: We cannot exclude that women from higher social classes, whose children presumably have a higher IQ due to positive environmental stimulation, have dietary habits that result in milk with higher DHA levels. Again, we do not know the start and the end of this 'virtuous' circle: what is the cause and what is the effect.

References

1   Agostoni C, Massetto N, Biasucci G, et al: Effects of long-chain polyunsaturated fatty acid supplementation on fatty acid status and visual function in treated children with hyperphenylalaninemia. J Pediatr 2000;137:504–509.
2   Giovannini M, Banderali G, Radaelli G, et al: Monitoring breastfeeding rates in Italy: national surveys 1995 and 1999. Acta Paediatr 2003;92:357–363.
3   Gokcay G, Baykal T, Gokdemir Y, et al: Breast feeding in organic acidaemias. J Inherit Metab Dis 2006;29:304–310.
4   Amre DK, Lambrette P, Law L, et al: Investigating the hygiene hypothesis as a risk factor in pediatric onset Crohn's disease: a case-control study. Am J Gastroenterol 2006;101:1005–1011.
5   Der G, Batty GD, Deary IJ: Effect of breast feeding on intelligence in children: prospective study, sibling pairs analysis, and meta-analysis. BMJ 2006;333:945.
6   Jacobson SW, Chiodo LM, Jacobson JL: Breastfeeding effects on intelligence quotient in 4- and 11-year-old children. Pediatrics 1999;103:e71.
7   Hollander D: Intestinal permeability in patients with Crohn's disease and their relatives. Dig Liver Dis 2001;33:649–651.
8   Kramer MS, Chalmers B, Hodnett ED, et al: Promotion of Breastfeeding Intervention Trial (PROBIT): a randomized trial in the Republic of Belarus. JAMA 2001;285:413–420.

Agostoni C, Brunser O (eds): Issues in Complementary Feeding.
Nestlé Nutr Workshop Ser Pediatr Program, vol 60, pp 43–63,
Nestec Ltd., Vevey/S. Karger AG, Basel, © 2007.

Traditional Foods vs. Manufactured Baby Foods

Elaine L. Ferguson[a], *Nicole Darmon*[b]

[a]Department of Human Nutrition, University of Otago, Dunedin, New Zealand;
[b]Human Nutrition Research Unit Inserm U476/Inra, Faculté de Médecine de la Timone,
Marseille, France

Abstract

The provision of nutrient-dense complementary foods is essential to ensure an infant's nutrient requirements are met. Yet often, relative to recommendations, traditional complementary foods have low levels of nutrients, suggesting a role, for fortified manufactured baby foods, in ensuring dietary adequacy. In this review, the potential benefits and safety of using fortified manufactured baby foods versus traditional foods alone are evaluated based on evidence from food composition data, diet modeling and intervention studies. Results from the food composition data and diet modeling suggest that ensuring a nutritionally adequate complementary feeding diet based on traditional foods alone is difficult. Conversely, except for biochemical iron status, intervention trials do not show consistent benefits, for growth or biochemical zinc or riboflavin status, with the use of fortified manufactured baby foods versus traditional foods alone. The safety of manufactured baby foods will depend on food preparation practices and the presence of effective governmental regulatory infrastructures. Hence, in environments where fortified manufactured baby foods are expensive, unavailable or where there is an absence of effective governmental regulatory infrastructures, the use of traditional foods is advised. Conversely, where affordable manufactured baby foods are available, marketed safely and fortified appropriately, their use is likely to result in improved nutrient intakes and infant biochemical iron status. In all environments, the promotion of breastfeeding, active feeding and high levels of hygiene is essential to ensure optimal nutritional status.

Introduction

The complementary feeding period is when children are most vulnerable to malnutrition and its associated adverse affects on health, growth and development [1]. Infants and young children, living in resource-limited environments, are particularly vulnerable to malnutrition, which is reflected in growth faltering between 6 and 24 months of age [1]. Consequently, international organizations, such as the World Health Organization (WHO), emphasize the importance of providing sufficient quantities of safe, nutritionally adequate and age-appropriate foods to complement breast milk intakes [1]. Nevertheless, for some nutrients, the amounts required from complementary foods are high relative to their contents in traditional foods, and antinutrients in these foods may modify nutrient absorption or digestion [1, 2]. Hence, strategies, such as fortification, may be necessary to increase the nutrient density of complementary feeding diets, suggesting a role, for fortified manufactured baby foods, in reducing rates of malnutrition. Furthermore, the processing of manufactured baby foods may reduce cooking times or levels of pathogenic micro-organisms, as well as inactivate enzymes or antinutrients to enhance the convenience, taste, digestibility or nutritional quality of the foods [1]. Consequently, for improving infant nutritional status, the use of fortified manufactured baby foods, in comparison with traditional foods alone, may be advantageous. However, evidence of such advantages, especially in resource-constrained and contaminated environments, is required. This review will, therefore, evaluate the potential benefits and safety of using fortified manufactured baby foods versus traditional foods alone, in resource-constrained environments, by examining evidence from food composition data, diet modeling, and intervention studies. It will begin with a description of traditional complementary feeding diets, in resource-constrained environments, and the extent to which manufactured baby foods are currently being used. It will then evaluate whether the use of fortified manufactured baby foods versus traditional foods alone is likely to improve dietary adequacy or infant nutritional status. Finally, safety considerations, for the use of manufactured baby foods versus traditional food alone, in resource-constrained environments, will be discussed.

Complementary Feeding Diets and the Use of Manufactured Baby Foods

In resource-constrained environments, complementary feeding diets are generally low in fruits, vegetables and animal source foods, and in comparison with affluent environments, the staple foods provide a high percentage of dietary energy (e.g., 73% in Malawi vs. 13% in New Zealand [3; unpubl. data]). In many countries, these staple foods are served as thin gruels prepared from cereals, roots or tubers, which have low densities of energy and nutrients [4, 5]. Their nutritional quality can be improved, however, via the use of nutrient-dense traditional foods, which depending on the country and population's affluence may include legumes, vegetables, fruits, milk, yoghurt, meat, liver, eggs or fish [2, 4, 5].

In some resource-constrained environments, manufactured baby foods, whether they are commercially available or freely distributed as food aid, are regularly consumed [2, 4–10]. For example, over 20 years ago, close to 20% of 6-month-old periurban and rural Northern Thai infants [8], and 21% of 4- to 6-month-old low- to middle-income infants in Nairobi were consuming commercial infant cereals [10]. More recently, in Guatemala, an estimated 80% of high-income and 50% of low-income infants were consuming Incaparina, a fortified commercial manufactured cereal-legume blend actively promoted to improve infant nutrition [9]. Similarly, in South Africa, 80% of black and 70% of colored 6- to 12-month-old urban infants and 55% of rural infants regularly consumed commercially manufactured baby foods [6, 7]. The types of manufactured foods these infants consumed included jarred baby foods, in some countries [6, 7], and, in most countries, roasted or extruded mixtures of cereal and legumes flours, some of which include oil, milk powder, dried fruits/vegetables or vitamin/mineral mixes [4, 9, 11]. Furthermore, in South Africa, commercial infant cereals were consumed more often than nutrient-dense nondairy animal source foods (i.e., 17% of infants consumed animal source foods vs. 55% for commercial infant cereals) [6]. Indeed, a low consumption of nondairy animal source foods is characteristic of complementary feeding diets in many countries, including resource-affluent countries (median 5% energy from animal source foods in the diets of 6- to 24-month-old breastfeeding New Zealand infants; unpubl. data). Similar to South Africa, in New Zealand complementary feeding diets, more dietary energy was obtained from manufactured baby foods than from nondairy animal source foods (median 46 vs. 5% energy; unpubl. data). Thus, based on studies from diverse countries, it appears that as long as manufactured baby foods are available and affordable, they are well-accepted; presumably for reasons of convenience, ease of preparation, organoleptic qualities or perceived health benefits, i.e. factors that motivate food choices a caregiver makes [2].

Nutrient Density and Dietary Adequacy

To evaluate the nutrient adequacy of complementary feeding diets, when breast milk intakes are not quantified, nutrient densities can be used to identify potential 'problem nutrients' [12]. Using this index, dietary data from Africa (Malawi, South Africa), the Asian-Pacific region (Indonesia, Bangladesh, the Philippines) and the Americas (Peru, Guatemala) consistently show low densities of calcium, iron and zinc, i.e. often <50% of the WHO recommended levels [6, 12, 13; unpubl. data]. In some countries, marked deficits were also apparent for vitamin A, thiamine, riboflavin and niacin, and, for younger infants, vitamin B_6 [13; unpubl. data]. Even in the USA and New Zealand, the iron densities of complementary feeding diets are well below the WHO recommendations [12; unpubl. data].

These results are not surprising, when the nutrient densities of complementary foods fed to 6- to 11-month-old infants, in Asia, Africa or Latin America [14–16], are compared with WHO recommended levels [12]. As shown in table 1, less than 15% of the 115 foods examined achieved the recommended nutrient density levels for calcium, iron and zinc. Furthermore, when all 12 nutrients were examined by food groups, except for protein and copper, less than 30% of cereals, which are the staple foods in many countries [4, 5], achieved the recommended density levels [12]. Even traditional recipes that were enriched with nutrient-dense foods rarely achieved the WHO recommended densities of iron, calcium, zinc, niacin and vitamin A (table 1; <20% of 23 recipes from Ghana, Malawi, Ethiopia, India, Papua New Guinea, the Philippines or Thailand [14]). Likewise, recipe trials from Haiti showed that to achieve WHO recommended nutrient densities, for iron and zinc, it was necessary to use a fortified manufactured cereal blend, and the recommended levels were only achievable for the older 12- to 23-month infants [2]. Clearly, based on food composition data alone, these analyses suggest that, for complementary feeding diets, it will be difficult to achieve WHO recommended nutrient density levels [12] using traditional foods alone.

Dietary surveys and diet modeling have shown similar results. Dietary data (24-hour recall) collected from 6- to 12-month-old rural South African infants (n = 475) showed significantly higher nutrient intakes among infants consuming fortified manufactured baby cereals compared with infants not consuming them [6]. Nevertheless, because intergroup differences, in overall diet composition, may have influenced diet quality, it is also noteworthy that similar results were shown via diet modeling. Indeed, a detailed study, using linear programming analysis and dietary data collected from 6- to 11-month-old Ghanaian, Bangladeshi and Latin American infants, showed that without the use of fortified foods or unrealistic amounts of animal source foods, recommended dietary nutrient intakes are difficult to achieve [15]. In these models, for nonbreastfed infants, the calcium, iron and zinc constraints were the most difficult to achieve. Similar results, for modeled diets of breastfed and nonbreastfed infants, were also found elsewhere [17, 18; Ferguson and Darmon, unpubl. data].

Dietary surveys and diet modeling, therefore, strongly suggest that the use of fortified manufactured baby foods versus traditional foods alone will improve dietary adequacy. However, because the nutrient requirements of infants are not well-established, errors exist in food composition tables and interactions among dietary and nondietary factors influence nutritional status [1, 12]; biochemical or functional evidence of improved nutritional status with the use of fortified manufactured baby foods versus traditional foods alone is required from randomized controlled intervention trials. Furthermore, dietary data from South Africa [6] indicate that, as a cost-saving measure, inappropriate dilutions of commercial manufactured baby foods may occur, in resource-constrained environments, which will reduce their potential nutritional benefits.

Table 1. Percentage of foods[1] within selected food groups achieving the WHO recommended nutrient density levels [12] expressed by age group

	n^2	Protein %	Ca %	Fe %	Zn %	Cu %	B_1 %	B_2 %	B_3 %	B_6 %	Vitamin A %	Vitamin C %	Folate %
For infants 6–8 months of age													
All foods	115	91	14	3	3	90	46	40	22	37	27	43	44
Cereals	21	100	0	0	0	81	19	0	0	5	0	5	14
Roots/tubers	6	67	0	0	0	100	67	17	17	100	33	100	83
Animal	21	100	19	5	14	81	24	62	38	29	24	19	14
Legumes	14	100	14	7	0	100	64	50	14	21	0	14	93
Fruit and veg	30	80	30	3	0	90	67	53	47	70	70	87	77
Enriched[3]	23	91	4	0	0	100	48	39	0	22	13	43	13
For infants 9–11 months of age													
All foods	115	91	15	8	14	91	52	47	28	64	27	41	45
Cereals	21	100	0	0	0	81	19	0	0	29	0	5	14
Roots/tubers	6	67	0	0	0	100	83	17	17	100	33	100	100
Animal	21	100	19	10	29	86	29	81	48	71	24	14	19
Legumes	14	100	14	14	43	100	79	50	21	64	0	14	93
Fruit and veg	30	80	33	17	13	90	73	67	57	77	70	87	77
Enriched[3]	23	91	4	0	0	100	52	39	4	65	13	39	13

[1] Foods from Ghana, Bangladesh or Latin America [15]; the Philippines [16]; Ghana, Malawi, Ethiopia, India, Papua New Guinea, the Philippines or Thailand [14], and unpublished data from Indonesia.
[2] The number of foods examined within each food group.
[3] Gruels enriched with nutrient-dense foods using recipes from Ghana, Malawi, Ethiopia, India, Papua New Guinea, the Philippines or Thailand [14].

Evidence from Intervention Trials

Four types of community-based intervention trials were reviewed, which were studies that evaluated the biochemical or functional benefits of using (a) a fortified manufactured baby food, (b) modified food preparation practices, (c) vitamin A-rich foods, or (d) education-supported dietary diversification (see tables 2–4). Of the 19 studies reviewed [19–37], 14 used a randomized control design and 5 used a quasi-experimental design. They were carried out in Africa (n = 7), Asia (n = 5), Latin America (n = 6) or in multiple areas (n = 1). In all studies, except 2 [28, 29], the participants were less than 3 years of age (see tables 2–4).

Fortified Manufactured Baby Foods
Of the 19 intervention studies, 8 investigated the nutritional benefits of using a fortified manufactured baby food versus traditional foods alone (see table 2), although only one makes comparisons with a traditional diet enriched with a nutrient-dense food [19]. In this latter 6-month randomized control intervention trial, 6-month-old Ghanaian infants were randomly assigned to one of four intervention diets, including a fortified infant cereal (fortified Weanimix, a maize-soybean-groundnut blend) and an enriched traditional diet (fermented maize + fish powder) [19]. At 7 months of age, marked improvements in intakes of iron, zinc, vitamin A and riboflavin were observed in the fortified group but not in the other groups (8–25 times vs. 0–2.1 times higher). Similarly, at 12 months of age, the consumption of a fortified infant cereal prevented an increase from baseline, in the prevalence of suboptimal biochemical iron and vitamin A status (i.e., 18–11% for ferritin and 35–10% for plasma retinol in the fortified group vs. 14–57 and 22–28%, respectively, in the enriched traditional diet group; p < 0.05). There were no significant intergroup differences in growth or biochemical zinc or riboflavin status [19].

Similar results were observed in South Africa. In a 6-month, randomized controlled trial, 6- to 12-month-old South African infants were randomly assigned to either a fortified or an unfortified maize porridge group. After 6 months, significantly higher biochemical indices of iron and vitamin A status were observed in the fortified versus the unfortified group (intervention effects of 9.4 μg/l, p = 0.001 for ferritin; of 9 g/l, p = 0.001 for hemoglobin, and of 0.14 μmol/l, p = 0.02 for serum retinol), without corresponding intergroup differences in growth or biochemical zinc status [20]. Likewise, in the other four trials reviewed, which examined biochemical iron status [21–23, 26], all trials except one (table 2) [23] showed that the use of an iron-fortified manufactured food positively affected hemoglobin concentrations via either improved status [22, 26] or the prevention of a decline in levels [21], although a corresponding response in ferritin was not always observed [22, 23]. In the one negative trial, participants were older and the intervention period was

Table 2. Summary of community-based intervention trials using a fortified manufactured baby food

Country	Design	Intervention	Length	Age[1] months	n	Effects with FMBF	No effects
Ghana [19]	RCT	Weanimix Fortified Weanimix Weanimix and fish Koko and fish	6 months	6	208	↑ Fe, Zn, B$_2$ and vitamin A intakes ↑ mean plasma retinol; ↓ % with low plasma retinol % with low ferritin did not ↑ as in other groups	Length, weight, skinfolds and head circumference Zn and B$_2$ status Morbidity BF frequency
South Africa [20]	RCT	Fortified maize flour Maize flour	6 months	6–12	361	↑ ferritin ↑ hemoglobin; ↑ serum retinol in phase I ↑ motor score	Length and weight Serum Zn Mental score BF prevalence
China [21]	RCT	Fortified rusk Rusk	3 months	6–13	226	No ↓ hemoglobin Plasma vitamin E ↓	Ferritin, ZPP, EGRAC, plasma vitamin A
Chile [22]	RCT	Fortified rice cereal Rice cereal	11 months	4	173	↑ hemoglobin ↓ % IDA	Ferritin, ZPP, MCV, TS morbidity
Guatemala [23]	RCT	FeSO$_4$ fortified beans Heme fortified beans Beans	10 weeks	12–36	110		Hemoglobin Ferritin

49

Table 2. (continued)

Country	Design	Intervention	Length	Age¹ months	n	Effects with FMBF	No effects
Senegal, Congo, Bolivia, New Caledonia [24]	Quasi-expt	Fortified enriched porridge No intervention	4 months	3	447	Senegal – ↑ length	Weight in all countries Length in Congo, Bolivia and New Caledonia
India [25]	RCT	Fortified milkcereal Counseling Visitation No intervention	8 months	4	481	↑ weight gain only at 26–38 weeks; ↑ morbidity and ↓ BF	Length Weight gain at 16–26 weeks and at 38–52 weeks
Mexico [26]	Quasi-expt	Fortified milk USD 25/month	2 years	<12	650	↑ hemoglobin; ↓ % low hemoglobin; ↑ height in poorest and youngest	Weight Height in other groups

FMBF = Fortified manufactured baby food; RCT = randomized control trial; ZPP = zinc protoporphyrin; EGRAC = erythrocyte glutathione reductase activation coefficient; IDA = iron deficiency anemia; MCV = mean cell volume; TS = transferrin saturation; Quasi-expt = quasi-experimental.
¹Age at the beginning of the intervention period.

Table 3. Summary of the community-based intervention trials using improved traditional foods or food processing/preparation

Country	Design	Intervention	Length months	Age[1]	n	Effects of improved food	No effects
Burkino Faso [27]	Quasi-expt	Red palm oil	24	12–36 months	210	↓ % low serum retinol; ↑ vitamin A intakes	
Gambia [28]	RCT	Mango; Mango and fat; Vitamin A supplement; Placebo	4	2–7 years	176	↑ plasma retinol in mango + fat and vitamin A supplement groups	
Ethiopia [29]	RCT	Iron pot; Aluminium pot	12	2–5 years	407	↑ Fe content in foods; ↑ available[2] Fe in meat and vegetables; ↑ hemoglobin; ↑ ferritin; ↑ length	Weight; Available Fe in legumes
Brazil [30], premature infants	RCT	Iron pot; Aluminium pot	8	4 months	45	↑ hemoglobin; ↑ MCV and ↑ TS	Length and weight; Ferritin
Congo [31]	RCT	Maize-soy flour + amylase (AG); Maize-soy flour	3	18 weeks	80	↑ respiratory disease; Adjusted length velocity > in AG	Daily energy intakes; BF; Weight velocity; Diarrhea

Table 3. (continued)

Country	Design	Intervention	Length months	Age[1]	n	Effects of improved food	No effects
Tanzania [32]	RCT	Germinated gruel[3] Ungerminated gruel	6	6 months	309	↓ phytate ↑ soluable Fe	Intakes energy and nutrients Growth and Fe status

Quasi-expt = Quasi-experimental; RCT = randomized control trial; MCV = mean cell volume; TS = transferrin saturation.
[1]Age at the beginning of the intervention period.
[2]Available iron assessed via an in vitro dialysis assay.
[3]Gruel = Finger millet (germinated or not), kidney beans (germinated or not), roasted groundnuts, dried mango purée.

Table 4. Summary of the community-based education-supported intervention trials

Country	Design	Intervention	Length months	Age[1]	n	Effects of education	No effects
Brazil [33]	RCT health centers	Counseled to BF Give > ASF, thick gruel, oil, beans Hygiene	6	4–18 months	422	↑ knowledge ↑ recommended foods ↑ weight gain for those ≥12 months old	Diet energy and nutrient intakes Length Weight gain for those <12 months old
Peru [34]	RCT health facilities	Thick purée ASF Feeding behavior	18	Birth	377	↑ knowledge ↑ length ↑ animal source foods, thick gruel	Diet Fe and Zn densities
India [35]	RCT village	Advise on BF, CF (milk, thick dahl, snacks), feeding behavior and hygiene	18	Birth	1,025	↑ length for males Energy intakes > from recommended foods	Weight Morbidity
Bangladesh [36]	Quasi-expt	Advise on BF, CF (milk, fish, lentils, oil, molasses, vegetables and fruits) and hygiene	5	4–14 months	117	↑ weight gain; ↓ % underweight; ↑ diet energy and protein adequacy; ↑ animal source foods, vegetables/ fruit, oil	Morbidity Diet vitamin A and Fe intakes

Table 4. (continued)

Country	Design	Intervention	Length months	Age[1]	n	Effects of education	No effects
China [37]	Quasi-expt	Monthly growth monitoring and advise on BF, CF (egg yolk, thick rice gruel and snacks) and hygiene	4–12	Birth	495	↑ knowledge and practices ↑ intakes of nutrient dense foods; ↑ breastfeeding ↑ hygiene ↑ hemoglobin; ↓ anemia ↓ stunting and underweight	Wasting

RCT = Randomized control trial; BF = breastfeed; ASF = animal source foods; CF = complementary feeding; Quasi-expt = quasi-experimental.
[1]Age at the beginning of the intervention period.

shorter than in other trials, and a legume instead of a cereal was fortified (see table 2). Such interstudy differences, particularly the length of the intervention period, may have contributed to the lack of a response in Guatemala. Similarly, two of the three studies that examined vitamin A status [19–21] showed an associated improvement in biochemical vitamin A status with the use of a manufactured baby food fortified with vitamin A. Again, compared with the two trials that showed positive results [19, 20], the one trial with negative results [21] had a shorter intervention period (see table 2).

In contrast, for all trials reviewed, the use of a fortified manufactured baby food was not associated with consistent improvements in growth (table 2) [24–26], which, in India, was partially attributable to higher levels of dysentery and fever in the intervention compared with the control group [25]. In the Indian study, an instant fortified manufactured baby food was used, cautioning against its use in a contaminated environment. Clearly, in these environments or under the intervention trial study conditions, other dietary or nondietary factors were limiting growth.

Similar to growth, biochemical zinc or riboflavin status did not respond to the use of a fortified manufactured baby food in the trials in which they were examined [19–21]. For zinc, plasma zinc levels at baseline were high in the Ghanaian trial (around $15 \mu mol/l$) [19], indicating the participants were not zinc deficient, and, in the South African study, a high phytate content of maize-meal porridge may have compromised zinc absorption [20, 38].

Overall, the evidence suggests that the use of a fortified manufactured baby food will benefit infant iron and vitamin A status. Nevertheless, the content of bioavailable iron and vitamin A, in the traditional diets that acted as control diets, may not have been optimal, because, except for the Ghanaian study [19], they were not enriched with iron- or vitamin A-dense traditional foods. Because the nutritional benefits of using a fortified manufactured baby food compared with traditional foods alone are not confirmed, the trials evaluating the nutritional benefits of dietary diversification or modified food processing/preparation techniques were examined.

Dietary Diversification or Modified Food Processing/ Preparation Techniques

The benefits of using traditional diets that have been improved via dietary diversification or the use of traditional food processing/preparation techniques have been evaluated in 11 community-based intervention trials, using either quasi-experimental or randomized control designs (see tables 3 and 4). For vitamin A, results suggest that traditional foods will ensure adequate status as long as dietary fat intakes are sufficient. For example, in Burkino Faso, 2 years after the introduction of red palm oil, the vitamin A intakes of 12- to 36-month-old infants increased from 41 to 120% of safe intake levels, with a corresponding increase in mean serum retinol levels (0.55 vs. $0.64 \mu mol/l$; $p = 0.012$) and a decrease in the proportion of low serum retinol values (13.0 vs. 7.6%

serum retinol <0.35 μmol/l; p = 0.04) [27]. Similarly, using a stronger random-ized control study design, after 4 months, significantly higher plasma retinol concentrations were observed in 2- to 7-year-old Gambian children consuming rehydrated dried mango with sunflower oil 5 days/week compared with chil-dren in the control group or the mango without added fat group [28].

In two studies, the use of an iron versus an aluminium cooking pot has been shown to successfully improve infants' iron status. After 8 months [30] or 12 months [29] of cooking foods in an iron versus an aluminium pot, improvement in biochemical iron status (intervention effect of 13 g/l for hemoglobin and 12.7 μg/l for ferritin among 407 Ethiopian children [29] and 1.3 g/l for hemoglobin, 6.8% for transferrin saturation and 7.9 fl for MCV among 45 Brazilian preterm infants [30]) was observed with a corresponding increase in food iron content [29]. However, the rusting of iron pots was iden-tified as a significant barrier against their long-term use [29], and one can imagine that their heavy weight could also become a barrier. Furthermore, an increase in available iron was not observed for legumes cooked in an iron pot [29], suggesting that, when traditional foods contain high levels of phytate, the strategy may be less effective.

Several trials have examined the benefits of using α-amylase to reduce the viscosity of thick gruels, which allows increased intakes of flour at one meal [31, 32, 39–41]. In carefully controlled, short-term crossover trials, significant increases in daily energy intakes (56–76%) were observed with amylase-treated versus nontreated infant gruels [39–41]. However, similar results were not shown in community-based trials conducted with infants in the Congo [31] and Tanzania [32], which was attributed to intergroup differences in meal fre-quency [32] or in the number of additional foods consumed [31]. Furthermore, after a 3-month [31] or a 6-month [32] intervention period, when compared with controls, the consumption of an amylase-treated gruel did not result in significant improvements in growth [31, 32] or biochemical iron or zinc status [32, 42]. Apparently, when energy intakes are not constrained, infants regu-late their daily energy intakes, which suggests that the nutritional benefits of consuming amylase-treated gruels will depend on their nutrient densities rel-ative to those of foods displaced. Conclusions would perhaps differ in circum-stances where infant energy intakes are constrained.

In contrast, to the above trials, those that have used an education-supported approach, which have promoted breastfeeding, the use of nutrient-dense tra-ditional foods, especially animal source foods, and improved behavioral or hygiene practices have generally shown a positive growth response to the intervention (see table 3) [33–37]. In these trials, local health workers were trained to deliver the education messages, and in two studies the Integrated Management of Childhood Illnesses protocols and counseling techniques were used [33, 35]. In the studies reporting a dietary outcome, there were sig-nificant increases in intakes of energy comparing the intervention versus con-trol groups, but not in intakes of iron, zinc or vitamin A [33–36], which often remained well below the WHO recommended levels [12]. Other important outcomes were improvements in maternal nutrition knowledge/practices and an increased consumption of nutrient-dense foods, especially animal source foods. Because nondietary as well as dietary changes were promoted in these studies, it is not known whether it was the use of nutrient-dense traditional foods alone or the adoption of other promoted practices that resulted in improved growth. The observed positive growth responses, despite small changes in energy and nutrient intakes, however, highlight the potential importance of promoting breastfeeding, good hygiene and behavioral practices in any intervention program.

The Safety of Using Manufactured Baby Foods Compared with Traditional Foods

During infancy, an important route of pathogen transmission, for diarrheal disease, is via the consumption of complementary foods that have been contaminated by flies/pests/animals, the food handler or contaminated eating utensils or water [1]. Risks, for food-borne illness, are particularly high when leftover foods are stored at ambient temperatures, for more than 3–4 h, without adequate reheating [1]. Thus, similar risks of exposure to food-borne contamination are likely for traditional foods and noninstant manufactured baby foods, and they may even be lower for noninstant manufactured baby foods packaged in single meal-sized sachets that avoid leftovers. A notable exception is when traditional foods are fermented, and the leftover manufactured baby foods or traditional foods are eaten without adequate reheating, because the low pH of fermented foods inhibits pathogenic bacterial growth [1]. In environments where water sources are contaminated, instant manufactured baby foods, which are prepared using water, are not safe.

The safety of locally produced manufactured baby foods will also rely on the presence of adequate government regulatory infrastructures to ensure the quality of the manufactured food [12]. Likewise, to avoid excessively high or inadequate levels of absorbed nutrients, the levels of fortification and their forms (i.e., bioavailable) must be strictly monitored. With the use of fortified manufactured baby foods, unlike traditional foods, there is also an increased risk of excessive nutrient intakes, especially of iron intakes, because fortification levels appropriate for 6- to 8-month-old infants exceed those of older infants [12].

The safety of commercial manufactured baby foods also relies on the presence of effective government regulatory infrastructures to enforce the Code of Marketing Breast-Milk Substitutes and the Codex Alimentarius for Canned Baby Foods and for Processed Cereal-Based Foods for Infants and Children [43]. The safety of manufactured baby foods is compromised when they are marketed in ways that interfere with sustained breastfeeding or discourage the use of a variety of foods, which is important to facilitate a smooth transition to the family diet.

Finally, the higher cost of commercial manufactured baby foods compared with traditional foods may also compromise safety. For example, in situations where, as a cost-saving measure, manufactured baby foods are excessively diluted, this may result in very low densities of energy or nutrients compared with traditional foods and compromise nutritional status.

Conclusions

The provision of sufficient quantities of safe, nutritionally adequate and age-appropriate foods to complement breast milk intakes is essential. Evidence from food composition data, diet modeling and dietary surveys suggest that complementary feeding diets based on traditional foods alone will not achieve recommended nutrient density levels, especially for iron, calcium and zinc, because relative to estimated infant nutrient requirements, their contents in traditional foods are low. Thus, manufactured baby foods, if fortified, may have an important role to play in ensuring the nutrient adequacy of complementary feeding diets.

In both resource-constrained and affluent environments, studies show that manufactured baby foods are readily accepted. Likewise, randomized controlled intervention trials indicate that their use will likely result in improved biochemical iron status in comparison to traditional foods, although their effectiveness, if not freely available, will diminish, if as a cost-saving measure, they are overdiluted. Contrary to iron, both vitamin A-fortified manufactured baby foods and vitamin A-rich traditional foods with added fat were efficacious in improving vitamin A status, whereas the use of fortified manufactured baby foods, in comparisons with traditional foods alone, did not consistently improve growth, biochemical zinc or riboflavin status. Indeed, a consistent growth response was only observed in education-supported intervention trials, which promoted breastfeeding, active infant feeding, hygiene and diet quality; this emphasizes the importance of understanding the underlying etiology of growth faltering and the benefits of a holistic approach.

Overall, as long as manufactured baby foods are available, affordable, fortified at appropriate levels with bioavailable fortificants and marketed safely, they potentially have an important role to play in improving the nutrient density of traditional complementary feeding diets and the iron status of infants. In urban environments, where there has been a shift away from traditional foods to street foods, there are distinct advantages in using low-cost fortified manufactured baby foods because of the associated health hazards or low nutritional quality of 'street foods' [44]. Conversely, in environments where affordable manufactured baby foods are not available or where there is an absence of effective governmental regulatory or distribution infrastructures, the use of nutrient-dense traditional foods is advised. In all environments, the promotion of breastfeeding, active feeding and high levels of hygiene is essential to ensure optimal nutritional status.

References

1 WHO: Complementary Feeding of Young Children in Developing Countries: A Review of Current Scientific Knowledge. Geneva, World Health Organization, 1998.
2 Ruel M, Menon P, Loechl C, Pelto G: Donated fortified cereal blends improve the nutrient density of traditional complementary foods in Haiti, but iron and zinc gaps remain for infants. Food Nutr Bull 2004;25:361–376.
3 Hotz C, Gibson RS: Complementary feeding practices and dietary intakes from complementary foods amongst weanlings in rural Malawi. Eur J Clin Nutr 2001;55:841–849.
4 Dop M-C, Benbouzid D: Regional features of complementary feeding in Africa and the Middle East; in Dop MC, Trèche S, de Benoist B, et al (eds): Complementary Feeding of Young Children in Africa and the Middle East. Geneva, World Health Organization, 1999.
5 Pelto G, Levit E, Thairu L: Improving feeding practices: current patterns, common constraints, and the design of interventions. Food Nutr Bull 2003;24:45–82.
6 Faber M: Complementary foods consumed by 6–12-month-old rural infants in South Africa are inadequate in micronutrients. Public Health Nutr 2004;8:373–381.
7 Oelofse A, Van Raaij JMA, Benadé AJS, et al: Disadvantaged black and coloured infants in two urban communities in the Western Cape, South Africa differ in micronutrient status. Public Health Nutr 2002;5:289–294.
8 Jackson D, Imong SM, Wongsawasdii L, et al: Weaning practices and breast-feeding duration in Northern Thailand. Br J Nutr 1992;67:149–164.
9 Tartanac F: Incaparina and other Incaparina-based foods: experience of INCAP in Central America. Food Nutr Bull 2000;21:49–54.
10 Huffman S, Oniang'o R, Quinn V: Improving young child feeding with processed complementary cereals and behavioural change in urban Kenya. Food Nutr Bull 2000;21:75–81.
11 López de Romana G: Experience with complementary feeding in the FONCODES Project. Food Nutr Bull 2000;21:43–48.
12 Dewey K, Brown KH: Update on technical issues concerning complementary feeding of young children in developing countries and implications for intervention programs. Food Nutr Bull 2003;24:5–44.
13 Gibson R, Hotz C, Perlas LA: Influence of food intake, composition and bioavailability on micronutrient deficiencies of infants during the weaning period and first year of life; in Pettifor J, Zlotkin S (eds): Micronutrient Deficiencies during the Weaning Period and the First Years of Life. Basel, Nestec, 2004, pp 83–103.
14 Gibson R, Ferguson EL, Lehrfeld J: Complementary foods for infant feeding in developing countries: their nutrient adequacy and improvement. Eur J Clin Nutr 1998;52:1–7.
15 Dewey K, Cohen RJ, Rollins NC: Feeding of nonbreastfed children from 6 to 24 months of age in developing countries. Food Nutr Bull 2004;25:377–406.
16 Perlas L, Gibson RS, Adair L: Macronutrient and selected vitamin intakes from complementary foods of infants and toddlers from Cebu, Philippines. Int J Food Sci Nutr 2004;55:1–15.
17 Ferguson E, Devlin M, Briend A, Darmon N: How achievable are recommended dietary allowances for 12–24 month old New Zealand children. Asia Pac J Clin Nutr 2004;13:S62.
18 Briend A, Darmon N: Iron and zinc: are they likely to be problem nutrients in children receiving complementary foods? Pediatrics 2000;5:1288–1290.
19 Lartey A, Manu A, Brown KH, et al: A randomised, community-based trial of the effects of improved, centrally processed complementary foods on growth and micronutrient status of Ghanaian infants from 6 to 12 mo of age. Am J Clin Nutr 1999;70:391–404.
20 Faber M, Kvalsvig JD, Lombard CJ, Spinnler Benade AJ: Effect of a fortified maize-meal porridge on anemia, micronutrient status, and motor development of infants. Am J Clin Nutr 2005;82:1032–1039.

21 Liu D, Bates CJ, Yin T, et al: Nutritional efficacy of a fortified weaning rusk in a rural area near Beijing. Am J Clin Nutr 1993;57:506–511.
22 Walter T, Dallman PR, Pizarro F, et al: Effectiveness of iron-fortified infant cereal in prevention of iron deficiency anemia. Pediatrics 1993;91:976–982.
23 Schumann K, Romero-Abal ME, Maurer A, et al: Haematological response to haem iron or ferrous sulphate mixed with refried black beans in moderately anaemic Guatemalan pre-school children. Public Health Nutr 2005;8:572–581.
24 Simondon K, Gartner A, Berger J, et al: Effect of early, short-term supplementation on weight and linear growth of 4–7-mo-old infants in developing countries: a four-country randomised trial. Am J Clin Nutr 1996;64:537–545.
25 Bhandari N, Bahl R, Nayyar B, et al: Food supplementation with encouragement to feed it to infants from 4 to 12 months of age has a small impact on weight gain. J Nutr 2001;131: 1946–1951.
26 Rivera J, Sotres-Alvarez D, Habicht JP, et al: Impact of the Mexican Program for Education, Health, and Nutrition (Progresa) on rates of growth and anemia in infants and young children. A randomised effectiveness study. JAMA 2004;291:2563–2570.
27 Zagré N, Delpeuch F, Traissac P, Delisle H: Red palm oil as a source of vitamin A for mothers and children: impact of a pilot project in Burkino Faso. Public Health Nutr 2003;6:733–742.
28 Drammeh B, Marquis GS, Funkhouser E, et al: A randomised, 4-month mango and fat supplementation trial improved vitamin A status among young Gambian children. J Nutr 2002;132: 3693–3699.
29 Adish A, Esrey SA, Gyorkos TW, et al: Effect of consumption of food cooked in iron pots on iron status and growth of young children: a randomised trial. Lancet 1999;353:712–716.
30 Borigato E, Martinez FE: Iron nutritional status is improved in Brazilian preterm infants fed food cooked in iron pots. J Nutr 1998;128:855–859.
31 Moursi M, Mbemba F, Trèche S: Does the consumption of amylase-containing gruels impact on the energy intake and growth of Congolese infants? Public Health Nutr 2002;6:249–257.
32 Mamiro P, Kolsteren PW, van Camp JH, et al: Processed complementary food does not improve growth or hemoglobin status of rural Tanzanian infants from 6–12 months of age in Kilosa district, Tanzania. J Nutr 2004;134:1084–1090.
33 Santos I, Victora CG, Martines J, et al: Nutrition counseling increases weight gain among Brazilian children. J Nutr 2001;131:2866–2873.
34 Penny M, Creed-Kanashiro HM, Robort RC, et al: Effectiveness of an educational intervention delivered through the health services to improve nutrition in young children: a cluster-randomised controlled trial. Lancet 2005;365:1863–1872.
35 Bhandari N, Mazumder S, Bahl R, et al; Infant Feeding Study Group: An educational intervention to promote appropriate complementary feeding practices and physical growth in infants and young children in rural Haryana, India. J Nutr 2004;134:2342–2348.
36 Brown L, Zeitlin MF, Peterson KE, et al: Evaluation of the impact of weaning food messages on infant feeding practices and child growth in rural Bangladesh. Am J Clin Nutr 1992;56: 994–1003.
37 Guldan G, Fan H-C, Ma X, et al: Culturally appropriate nutrition education improves infant feeding and growth in rural Sichuan, China. J Nutr 2000;130:1204–1211.
38 Gibson R, Perlas L, Hotz C: Improving the bioavailability of nutrients in plant foods at the household level. Proc Nutr Soc 2006;65:160–168.
39 Bennet V, Morales E, González J, et al: Effects of dietary viscosity and energy density on total daily energy consumption by young Peruvian children. Am J Clin Nutr 1999;70:285–291.
40 Islam M, Peerson JM, Ahmed T, et al: Effects of varied energy density of complementary foods on breastmilk intakes and total energy consumption by healthy, breastfed Bangladeshi children. Am J Clin Nutr 2006;83:851–858.
41 Traoré T, Vieu M-C, Traoré AS, Trèche S: Effects of the duration of the habituation period on energy intakes from low and high energy density gruels by Burkinabè infants living in free conditions. Appetite 2005;45:279–286.
42 Lachat C, Van Camo JH, Mamiro PS, et al: Processing of complementary foods does not increase hair zinc levels and growth of infants in Kilosa district, rural Tanzania. Br J Nutr 2006;95:174–180.
43 Clark D, Shrimpton R: Complementary feeding, the code, and the codex. Food Nutr Bull 2000;21:25–29.

44 Ruel M: Urbanization in Latin America: constraints and opportunities for child feeding and care. Food Nutr Bull 2000;21:12–24.

Discussion

Dr. Guno: In your slide where you showed that there was increased consumption of fortified manufactured baby food over enriched foods and non-fortified foods, what were the factors that lead to the increased consumption? Was it palatability or was it the ease and convenience of preparation for the mothers?

Dr. Ferguson: I was not involved in these studies but from the literature I suspect that the ease of preparation and the perceived nutritional or health benefits of fortified manufactured baby foods may have contributed to their frequency of consumption in South Africa [1, 2].

Dr. Kruger: I am from South Africa, and there is a perception among mothers that modern foods are better, which is an important factor.

Dr. Giovannini: In all the papers you looked at, did you find any correlation between education and intervention for the food, because education is important. In southeast Asia, for example in Cambodia, colostrum was thrown away because it was a different color from human milk, and in this case we found good education to be very useful. It is very important to educate public health workers in every part of developing countries. The other problem is conservation. When we speak about not home-prepared food, industrialized products may be safe and useful, but conservation may be very difficult. We have good results in using sprinkles due to good compliance. I think that compliance is the important thing. This is why we have to work in developing countries and publish the results. There are many studies in Africa but we don't have too much data from around the world, and it is very important to compare what happens in Asia, southeast Asia and Africa because the spirit of this is not only to give something but to teach, which is the hardest thing. We are now educating public health workers, which is sometimes very hard, but I think this may be the best way in these countries: teach the people to fish, do not give them a fish.

Dr. Ferguson: These are important comments. Of the intervention studies reviewed, those showing a positive growth response generally included an education component. Also, manufactured baby foods may benefit urban more than rural populations because of urban-rural differences in terms of education, food availability and working mothers' time. In rural areas, your experience with the use of sprinkles is of interest because it suggests that it may be easier to achieve high compliance with sprinkles than with foods.

Dr. Giovannini: The last is the cost.

Dr. Ferguson: And the cost, yes.

Dr. Ibe: The socioeconomic status of the mother has an effect on the use of manufactured food or even the use of traditional foods, and also traditional food is part of the local environment, that also has an effect.

Dr. Ferguson: Most studies reviewed were conducted in poor rather than affluent environments, which would have limited the acceptability of some foods. The education-supported studies put considerable effort into the selection of appropriate local foods, for example, eggs, chicken livers and shredded meat. However, in addition to the barriers of cost and availability, the amount of animal source foods, especially meat, an infant can consume is low [3], which is perhaps another reason why improvements in dietary nutrient density, particularly for iron and zinc, were not seen.

Dr. Domellöf: As you said there are a number of studies now suggesting that it is very difficult to achieve the theoretical nutrient requirements using unfortified complementary foods. I wonder how you would explain that in terms of evolution and has this been described for animals?

Dr. Ferguson: Yes, it does seem unusual that it is difficult to achieve the theoretical iron nutrient requirements without the use of fortified foods. This raises the question of whether they have been overestimated. Theoretical iron requirements are estimated using a factorial approach [4] which relies on a limited number of studies, an assumed level of iron absorption, and an allowance for increased body iron stores. Thus estimated levels are set to exceed functional iron needs, and the data upon which they are based are limited. A second possibility is that prehistoric complementary feeding diets, which were consumed when nutrient requirement levels evolved, differed substantially in their contents of bioavailable iron from those of today. Modern diets, for example, are often based on cereals which can have a high phytate content, i.e., a potent inhibitor of iron absorption, especially if unrefined. Interestingly, in the studies reviewed, the use of iron-fortified foods generally had a beneficial effect on iron status, indicating that dietary iron requirements are indeed high.

Dr. Solomons: You mentioned a study that I was a part of by Schumann et al. [5]. After we tortured the data we did find a difference, we didn't find it in the whole sample, and it was for people who apparently had a low iron status that we found an effect. But what is important in evaluating so many studies is that there is a mixed population, some of whom cannot respond with benefit because they are already there, and that is one of the problems of looking at whole samples. With regard to evolution, clamping the cord is a relatively new human evolution. Births that are attended in the traditional way, that is where the placenta was born along with the child before separation and provided about 2 months more support of iron status; so getting to 6 months without developing anemia was easier if you didn't have your umbilical cord clamped immediately. The other thing on evolution is the work by Cordain et al. [6] in Colorado who say that we have only been agriculturists for the last 10,000 years. Before that we were pastoralist from 40,000 to 10,000 years and before that, from the beginning of evolution, we were hunter-gathers. In that culture, pre-masticated meat was presumably the complementary food; so it was our seeking stability to agriculture which prejudiced against our youngest children, and presumably that is a very new and cultural evolution in a very long human evolution. So where we went wrong was to become agriculturists according to Cordain et al. and rely on grains. It is great for older people but it doesn't get us from 6 to 24 months.

Dr. Ferguson: Also of interest, in New Zealand we observed a decline in serum ferritin levels across the 6- to 24-month age range which was negatively associated with cow's milk consumption (low iron food) and positively associated with iron-fortified milk consumption [7]. Thus even in affluent environments, where complementary feeding diets are not based on unrefined cereals, modern diets do not ensure optimal iron status.

Dr. Brown: I was impressed with the differences that you were showing when you compared the home-prepared diet versus the manufactured foods particularly with regard to growth outcomes. Could you speculate on why those two sets of studies may be producing two different sets of results? Just to describe the degree of skepticism I am always faced with when I try to promote traditional food-based interventions, and that is that the public health community simply doesn't believe that these are feasible in terms of being able to scale them up because of the intensity of formative research that is required and the intensity of the educational intervention itself. So I just wonder if you could speak on some of those feasibility issues.

Dr. Ferguson: These are two important issues to raise. The education-supported studies promoted dietary as well as non-dietary factors (e.g., hygiene, behavioral practices), which suggests that a holistic approach will improve growth more than a single food alone. In addition, several of the fortified foods evaluated (i.e., unrefined maize flours or cereal-soy blends) were probably high in phytate which may have inhibited zinc absorption and limited growth. Alternatively, as Dr. Solomons emphasized earlier, the children participating in these studies may have been unresponsive to a micronutrient intervention. In relation to your second comment, our work in Indonesia has also found that feasibility, availability and affordability were important barriers to a food-based approach. However, rather than discounting it as an important strategy, perhaps a combined approach including, for example, sprinkles and a food-based approach will result in more sustainable improvements.

References

1   Faber M, Benade AJ: Perceptions of infant cereals and dietary intakes of children aged 4–24 months in a rural South African community. Int J Food Sci Nutr 2001;52:359–365.
2   Dewey K: Success of intervention programs to promote complementary feeding; in Black R, Michaelsen KF (eds): Public Health Issues in Infant and Child Nutrition. Nestlé Workshop Series Pediatric Program. Vevey, Nestec/Philadelphia, Lippincott Williams & Wilkins, 2002, vol 48, pp 199–216.
3   Fox MK, Reidy K, Karwe V, Ziegler P: Average portions of foods commonly eaten by infants and toddlers in the United States. J Am Diet Assoc 2006;106(suppl 1):S66–S76.
4   Institute of Medicine, Food and Nutrition Board: Dietary Reference Intakes Vitamin A, Vitamin K, Arsenic, Born, Chromium, Copper, Iodine, Iron, Manganese, Molybdenum, Nickle, Silicon, Valadium and Zinc. Washington, National Academy Press, 2000.
5   Schumann K, Romero-Abal ME, Maurer A, et al: Haematological response to haem iron or ferrous sulphate mixed with refried black beans in moderately anaemic Guatemalan pre-school children. Public Health Nutr 2005;8:572–581.
6   Cordain L, Eaton SB, Sebastian A, et al: Origins and evolution of the Western diet: health implications for the 21st century. Am J Clin Nutr 2005;81:341–354.
7   Soh P, Ferguson EL, McKenzie JE, et al: Dietary intakes of 6–24-month-old urban South Island New Zealand children in relation to biochemical iron status. Public Health Nutr 2002;5:339–346.

Agostoni C, Brunser O (eds): Issues in Complementary Feeding.
Nestlé Nutr Workshop Ser Pediatr Program, vol 60, pp 65–78,
Nestec Ltd., Vevey/S. Karger AG, Basel, © 2007.

Potential Contaminants in the Food Chain: Identification, Prevention and Issue Management

Francis P. Scanlan

Nestlé Research Center, Quality and Safety Department, Lausanne, Switzerland

Abstract

Contaminants are a vast subject area of food safety and quality. They are generally divided into chemical, microbiological and physical classes and are present in our food chain from raw materials to finished products. They are the subject of international and national legislation that has widened to cover more and more contaminant classes and food categories. In addition, consumers have become increasingly aware of and alarmed by their risks, whether rightly or not. What is the food industry doing to ensure the safety and quality of the products we feed our children? This is a valid question which this article attempts to address from an industrial viewpoint. Chemical food safety is considered a complex field where the risk perception of consumers is often the highest. The effects of chronic or acute exposure to chemical carcinogens may cause disease conditions long after exposure that can be permanently debilitating or even fatal. It is also a moving target, as knowledge about the toxicity and occurrence data of new chemical contaminants continues to be generated. Their identification, prevention and management are challenges to the food industry as a whole. A reminder of the known chemical hazards in the food chain will be presented with an emphasis on the use of early warning to identify potential new contaminants. Early warning is also a means of prevention, anticipating food safety concerns before they become issues to manage. Current best management practices including Hazard Analysis and Critical Control Points relating to the supply chain of baby foods and infant formulae will be developed. Finally, key lessons from a case study on recent contamination issues in baby food products will be presented.

Introduction

Contaminants are a vast subject area of food safety and quality. They are generally divided into chemical, microbiological and physical classes and are present in our food chain from raw materials (RMs) to finished products. They are the subject of international and national legislation that has widened to cover more and more contaminant classes and food categories. In addition, consumers have become increasingly aware of and alarmed by their risks, whether rightly or not. What is our food industry doing to ensure the safety and quality of the products we feed our children? This is a valid question which this article attempts to address from an industrial viewpoint.

Stomach upsets and incidences of food poisoning have mainly been attributed to microbiological hazards such as *Campylobacter*, *Salmonella*, *Escherichia coli* 0157, etc. Infections of these and other pathogens can be food-borne, due to poor hygiene or even contracted from domestic or farm animals. Hazard Analysis and Critical Control Points (HACCP) is a very well established risk management tool in the food industry that has certainly led to an overall decrease in gastrointestinal infections from processed food. Physical contaminants like foreign bodies, glass and metallic fragments can be avoided by a strict management of supply chain and manufacturing processes and also by the use of instruments like X-ray detectors. Microbiological and physical contaminants have been the historical focus of the food industry for many decades and will continue to be the focus of attention and new approaches for their elimination. Indeed, this article could be solely dedicated to these types of contaminants. However, the purpose here is to focus on chemical contaminants.

Chemical food safety is considered a complex field where the risk perception of consumers is often the highest. The effects of chronic or acute exposure to chemical carcinogens may cause disease conditions long after exposure that can be permanently debilitating or even fatal. It is also a moving target, as knowledge about the toxicity and occurrence data of new chemical contaminants is continuing to be generated. Their identification, prevention and management are challenges to the food industry as a whole.

Identification

The field of chemical contaminants has undergone a certain evolution. In the early days and up to about two decades ago, research in food safety was mainly focused on the analysis and toxicity of active compounds like the class of organochlorine pesticides. Then it became understood that the degradation products or metabolites of some compounds could equally be found in foodstuffs and could have an even higher toxicological risk. Examples are, ethylenethiourea and propylenethiourea originating from dithiocarbamates or desulfylfipronil and fipronil sulfone from fipronil. More recently attention has been turned to understanding the fate of contaminants produced from industrial thermal processes, enzymatic processes, and those that can exist in a bound form linked to other constituents of the foodstuff such as proteins or

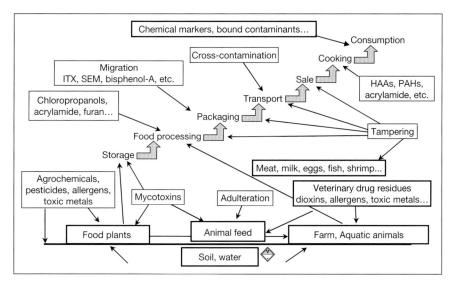

Fig. 1. Chemical hazard identification in the food chain.

carbohydrates. Examples are: bound deoxynivalenol glucoside in fusarium-infected wheat and maize [1]; enzymatically formed 3-monochloropropanediol [2], and heat-induced acrylamide [3]. Andrews et al. [4], in Safety and Quality Research Priorities in the Food Industry, provide a good overview of the main areas of contaminants highlighting new avenues for research.

As an overview, the field of chemical contaminants can be broken down into several subclasses as presented in figure 1. The scope is quite large ranging from plant protection products to veterinary drugs and packaging migration compounds. Also, the points where a potential contamination could occur are all along the food chain. This gives an idea of the complexity involved when implementing a contaminant management program. Classical contaminants like pesticide residues, mycotoxins, heavy metals, etc., are well described in the literature and are routinely monitored in food analysis laboratories. To ensure low or the absence of contaminant residues in baby foods and infant formulae, agricultural RMs are or should be monitored. We will see later that combined with a strict upstream control of the supply chain is the best means to avoid contaminant residues from entering infant food.

In addition to batch-to-batch analysis for infant food manufacturers, most governmental agencies also carry out yearly monitoring programs to assess the levels and risks associated with known contaminants in these sensitive food products. Today, baby food and infant formulae are the most tested of all food categories. Increased awareness and surveillance has led to improvements in agricultural practices and supply chain control leading to minimized

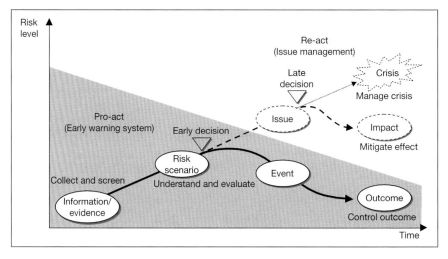

Fig. 2. Philosophy of Nestlé's early warning system.

and safe levels in RMs. Published official surveys in developed countries have shown a consistent decline in contamination levels in both RMs and finished products. The British Food Standards Agency released results from a 2003 survey on dioxins and dioxin-like PCBs in 124 retail samples of baby foods and concluded a continued decrease of 85% in dietary intakes since they first started the surveys in 1989 [5]. Furthermore, for the food types where EU limits are in force, i.e. milk-, meat-, egg- and fish-based products, all concentrations of dioxins were within the appropriate EU limits.

What about emerging or unknown contaminants? For the last 2–3 years early warning has been the current trend where food companies and authorities attempt to take a proactive approach anticipating food safety issues rather than being obliged to work reactively when faced with a declared problem. Within Europe the European Food Safety Authority (EFSA) has commissioned a project to develop an early warning system, described in the EFSA Journal [6]. This is called the EU EMRISK Project.

Early warning systems if well designed and of high quality can identify new chemical risks before they become issues to manage. Figure 2 shows this underlying philosophy upon which Nestlé's Early Warning System has successfully been built. Our early warning system proceeds through three main stages. Firstly, there is the collection of information. The outcome of early warning is only as good as the input to the system. In addition to other areas of importance to food safety like microbiology, in the case of contaminants the system mobilizes our key scientists in all fields of contaminant expertise corresponding to the scope along the food chain as shown in figure 1. They do not act alone, as toxicologists, agronomists, RM buyers, analytical experts from testing laboratories, and our external consultants all contribute to enrich the quality and quantity of information that feeds the system. The second stage is to scientifically evaluate the information, weeding out the useful from the rest. The relevant valid information is then used to elaborate possible solution strategies for prevention or mitigation actions in the operational environment. Senior management commitment and their decisions on proposed recommendations is necessary for this system to function effectively. The system is based on a network approach where the company leverages all its resources to bring benefit to the company and to the consumer.

Prevention

Above, it was shown that an effective early warning system for food safety can be an instrument in the work of prevention. However, on a daily basis the greatest measures of prevention belong to the operational procedures used to control the industrial supply chain and production of baby foods and infant formulae. This is part of the overall quality assurance system that starts with written documents describing the controls on all the following critical areas:

- Selection of suppliers, farms, fields
- Agricultural practices (seeds, fertilizers, plant protection products)
- Harvesting
- Transport
- Storage
- Sampling procedures
- Analytical and monitoring programs
- Product release procedures
- Supplier audits, corrective actions
- Laboratories, performance tests, accreditation
- HACCP plan
- Distribution

It is quite an extensive program that encompasses all aspects related to the infant nutrition supply chain, production and distribution. For more information, Vasconcellos [7] provides a comprehensive review of all quality assurance aspects in the food industry. Finished products must also be compliant with national or international legislation. In this respect, standards and norms are also a means of prevention, obliging the producer to respect specific limits in finished products and taking the necessary actions to ensure those limits are respected through the entire industrial process. As mentioned earlier, for infant nutrition products, control of the supply chain is crucial.

Different sourcing strategies exist depending on the nature and safety risk of the RM. Some RMs are sourced through the trade channels, others directly from farmers. The Nestlé approach involves adaptation of growing systems, contract growing and development of full traceability meeting legislation and internal norms. Contract growing is used for sensitive RMs with high risk and difficult supply; supplier contract growing for relatively high risk RMs where the supplier guarantees supply and safety through their own competence. Selective purchasing is used where risk is relatively low and the supplier guarantees supply and safety from their own controls. Finally open market trading can be used for relatively low risk RMs and where availability is high. This entails a methodological work of selecting suppliers, farmers and farms applying restrictive instructions with contractors and farmers. It can also involve contracting before start of season. Application of good agricultural practices is key. For example, an approach to avoid mycotoxin problems in cereals involves:

- Selection of growing areas
- No maize in crop rotation
- Control of fusarium toxins (implies choice of fungicides)
- Choice or resistance varieties
- Correct grain drying before storage
- Selection of storage facilities
- Analyses to identify critical control points

Consequences of this approach encourages suppliers and farmers to act as experts guaranteeing measurable quality and safety, participating in sustainable agricultural programs, increasing added value if requirements are met. These measures will in turn increase the responsibility of the primary production sector.

Agronomists follow up with agricultural advise and control during the growing season using defined analytical procedures that meet analytical specifications on representative samples taken from homogeneous lots. Representative samples are the key to quality assurance. These need to be obtained taking all risks into account. These may be taken over different stages, e.g. cereals at the field, storage, transport, or vegetables at the field and harvest. The range of contaminants analyzed depends on the reliability of information. Taking pesticides for example, information on registered pesticides, spray plans and illegal use allow a hit list of pesticides to be identified. This can then be used to establish analytical programs carried out in the Nestlé laboratories.

Processing RMs into finished products is considered a safety factor but, on its own, not a solution. Careful management of growing systems aims to reduce the range of contaminants. Once within the factory environment HACCP is 'the' tool for assisting in the prevention of safety issues. It requires an in-depth knowledge of processes and products from start to finish. Simply put, potential hazards are identified by specialists (in cross-functional teams) and controls are implemented to monitor them with the system documented and continuously improved. More information on HACCP can be found in Mortimore and Wallace [8].

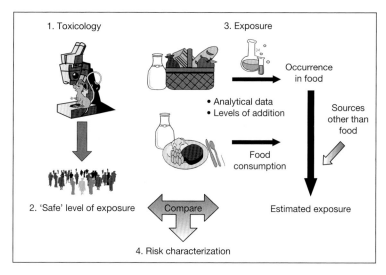

Fig. 3. Risk assessment approach.

The above measures are designed to give confidence that food safety is being managed properly and professionally allowing the manufacturer to focus on producing a safe product.

Issue Management

Zero risk does not exist! Food companies and legislators are obliged to manage the issues in order to minimize risks. Chemical risk assessment is a tool for issue management. The principles of risk assessment of food and human health care are well described in the ILSI monograph series [9]. Schilter [10] also described the risk assessment approach in the 'Assessment and Management of Pesticides Toxicological Risk in Baby Food Manufacturing and New Product Development'. Figure 3 shows the approach used to perform a risk assessment.

One of the first tasks is to establish safe levels. Paracelsus is attributed with stating that the poison is in its dose. The identification of a chemical hazard has to be based on scientific facts that either declare the potential hazard to be real or not. If toxicological and occurrence data exist for a known contaminant in a RM or finished product then assessing the risk is reasonably straightforward (fig. 4). However, when confronted by new chemical molecules for which there are no toxicity data then estimations have to be made (fig. 5). These are usually based on molecular structure and calculated reactivity. Modelization tools, such as quantitative structure activity relationships or computational toxicology, are useful for estimating toxicity. Once past this

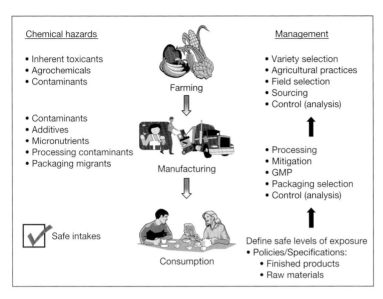

Fig. 4. Ensuring food safety in existing products.

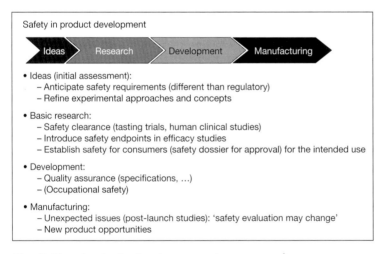

Fig. 5. Ensuring food safety in new products.

filter then the job of assessing its occurrence in food is required. Risk assessors then use experimental or modeled exposure data. Most available toxicological data on contaminants is often at high doses. Due to the general low levels found in food, a current area of research is to develop risk assessment approaches for contaminants at low doses and over long periods of time.

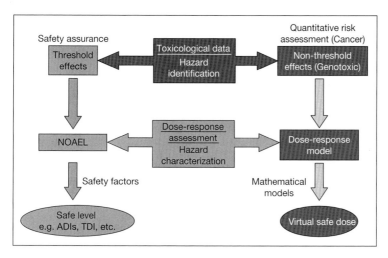

Fig. 6. Safety assessment of semicarbazide (SEM).

A conservative approach often used in Europe for contaminants of unknown toxicity is the threshold of toxicological concern [11]. In risk assessments for infants and children the nature of their food consumption is most important. Infants are restricted to similar diets everyday offering little variety when compared to adults, and this consumption is very high when related to body weight. Furthermore, their diet is consumed for a relatively short time period until the infant starts to consume a greater variety of foods.

The recent case of the hydrazine compound semicarbazide (SEM) found in baby food jars in 2003–2005 illustrates an example of issue management. SEM is a known metabolite of nitrofuran antibiotics which are prohibited in the EU and should not be found in baby foods. These antibiotics are allowed for veterinary use and residues can be found in animal products such as meat, eggs, shrimp, honey, etc. In early 2003, SEM was found in baby foods not containing animal RMs. At first difficult to understand, the presence of SEM in the vegetable-containing baby food was attributed to the migration from the azodicarbonamide blowing agent used to manufacture the air-tight seal of the jar closure. IARC classifies SEM as group 3 meaning 'not classifiable as to its carcinogenicity to humans'. As there was a concern about possible carcinogenicity risk, a safety assessment was performed. The approach is shown in figure 6. From the literature there were some indications that SEM has a weak genotoxicity and a weak carcinogenicity. Therefore during June–July 2003 the Nestlé Research Center focused on the safety assessment on non-threshold, carcinogenic effects. The basis of the exposure assessment was the following:

- A lifetime exposure was assumed with variations according to life stages
- Highest exposure was assumed in infants with a peak at 6–12 months
- 95th percentile intake of baby foods was taken
- 20 ppb level was taken for all products
- Highest exposure = 1.05 µg/kg birth weight/day in 9-month-old infants.
- Such an exposure is likely to decrease over time, e.g. a 60-kg adult consuming 100 g products (e.g. sauces, dressings) contaminated at 15 ppb, is exposed to SEM at about 0.025 µg/kg body weight/day.

Exposure to 1.05 µg/kg body weight/day is unlikely to be of concern for non-cancer threshold toxicity (i.e. osteolathyrism, vasculopathy, neurotoxicity) since the reported lowest observed adverse effect levels for these effects are about 50–100 mg/kg body weight/day.

The assumptions for non-threshold carcinogenicity were:

- No safe level assumed, use of quantitative risk assessment
- Quality risk assessment models express risk (i.e. probability) as function of dose
- When assuming simple linear proportionality of risk as a function of dose and extrapolating this risk at the highest estimated SEM exposure
- SEM exposure of 1.05 µg/kg body weight/day leads to a theoretical increased risk of about 2.3 extra cancer cases in a million persons exposed over lifetime
- Conservative assumptions: (1) linear dose-response (several authors note that use of simple linear models to low-dose extrapolation is very conservative and may exaggerate risk by about 2 orders of magnitude); (2) absence of detoxification and repair processes, and (3) constant upper-bound exposure over lifetime

Therefore, the theoretical risk was considered low – it is usually considered that exposures resulting in risk $<10^{-6}$ are virtually safe. SEM from food in jars is unlikely to present appreciable carcinogenic risk to human health.

At that time in July 2003, the EFSA was informed through the European Confederation of Food Industries. The food and packaging industry started a joint working group to find solutions to the potential problem. The EFSA also commissioned a genotoxicity study. In October 2003, EFSA publicly recommended reducing SEM in baby foods but also advised not to change eating habits. In January 2004, an EU directive was published banning the use of azodicarbonamide as a blowing agent in seals. Then in March 2004, the EFSA study revealed SEM not to be genotoxic. The joint industry group was starting to have promising results and by November 2004 was praised by EFSA and the EU for their progress. In February 2005, commercial alternatives existed to replace azodicarbonamide. Finally, in July 2005, the EFSA scientific panel concluded that there is no health concern from SEM at levels currently found in food, even for infants. SEM acts through a genotoxic threshold effect.

- SEM-induced genotoxicity has been shown to be mediated by reactive oxygen species, and inhibited by antioxidants or metabolic systems.

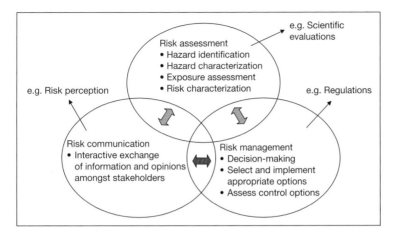

Fig. 7. Widely recognized framework for risk management (Codex, EU, US, etc.).

- Therefore, a practical/apparent threshold for carcinogenicity may be applied, suggesting that SEM is unlikely to be of concern for carcinogenicity [12, 13].

It is generally considered that issue management is a combination of three factors: risk assessment, risk management and risk communication (fig. 7). While important to assess the safety of contaminants in foods, the SEM case shows that it is important to keep into perspective the relevance of the risk and weigh it against the benefits. In the SEM case, the blowing agent was providing a microbiologically safe product whose benefits far outweighed any potential risk of adverse effects.

Acknowledgements

The author wishes to thank his colleagues, B. Schilter, L.A. Tran, M.D. Estevez, D. O'Connor, and A. Huggett, for their kind contributions.

References

1 Berthiller F, Dall'Asta C, Schuhmacher R, et al: Masked mycotoxins: determination of a deoxynivalenol glucoside in artificially and naturally contaminated wheat by liquid chromatography-tandem mass spectrometry. J Agric Food Chem 2005;53:3421–3425.
2 Robert MC, Oberson JM, Stadler RH: Model studies on the formation of monochloropropanediols in the presence of lipase. J Agric Food Chem 2004;52:5102–5108.
3 Stadler RH, Blank I, Varga N, et al: Acrylamide from Maillard reaction products. Nature 2002; 419:449–450.
4 Andrews G, Penman A, Hart C: Safety and quality research priorities in the food Industry; in Hester RE, Harrison RM (eds): Issues in Environmental Science and Technology. No 15: Food Safety and Food Quality. London, Royal Society of Chemistry, 2001.

5 UK Food Surveillance Information Sheets 60/04, http://www.foodstandards.gov.uk; June 2004: Dioxins and Dioxin-like PCB's in Baby Foods.
6 Opinion of the Scientific Committee on a request from EFSA related to the early identification of emerging risks. http://www.efsa.europa.eu EFSA J 2006;375:1–14.
7 Vasconcellos JA: Quality Assurance for the Food Industry. Boca Raton, CRC Press, 2004.
8 Mortimore S, Wallace C: HACCP: A Practical Approach. Chapman & Hall Food Science Book. Gaithersburg, Aspen Press, 1998.
9 Benford D (ed): Principles of Risk Assessment of Food and Drinking Water Related to Human Health. ILSI Europe Concise Monogr Ser. Brussels, ILSI Press, 2001.
10 Schilter B: Assessment and management of pesticides toxicological risk in baby food manufacturing and new product Development; in Aggett PJ, Kuiper HA (eds): Risk Assessment in the Food Chain of Children. Nestlé Nutr Workshop Ser Pediatr Program. Vevey, Nestec Ltd./Philadelphia, Lippincott Williams & Wilkins, 2000, vol 44, 209–224.
11 Barlow S (ed): Threshold of Toxicological Concern (TTC). A Tool for Assessing Substances of Unknown Toxicity Present at Low Levels in the Diet. ILSI Europe Concise Monogr Ser. Brussels, ILSI Press, 2005.
12 Hirakawa K, Midorikawa K, Oikawa S, Kawanishi S: Carcinogenic semicarbazide induces sequence-specific DNA damage through the generation of reactive oxygen species and the derived organic radicals. Mutat Res 2003;536:91–101.
13 Nestmann ER, Lynch BS, Musa-Veloso K, et al: Safety assessment and risk-benefit analysis of the use of azodicarbonamide in baby food jar closure technology: putting trace levels of semicarbazide exposure into perspective – a review. Food Addit Contam 2005;22:875–891.

Discussion

Dr. Haschke: For most pediatricians this is new, but not for me because I have been involved several times. It shows how a company, and I think Nestlé is not alone, takes care in the safety of food. You showed us the case of semicarbazide where you could manage the risk from the first to the last step. There was only one critical issue when an issued statement was a little bit preliminary, but there are other issues which are more or less not manageable that way, they end up being an emotional issue. You have mentioned the ITX issue; it was clear from the beginning that there would be no health risk, but on the other hand it ended up as a highly emotional thing which appeared on the internet within a few days and of course was used by several organizations to criticize the quality of commercial products. What is the percentage of the problems which become emotional, where you really have a comparison tool with which you can manage the whole value chain of risk management? In the case of ITX, was there no chance to come up with a sound scientific statement before it became emotional and politicians picked up the issue and brought it to the surface? Would there not have been a chance to handle that differently?

Dr. Scanlan: I don't have a value or any figures about the number of incidences that occur where there is the emotional side to it. For the last few years the handling of these issues has become more professional, and because there is more awareness on the regulator side, they are being managed better. Remember the case of acrylamide a few years ago that went directly to the media, and it created a real snowball effect. In the case of furan, the most recent one, there has been no snowball effect. It has been handled much better. There has been an improvement in that but different people, journalists for example, have their own interest, they want to sell newspapers, so when it comes to things like ITX they will jump on the wagon and create a big issue. At the time of the ITX story, we actually did a risk assessment which was provided to the Italian authorities, but it didn't lead to resolving the problem at the time. We shared all our information about any potential concern with them, and actually it wasn't found to be any kind of threat; this was also communicated to European Food Safety

Association (EFSA) at the time, and they agreed with us by the way. I don't know if you know this, but the EFSA actually came out and said that our risk assessment was correct and there was no concern about ITX but the Italian authorities decided otherwise. Of course it was in the hands of the judges who were applying a very black and white approach to it, presence, no presence; they weren't really concerned with the state of the assessment.

Dr. Calçado: I think people have a lot of misconception about food, not only in Brazil but worldwide. They think that non-processed foods are all healthy and not contaminated by bacteria or toxins. Otherwise, industrialized foods are thought to be not the best and full of dangerous additives.

Dr. Scanlan: That is true, processing is healthy, it is not the only means of course but it is healthy. The statement can be made that processed foods today have never been as safe; if you go back 100 years, today the food is far safer than it was then. I hope the next speaker will talk about the microbiological aspects and bring that up.

Dr. Jongpiputvanich: According to the actual WHO recommendations the sugar content should be less than 10% of the total calories. But in commercial baby food or commercial complementary food, the sugar content is more than 10% of the total calories. Why do the manufacturers do that? Are they only concerned about the taste of the food rather than healthy food?

Dr. Scanlan: I would imagine that there are regulations about how much sugar can be put in the food. Dr. Gailing, do you want to comment?

Dr. Gailing: Yes, a specific regulation in Thailand asks that sucrose not be added to infant formula. In the new Codex standard for infant formula it is the same, but for cereal-based baby food the new Codex standard allows up to 20% of added sugar in the components because there is no scientific base to ban sugar from the food of children, they need some calories. We just probably need to limit the consumption of sugar, but nevertheless the higher level is 20% of the total calorie intake in the cereal formula. Globally in our products we are between 10 and 15% when we add sugar.

Dr. Turck: It is generally considered that risk assessment and risk management at the regulatory level should be conducted by two different institutions. In my experience at the French Food Safety Agency, I am not sure that this is the ideal solution. What is your opinion on the experience of the EFSA which finally has a quiet opinion on the contaminant whereas DG Sanco decides exactly the reverse?

Dr. Scanlan: I would agree with you that the two bodies should act independent from one another in the sense that there are two different bodies; there are the risk assessors and the risk managers, but they need to have a very good communication. Don't forget that in 2003 EFSA was brand new and had just started their operations, and they were also engaged in a learning curve on how to deal with these types of issues, not only with DG Sanco but also with the different national regulators in the different countries of the EU. I remember discovering at the time that there wasn't very good communication between EFSA and France, UK, Germany, it was quite scattered, and then we saw with DG Sanco that there was a very poor communication going on. I would hope that it has improved since then, but I think it was more to do with a learning curve.

Dr. Gailing: It is not the problem of having separate risk assessment and risk management because they can talk together. It is more a problem of the application of the precautionary principle that the risk managers very often use because they want to go very quickly to protection because it is the aim of the precautionary principle to protect the public, even if it is not useful.

Dr. Scanlan: That's a good remark.

Ms. Darira: There is a growing perception among consumers that organic foods are actually safer. In your opinion, as a chemist, is this true or not?

Scanlan

Dr. Scanlan: That is not a simple question. I wouldn't want to get into the debate between organic food and processed food. It all depends on the hazards in the food, whatever it happens to be, and how that is managed. I have seen a lot of surveys of naturally grown organic food where the pesticide residue levels were far higher than whatever is found in the processed food. I have also seen cases where it is very clean and very good. So it all depends on the supply chain, how it is managed, how the whole production is taken care of. So there is no easy answer to your question.

Agostoni C, Brunser O (eds): Issues in Complementary Feeding.
Nestlé Nutr Workshop Ser Pediatr Program, vol 60, pp 79–90,
Nestec Ltd., Vevey/S. Karger AG, Basel, © 2007.

The Microbiological Risk

Lorenzo Morelli

Istituto di Microbiologia, Università Cattolica del Sacro Cuore, Piacenza, Italy

Abstract

Microbiological risk in the first part of life is endowed with peculiar features when compared to the same risk in adulthood. The purpose of this review is to highlight these age-related traits. While pathogens harmful for neonates and infants have been reviewed, less attention has been paid to the role played by the infant gut as battle field between pathogens and protecting bacteria or between pathogens and the immune system. Immediately after birth a race for colonizing the gut begins; the main tool for neonates to select good bacteria is represented by mother's milk. Quite surprisingly, this milk carries potentially harmful bacteria, but antibodies, oligosaccharides and the whole breast milk composition provide a powerful selective tool. Nevertheless this selective action is deeply influenced by the type and/or time (i.e. premature) of delivery or in premature subjects; recent data also show that breast milk could have a different potential in selecting bacterial species. The hygienic conditions of parents and, more generally, of the surrounding environment play a role in the selection of the intestinal biota of infants. It is then possible to group neonates according to the composition of the microbiota. Results of ecological studies suggest that neonates with a different microbiota could have a different microbiological risk.

Copyright © 2007 Nestec Ltd., Vevey/S. Karger AG, Basel

Introduction

Once the germ theory of disease was accepted, microbes were considered to be pathogens if they met the stipulations of Koch's postulate [1]. However, it rapidly became apparent that bacteria that are harmless to adults can be harmful in different hosts, such as infants; virulence, despite being a microbial characteristic, is differentially expressed in a susceptible host [2]. Thus, the question, 'What is a pathogen?' begs the question, 'What is the outcome of the host-microbe interaction?'. This question is simple to raise but difficult to answer, as it is necessary to move our attention from the microbe to the environment.

Environment means, in the case of neonates, mainly the gut, which is to be considered as a battle field in which three armies are engaged: pathogens, commensal bacteria and the immune system. Additional factors are also relevant for the final outcome of the battle: whether the child is born by natural or cesarean section delivery, and the status of the intestinal tissues, mucus, etc.

However, the ultimate weapon of this war is represented by the type of food supplied to troops and this is why complementary feeding can have a relevant role in managing the microbiological risk in infants.

The Gut as a Bacterial Ecological Niche

I would like to start presenting some comments on the 'battle field', which at the beginning is totally germ-free; however, immediately after birth, a race starts in order to invade the 'new lands'. These lands are quite easy to be reached as in neonates there are very reduced barriers at the borders:

- Adults tend to eat three meals a day and between these meals gastric pH is low; in newborn babies there is frequent feeding with milk, which is a good buffer [3]. This leads to the pH of the gastric contents being raised for prolonged periods. Under these circumstances, the gastric barrier is not really working and can provide only a limited selective action; this situation closely resembles what happens in adults treated with antiacid compounds.

- In fetus the liver develops from progenitor cells into a well-differentiated organ in which bile secretion can be observed by 12 weeks' gestation. Full maturity takes up to 2 years after birth to be achieved and the real potential of bile salts of neonates in controlling the uptake of orally delivered bacteria is not clear [4]. It should be noted, however, that breast milk does contain some trace of bile salts [5] but it is unclear whether, in addition to the emulsifying activity, there is also an action of selection against sensitive bacteria.

- The intestinal mucosal immune system is fully developed after a full-term birth, but the actual protective function of the gut requires the microbial stimulation of initial bacterial colonization [6]; then it takes some time in between the end of the protective action of antibodies carried by mother's milk and full activation of the neonate's immune mucosal protection.

- The whole load of bacteria in the first days of life is low; in adults the presence of the so-called 'autochthonous' (meaning in this case already present) bacteria provides a powerful barrier to the persistence of newcomers; this barrier has been defined as 'colonization resistance' and it is possible to measure it in a objective way. Obviously, in neonates this resistance is very low [7]. In addition after a few months of life the gut microbiota is 'disturbed' by a revolution in feeding habits: weaning is a dramatic change for the intestinal microbiota which has to reach a new homeostasis [8].

The First Colonization

As a consequence of this reduced presence of barriers the first bacteria entering the human gut and reproducing in this environment are a mixture of enteric and nonenteric bugs. The first to arrive are not really 'good guys' for the host as they belong to *Enterobacteriaceae*, streptococci, staphylococci [9]. It takes some days for bifidobacteria, lactobacilli and possibly other, still less known anaerobic bacteria to take over from the first bacteria.

Most of the knowledge on microbiota composition of the first part of our life has been obtained by means of classical microbiological techniques such as plate counting, but recent papers have shown, by using a molecular biology approach, that it is probably time to make some changes. Several studies carried out using molecular methods have recently shown the presence of the genus *Ruminococcus*, described as an important component of the infant's intestinal microbiota [9, 10]. In fact, the bacterial genus *Ruminococcus* is recognized to have an important protective effect on the host since it produces ruminococcin A, a bacteriocin that can inhibit the development of many of species of *Clostridium* [11].

Molecular biology techniques have also allowed to detect the presence of members of the genus *Desulfovibrio* [12], which have previously only been found in adults. This genus is mainly present in bottle-fed babies but it was also detected in breastfed ones.

By means of both classical and molecular-based techniques it is known that in healthy babies, *Escherichia coli* or bacteria belonging to *Clostridium* spp. are the initial colonizers rapidly followed by *Bifidobacterium, Bacteroides, Clostridium, Streptococcus, Enterococcus* and *Actinomyces*. *Bifidobacterium* species appeared already after 5 days in breast-fed babies but with some delay in bottle-fed neonates.

The molecular biology approach now provides, however, a better understanding of the process leading to the formation of the first, stable microbiota in infants. It has been pointed out that, in addition to the bacteria cited above, strictly anaerobic ones are also present in the gut of neonates [12]. The real role of these bacteria in protecting the health of babies is far from being understood. As a consequence, while the concept that microbiota of breastfed babies is the 'golden standard' still holds, our feeling that more than 90% of this microbiota is composed of bifidobacteria needs to be revised. Just as an example in several breastfed babies ruminococci are present at the same level as bifidobacteria. However we have to point out that different techniques [denaturing gradient gel electrophoresis (DGGE), fluorescent in situ hybridization (FISH), quantitative polymerase chain reaction (Q-PCR), cloning] resulted in a determination of the microbiota composition which did not always match. More studies, performed on a large number of subjects to avoid the natural personal variation, are needed and therefore we have to be cautious in drawing conclusions. What seems clear is that molecular ecology of the gut microbiota of infants is rapidly accumulating new data.

Microbiota Composition and Infant-Specific Pathogens

Whatever the real composition of gut microbiota is in neonates, it is clear that it is managed by a few tools, when compared to the situation in adults. Moreover, this situation could lead to having an unstable environment where also bacteria with a low pathogenic potential could be harmful and even lethal. Just as an example I will here refer to *Enterobacter sakazakii*, the most recent and 'fashionable', infant-specific pathogen.

Pathogenesis of *E. sakazakii* involves bacteremia and/or sepsis, cerebrospinal fluid infection and meningitis, brain abscess or cyst formation, and has been associated with necrotizing enterocolitis [13]. Infant mortality rate for *E. sakazakii* meningitis was reported to be 40–80%. This bacterium seems to be able to breach the blood-brain barrier, as it has a tropism for the central nervous system. The real molecular mechanism of this tropism in neonates and infants, however, remains a mystery. Adhesion potential of this bacterium, a trait necessary for bacterial translocation, has been only recently assessed [14].

It is also surprising to note that, even though the first report of infection caused by this bacterium dates back to the 1960s and the first review of clinical aspects of the reclassified bacterium is dated 1988 [15], the first report on toxin production by *E. sakazakii* appeared only in 2003 [16] and up to now studies showing the real pathogenic features of these bacterium have been very few.

Enterotoxin production as well as adhesion potential have been shown; however these traits are not strong enough to be harmful for the adult, otherwise healthy, population.

We can probably conclude that this bacterium is mainly harmful because its stationary phase cells are remarkably resistant to osmotic and drying stresses compared with other species of the *Enterobacteriaceae* [16]; these technological features are the real 'pathogenic phenotype' at least for infants: if these cells arrive in sufficient number in the infant's gut, they can multiply to such a level to be dangerous. But it seems to be more a problem of poor defense barriers than a high level of toxicity.

Managing the Microbiota to Reduce Microbiological Risk

It is then possible to turn the attention to the main section of this review: how can we manage the gut environment of infants in order to reduce the microbiological risk. What has been outlined before has probably made clear that feeding could have a central role in this effort.

The gut microbiota of an adult is quite a stable environment and several factors contribute to its homeostasis: the selection done by the gastric environment, the lytic action of bile salts, the immune system, the mucus composition, and the colonization resistance. In contrast selection and maintenance of good bacteria in neonates can rely on only two main tools: type of feeding and mucus covering their intestinal tissues [17–19]. Breast milk also provides a strong selective action due to the mother's antibodies, but this action declines with time. I will only deal with the first of these tools, as there is stronger evidence available of the real impact of food on the microbiota composition.

As regards the food as bacterial selection agent it should be noted that the development of the bifidobacteria-dominant microflora has been related to the peculiar composition of human milk. In particular a bifidogenic effect has been ascribed to a low concentration of proteins and phosphorus, the presence of lactoferrin and nucleotides even if oligosaccharides of human milk have the best-documented bifidogenic action. A high percentage of such substances resist digestion in the gastrointestinal tract and reach the colon where they stimulate microbiota development. They are partially excreted with feces, representing the paradigm of the prebiotics [20]. Human milk oligosaccharides are synthesized in the mammary gland through the sequential action of specific glycosyltransferases that add monosaccharide units (galactose, fucose, sialic acid, N-acetyl-glucosamine) to lactose. Among these enzymes, the fucosyltransferases add one or more fucose moieties through specific bonds. Their presence is linked to the expression of the secretor and Lewis genes of the nursing mothers. Depending on the expression of these genes, one or more fucosyltransferases are present and, in turn, they significantly condition both the qualitative and the quantitative composition of fucosyloligosaccharides. Breast milk oligosaccharides have also been found to be analogues for microbial receptors preventing mucosal attachment, the initial step of most infections. As a result, breastfeeding significantly reduces the risk of neonatal septicemia, respiratory tract infections, otitis media, diarrhea and urinary tract infections.

Breast milk is then one of the best example of how potent the diet can be in influencing an ecological, bacterial niche such as the gut and, in turn, how the gut microbiota can have an impact on health and also on physiological functions.

The first defense mechanism to be influenced by gut microbiota is the immune system; data are available pointing out the role played by different microbiota in the early maturation of the gut immune system [21]. In addition, specific bacteria, could enhance different immunoresponses [22, 23]. It was shown [22] that bifidobacteria have species-specific effects on the expression of the dendritic-cell activation marker CD83 and the production of interleukin-10 (IL-10). Whereas CD83 expression was increased and IL-10 production was

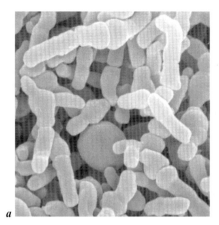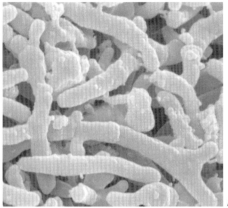

a *b*

Fig. 1. *B. infantis* (***a***) and *B. longum* (***b***) cells observed by scanning electron microscopy. These two species are highly phylogenetically related [31] but have totally different immune stimulation potential.

induced by *Bifidobacterium bifidum*, *B. longum*, and *B. pseudocatenulatum*, *B. infantis* failed to produce these effects. It was concluded that *B. infantis* does not trigger the activation of dendritic cells to the degree necessary to initiate an immune response but that *B. bifidum*, *B. longum*, and *B. pseudocatenulatum* induce a Th2-driven immune response. This observation, even if preliminary, clearly stimulates the need of further, more detailed investigation at the species and subspecies levels, as *B. longum* is known to be strictly related to *B. infantis* (fig. 1).

After these remarks on the protective action of breast milk, it is safe to add, however, that this activity is far from being completely understood, as recent data have also shown that breast milk taken from different mothers could have varying potential for selecting bacterial species [19]. The hygienic conditions of parents and, more generally, of the surrounding environment, could also play a role in selecting intestinal biota. It was shown that microbial profiles of babies and their parents could be quite similar, suggesting a vertical transmission determined by genetic and environmental factors [10].

An aberrant composition of gut microbiota between groups of healthy and allergic children has also been reported [24]. Quite interestingly, the serum total IgE concentration correlated directly with *E. coli* counts in all infants indicating that the presence of these bacteria is associated with the extent of atopic sensitization.

It has been proven by meta-analysis results that prevention of the typical gastrointestinal diseases such as diarrhea is possible by feeding the 'right' bacteria to infants; this action does not seem related to a specific bacterium, as the same positive results can be achieved using different probiotic preparations, containing bacteria or yeast. It seems then that the action could be related to a nonspecific, ecological action more than a strain-specific phenotype [25, 26].

Preterm Neonates as a 'Model System'

To conclude it could be worthwhile to stress that the relevance of the gut environment in managing the selection of 'good bugs' is also provided by a negative reference test, the microbiota of preterm neonates. In these subjects the number of bacteria is reduced but also the range of different bacterial species is kept at a minimum [27]. Comparisons between term and preterm neonates in terms of gut microbiota really suggest the relevance of the environment in selecting and sustaining the good bacteria. As an example, it is possible to focus on the need that bacteria have to adhere to intestinal mucus; it has been shown [19] that this feature is age-specific, but we still lack knowledge on the specific interactions between bacteria and mucus of neonates, especially for those delivered preterm and/or very low birth weight subjects.

A low presence of indigenous commensal bacteria could open the door to bacteria causing necrotizing enterocolitis.

Preterm babies have a very low potential in retaining in their gut bifidobacteria [28] but, after one century of investigations, we have now adopted an evidence-based nutritional approach to manage the well-being of infants.

Intervention on Microbiota Management

As a first step in this evidence-based nutritional approach we can now deal with intervention studies in which probiotics and/or prebiotics have been fed to neonates in order to mimic, as a final result, the microbiota composition of breastfed babies, which is believed to be the most protective microbiota.

A range of bacteria have been used in different types of formula milk as well as some prebiotic substances, as a mixture or as pure compounds.

It has been shown, in several instances, that probiotic strains, if selected according to scientific criteria, are able to survive, reproduce and persist in the gut of neonates. Colonization seems to be more easy to achieve if the initial numbers of bifidobacteria or lactobacilli are low. However, colonization of preterm neonates seems to be more difficult to achieve but when successful it seems to allow a certain degree of protection against opportunistic infections.

Prebiotics have been shown to be able to manage microbiota composition in both term and preterm neonates; some data on the positive effects of this prebiotic-mediated microbiota on allergy are becoming available. Work in the field is rapidly progressing and results seem promising but I feel it is more prudent to refer to the cautious approach taken by ESPGHAN in assessing the use of both probiotics and prebiotics [29, 30].

In the end it could be relevant to answer the following 'old' question: 'If we group neonates according to the composition of the microbiota, may we find a correlation with their resistance to disease?' This is the same question as the one raised by Tissier more than one century ago, 'Is there any direct link between bacteria in the stool and health?', but we have to admit that data are still scarce, even if extremely promising.

At the moment this is more an area of research than application, but I am confident that a significant reduction in the microbiological risk for neonates will be provided in the future by an ecological approach, exploiting the protective action of the gut as an ecological niche.

References

1 Casadevall A, Pirofski LA: Host-pathogen interactions: basic concepts of microbial commensalism, colonization, infection, and disease. Infect Immun 2000;12:6511–6518.
2 Casadevall A, Pirofski LA: Host-pathogen interactions: the attributes of virulence. J Infect Dis 2001;184:337–344.
3 Omari TI, Davidson GP: Multipoint measurement of intragastric pH in healthy preterm infants. Arch Dis Child Fetal Neonatal Ed 2003;88:F517–F520.
4 Beath SV: Hepatic function and physiology in the newborn. Semin Neonatol 2003;8:337–346.
5 Forsyth JS, Donnet L, Ross PE: A study of the relationship between bile salts, bile salt-stimulated lipase, and free fatty acids in breast milk: normal infants and those with breast milk jaundice. J Pediatr Gastroenterol Nutr 1990;1:205–210.
6 Macpherson AJ, Harris NL: Interactions between commensal intestinal bacteria and the immune system. Nat Rev Immunol 2004;4:478–485.
7 Vollaard EJ, Clasener HA: Colonization resistance. Antimicrob Agents Chemother 1994;38: 409–414.
8 Amarri S, Benatti F, Callegari ML, et al: Changes of gut microbiota and immune markers during the complementary feeding period in healthy breast-fed infants. J Pediatr Gastroenterol Nutr 2006;42:488–495.
9 Favier CF, Vaughan EE, De Vos WM, Akkermans AD: Molecular monitoring of succession of bacterial communities in human neonates. Appl Environ Microbiol 2002;68:219–226.
10 Favier CF, de Vos WM, Akkermans AD: Development of bacterial and bifidobacterial communities in feces of newborn babies. Anaerobe 2003;9:219–229.
11 Dabard J, Bridonneau C, Phillipe C, et al: Ruminococcin A, a new lantibiotic produced by a *Ruminococcus gnavus* strain isolated from human feces. Appl Environ Microbiol 2001;67: 4111–4118.
12 Hopkins MJ, Macfarlane GT, Furrie E, et al: Characterisation of intestinal bacteria in infant stools using real-time PCR and northern hybridisation analyses. FEMS Microbiol Ecol 2005; 54:77–85.
13 Lai KK: *Enterobacter sakazakii* infections among neonates, infants, children, and adults. Case reports and a review of the literature. Medicine (Baltimore) 2001;80:113–122.
14 Mange JP, Stephan R, Borel N, et al: Adhesive properties of *Enterobacter sakazakii* to human epithelial and brain microvascular endothelial cells. BMC Microbiol 2006;6:58–68.
15 Willis J, Robinson JE: *Enterobacter sakazakii* meningitis in neonates. Pediatr Infect Dis J 1988;7:196–199.
16 Lehner A, Stephan R: Microbiological, epidemiological, and food safety aspects of *Enterobacter sakazakii*. J Food Prot 2004;67:2850–2857.
17 Wold AE, Adlerberth I: Breast feeding and the intestinal microflora of the infant: implications for protection against infectious diseases. Adv Exp Med Biol 2000;478:77–93.

18 Lonnerdal B: Nutritional and physiologic significance of human milk proteins. Am J Clin Nutr 2003;77:1537S–1543S.
19 Ouwehand AC, Isolauri E, Kirjavainen PV, Salminen SJ: Adhesion of four *Bifidobacterium* strains to human intestinal mucus from subjects in different age groups. FEMS Microbiol Lett 1999;172:61–64.
20 Coppa GV, Bruni S, Morelli L, et al: The first prebiotics in humans: human milk oligosaccharides. J Clin Gastroenterol 2004;38(suppl):S80–S83.
21 Macpherson AJ, Harris NL: Interactions between commensal intestinal bacteria and the immune system. Nat Rev Immunol 2004;4:478–485.
22 Young SL, Simon MA, Baird MA, et al: Bifidobacterial species differentially affect expression of cell surface markers and cytokines of dendritic cells harvested from cord blood. Clin Diagn Lab Immunol 2004;11:686–690.
23 Mullie C, Yazourh A, Thibault H, et al: Increased poliovirus-specific intestinal antibody response coincides with promotion of *Bifidobacterium longum-infantis* and *Bifidobacterium breve* in infants: a randomized, double-blind, placebo-controlled trial. Pediatr Res 2004;56:791–795.
24 Kirjavainen PV, Arvola T, Salminen SJ, Isolauri E: Aberrant composition of gut microbiota of allergic infants: a target of bifidobacterial therapy at weaning? Gut 2002;51:51–55.
25 Huang JS, Bousvaros A, Lee JW, et al: Efficacy of probiotic use in acute diarrhea in children: a meta-analysis. Dig Dis Sci 2002;47:2625–2634.
26 Szajewska H, Mrukowicz JZ: Use of probiotics in children with acute diarrhea. Paediatr Drugs 2005;7:111–122.
27 Westerbeek EA, van den Berg A, Lafeber HN, et al: The intestinal bacterial colonisation in preterm infants: a review of the literature. Clin Nutr 2006;J25:361–368.
28 Magne F, Abely M, Boyer F, et al: Low species diversity and high interindividual variability in faeces of preterm infants as revealed by sequences of 16S rRNA genes and PCR-temporal temperature gradient gel electrophoresis profiles. FEMS Microbiol Ecol 2006;57:128–138.
29 Agostoni C, Axelsson I, Goulet O, et al; ESPGHAN Committee on Nutrition: Prebiotic oligosaccharides in dietetic products for infants: a commentary by the ESPGHAN Committee on Nutrition. J Pediatr Gastroenterol Nutr 2004;39:465–473.
30 Agostoni C, Axelsson I, Braegger C, et al; ESPGHAN Committee on Nutrition: Probiotic bacteria in dietetic products for infants: a commentary by the ESPGHAN Committee on Nutrition. J Pediatr Gastroenterol Nutr 2004;38:365–374.
31 Sakata S, Kitahara M, Sakamoto M, et al: Unification of *Bifidobacterium infantis* and *Bifidobacterium suis* as *Bifidobacterium longum*. Int J Syst Evol Microbiol 2002;52:1945–1951.

Discussion

Dr. Haschke: Thank you for a fascinating lecture on this neonatal balance between good and bad bacteria. Would you agree that today we can say that vaginal delivery is better than cesarean section in terms of promoting a good bacterial balance early in the gut? There are a lot of data supporting this. If bifidobacteria and lactobacilli are not found in the stool during the first day of life that doesn't mean that that they are not already present because the baby does not pass stool on the first day, it is meconium. The first day's stool is what was already in the fetus before birth, it just shows that the fetal gut was sterile. But the stool comes after 24 h, and in some infants after 48 h, and then from the first moment you see the bacteria. So the bacteria are going in by the mouth, probably at birth in most of them, and we have also learned that breast milk contains certain bifidobacteria and lactobacilli. And finally, the ruminococci story is new to me; would it be an advantage for very young infants to have more in the gut to stimulate growth by mechanisms such as the prebiotic approach?

Dr. Morelli: Cesarean delivery is a kind of nightmare for the gut microbiota of a newborn. There are some papers indicating that it took almost 2 years to obtain a normal balance after cesarean section [1, 2]. I have probably underrepresented the delivery system among the 6 points that are important but I have not tried to go into detail. I think that this field could be one of the most promising in which to have food intervention just to promote quicker recovery of the normal microbiota. I am not so sure that breast milk could be a relevant source of lactobacilli, even though there are papers showing the presence of bacteria in breast milk [3, 4], I would like to be cautious. It is obvious that there are bacteria in breast milk, this is not new. There are also good indications that there is a unique and single ecosystem between the mother and the mouth of the baby. The skin of the mother and the mouth of the baby are exchanging bacteria. The physiological mechanism allowing bacteria to pass into breast milk has recently been investigated [5]. But the total number of bacteria is estimated to be low. So this is an argument for the future.

I would like to draw attention to the presence of ruminococci that have been found in neonates by several groups [6–8]. We know that they have an important anticlostridial action, they are Gram-positive and are definitely not pathogenic bacteria. So it is possible that the ruminococci could play a positive role or nothing, but this is something new that must be taken into consideration.

Dr. Haschke: We know that the lactobacilli and bifidobacteria might come from the skin or might be transported into breast milk by a mechanism which we don't yet understand. But they come from the mother. Where do the ruminococci come from?

Dr. Morelli: From the mother also. There are some studies that have demonstrated exactly the same bonding pattern between the parents and the baby after the baby arrived home.

Dr. Giovannini: Compliments, very interesting, but I have a point to clarify: the problem of probiotics, because sometimes there is a bias between human milk oligosaccharide and prebiotics. All the papers on prebiotics are only about fecal consistence, and one paper about the lower incidence of atopic dermatitis between 3 and 6 months. We have known for many years and from long experience that probiotics may be in the food and we know that probiotics will arrive in the gut and are sometimes difficult to replicate. For this reason I think that after the first year of life children should perhaps receive probiotics in their food every day. But I am worried about the problem of prebiotics because sometimes it is not evidence-based and sometimes prebiotics may be a problem of marketing. We speak too much about fecal culture and not enough about bacterial DNA which is the best way, a little bit expensive, to detect a single bacterial strain.

Dr. Morelli: I totally agree with you. Microbiology has a lot of new tools, and as a science it was born when the microscope, a necessary tool, was invented. Microbiology is not like mathematics in which pencil and paper are used; without a microscope microbiology wouldn't exist. Now we have the genetic tools to obtain evidence-based information about the real impact of pre- or probiotics. There is now DNA fingerprinting of each single bacterial strain, so that we are in a position to say that these bacteria recovered from a fecal sample are exactly the same bacteria as those fed 2 days earlier, and this is important. It is a tool. I am not a clinician, I have no explanation for the clinical aspect, the impact and so on. I am in the position to provide diagnostic tools and information on diagnosis by means of these diagnostic tools.

Dr. Ribeiro: Using your analogy of war strategy and transportation, food, sources, what is your concern about timing for the use of pro- or prebiotics?

Dr. Morelli: I am not a clinician so I will respond as a microbiologist. The urgency to intervene, to add pro- or prebiotics, is really relevant in cesarean section or in babies who have received antibiotics for whatever reason. I feel that in naturally delivered and breastfed babies it is probably not as necessary in the beginning to support the microbiota. It is possible that within 2 years my answer will change because we will most likely have more information, but at this moment I think that babies born by cesarean section or with a special condition, such as preterm, probably really need support from point zero. Under normal conditions, normal delivery, natural delivery and breastfeeding, we can probably wait.

Dr. Delgado: Pathogenic bacteria are presented by lymphocytes and can produce proinflammatory cytokines. With probiotics this mechanism can be changed or modified. Is it possible to produce more anti-inflammatory cytokines with this substance or bacteria?

Dr. Morelli: Nestlé has produced a lot of papers about gut-associated lymphoid tissues, and the answer is definitely yes. From my point of view what we are lacking is knowledge about the molecule. In my group we are working on the surface layers, some proteins that are outside the bacteria or the metabolite that are able to crosstalk with intestinal tissue. There are a lot of papers coming out using genomic array, the human genomic array, and there is regulation of the genes involved in this kind of response. So the answer is yes.

Dr. Agostoni: You said that we only know 30% of the bacteria present in the gut, and that ruminococci are strong agents against clostridia. Could we speculate that lactobacilli and bifidobacteria and now ruminococci are just proxies for the decrease in clostridia? This is the key point of the probiotic story to take space from clostridia to reduce their numbers and maybe all around the clostridia.

Dr. Morelli: The 30% figure was published by a French group for adult microbiota. We do not have exactly the same figures for infants, but we can speculate that more or less we are in the same condition. I have no answer to the second part of your question, but we need more details about the gut microbiota of infants in order to really exploit the good groups in a cleverer way. Probably in the near future we will have prebiotics that will be ruminococci-specific, or whatever other group specific, in order to see their clinical relevance because there is still a kind of open question mark. More than a century ago it was said that bifidobacteria are present in healthy babies, but as far as I know there is not really a lot of clinical data showing that babies with a very high level of bifidobacteria have better health or clinically significant outcome due to the presence of very high levels of bifidobacteria. This is a kind of dogma.

Dr. Agostoni: But the reason for my question is that from a practical point of view, as far as I know, the major association for clostridia is gut cancer. An excess amount of meat in the diet is associated with an increased number of clostridia and a supposed predisposition to get cancer.

Dr. Morelli: I know what you are trying to suggest but I don't want to answer very clearly because I am prudent.

Dr. Haschke: I assume that the weaning period is more complex. I would not really agree with the conclusion that this good bacteria; might it be that *Lactobacillus* GG or *Bifidobacterium lactis* are contributing to health during the weaning period and later on? There are several data showing that they protect from diarrhea, and they are very important in terms of more rapid recovery from diarrhea, so there are a lot of data there. The bacteria when given either as a supplement or together with a formula have a beneficial effect. So there are health effects, would you agree? In a breastfed infant, how long would you suggest that the bifidogenic gut flora is beneficial, or when does it become trivial because solid foods are introduced anyway and the microbiota is moving towards the adult pattern? Perhaps you can only speculate, but how long would it be beneficial?

Dr. Morelli: About the first part of your question, I am not saying that adding selected bacteria will not be useful. I am wondering if a high level of naturally occurring bacteria of the same group of the selected bacteria is really useful or not, because we know that probiotic bacteria have been selected through a very thought-provoking selection scheme in the laboratory so we know that they are able to immune modulate and so on. This is not true for the naturally occurring bacteria. Then the 10^7 lactobacilli or 10^9 bifidobacteria, naturally occurring in the gut, have been selected simply because they are able to survive in saliva, in the stomach, in the bile, and then they use the food. This is something clever for them, I am not so sure that it is clever for me. In the laboratory we have selected bacteria that are able to do something for the human body. This is not a natural process. We are scientists, we must not presume that the natural selection scheme is able to select the best bacteria for our health. That is my point. Frankly, I can only speculate on the second point, so I would prefer to skip it.

Dr. Calçado: As the endosymbiotic theory from the 1920s shows that the mitochondria could be a bacterium that was incorporated by us ages ago, we know that many bacterial genes have important command over our body. In this way the bacterial flora could be called an organ, not a traditional organ like the heart or liver, but a pool of cells with a genetic expression.

Dr. Morelli: Microbiologists call the human gut microbiota the neglected organ, and so I really believe that it is an organ. But we have to learn how to exercise this organ, to train this organ in a better way, not for the organ itself but for the body, and that is the challenge for the future.

References

1   Gronlund MM, Lehtonen OP, Eerola E, Kero P: Fecal microflora in healthy infants born by different methods of delivery: permanent changes in intestinal flora after cesarean delivery. J Pediatr Gastroenterol Nutr 1999;28:19–25.
2   Salminen S, Gibson GR, McCartney AL, Isolauri E: Influence of mode of delivery on gut microbiota composition in seven year old children. Gut 2004;53:1388–1389.
3   Martin R, Olivares M, Marin ML, et al: Probiotic potential of 3 Lactobacilli strains isolated from breast milk. J Hum Lact 2005;21:8–17; quiz 18–21, 41.
4   Martin R, Heilig HG, Zoetendal EG, et al: Cultivation-independent assessment of the bacterial diversity of breast milk among healthy women. Res Microbiol 2007;158:31–37.
5   Perez PF, Dore J, Leclerc M, et al: Bacterial imprinting of the neonatal immune system: lessons from maternal cells? Pediatrics 2007;119:e724–e732.
6   Magne F, Hachelaf W, Suau A, et al: A longitudinal study of infant faecal microbiota during weaning. FEMS Microbiol Ecol 2006;58:563–571.
7   Favier CF, Vaughan EE, de Vos WM, Akkermans AD: Molecular monitoring of succession of bacterial communities in human neonates. Appl Environ Microbiol 2002;68:219–226.
8   Favier CF, de Vos WM, Akkermans AD: Development of bacterial and bifidobacterial communities in feces of newborn babies. Anaerobe 2003;9:219–229.

Agostoni C, Brunser O (eds): Issues in Complementary Feeding.
Nestlé Nutr Workshop Ser Pediatr Program, vol 60, pp 91–105,
Nestec Ltd., Vevey/S. Karger AG, Basel, © 2007.

Cereal Fortification Programs in Developing Countries

Saraswati Bulusu,[a] *Luc Laviolette,*[a] *Venkatesh Mannar,*[a]
Vinodini Reddy[b]

[a]Micronutrient Initiative, New Delhi, India, and [b]Ex-National Institute of Nutrition,
Hyderabad, India

Abstract

Malnutrition is a major problem among children especially in the developing world. In most developing countries children show growth faltering between 6 and 24 months of age due to inadequate complementary feeding. Complementary foods are transitional foods given in addition to breast milk, following exclusive breastfeeding during the first 6 months, to meet the full nutritional requirements of the infant. Strategies to improve the availability of and accessibility to low cost complementary foods can play an important role in improving the nutritional status of infants and young children. Cereals constitute the most suitable vehicle for delivering micronutrients to an at-risk population because of their widespread consumption, stability and versatility. To reduce the vulnerability to the health impacts of micronutrient deficiencies, several developed and developing countries have adopted various innovative, cost-effective strategies to fortify cereal-based complementary foods and to reach children through public programs. This article reviews cereal fortification programs in developing countries, with special reference to low cost fortified complementary foods, and emphasizes the need for public-private-civic sector initiatives to improve the health and wellbeing of people around the world.

Introduction

Malnutrition is one of the major problems of public health significance in developing countries; it tends to severely affect the most vulnerable groups such as women and young children in rural areas. The increasing migration of rural people to urban and semi-urban areas for economic pursuits is contributing to a third significant group in the form of slums in the urban areas. Malnutrition of children remains of particular concern in the developing

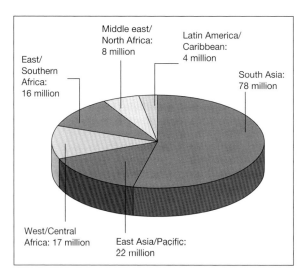

East/
Southern
Africa:
16 million

Middle east/
North Africa:
8 million

Latin America/
Caribbean:
4 million

South Asia:
78 million

West/Central
Africa: 17 million

East Asia/Pacific:
22 million

Fig. 1. Child malnutrition. Figures based on latest available estimates of underweight prevalence in 110 developing countries (1996–2005). Source: UNICEF.

world (fig. 1). The first 2 years of life are a critical window for mental and physical development. The damage that occurs during this period due to malnutrition is often irreversible even if corrective actions are taken later in life. Approximately one third of children less than 5 years of age in developing countries have low height-for-age ratio (≤2 SD with respect to reference data) [1]. It is estimated that around 5.6 million children die from malnutrition each year.

Nutritional Problems in Developing Countries

While being underweight or stunted is recognized as an important risk factor for the increased prevalence and severity of infection and high mortality rates, there is increasing evidence on the enhanced risks due to micronutrient deficiencies, and three key nutrients are well known to play a vital role [2]. The prevalence of iron deficiency among children is high in most developing countries and is particularly high in South Asian countries (especially India, Bangladesh, Pakistan and Nepal). During infancy and early childhood, iron deficiency is associated with increased infant mortality, impaired psychomotor development, cognitive function and reduced learning capacity that may be irreversible. Vitamin A deficiency has grave consequences for the survival and wellbeing of children. Improving vitamin A status has been shown to reduce child morbidity and mortality as well as pregnancy-related mortality. Iodine deficiency is the leading cause of preventable mental retardation among young children. Other effects of iodine deficiency in the mother range from stillbirths, birth defects to growth retardation and cretinism. The linkages between micronutrient deficiencies and the Millennium Development Goals are highlighted in table 1.

Increasing evidence on the role of zinc and folic acid for young child survival and growth is also being reported. Improving zinc status reduces stunting, morbidity and mortality from diarrheal and respiratory infections [3]. Each year folate deficiency near conception causes 250,000 unnecessary infant deaths or paralysis from folic acid-preventable spina bifida and anencephaly. Spina bifida is devastating as it manifests itself in newborn children as paralysis, bladder and bowel incontinence, bone deformities, or hydrocephalus. It is a significant socioeconomic burden in several developing countries, including India, where the incidence has been reported to be very high [4].

Infancy is a time of rapid physical growth and, therefore, nutritional requirements are at the highest during this period. Adequate nutrition during the first 2 years of life is critical to ensure optimal physical and mental development of infants and young children. Development of successful interventions to improve child feeding practices, in particular, is necessary to avoid serious adverse consequences in the future.

Fortification of Cereals

Fortification of foods has been practiced for several decades in developed countries. Foods that have been fortified with single or multiple micronutrients include margarine, milk, bread, sugar, wheat and other grains, tea, dairy foods, edible oils, formula foods, malted beverages, salt and other specialty items [5–9].

When micronutrient deficiencies are population-wide and result from a combination of low intake and/or low bioavailability, fortification of commonly consumed cereal flours with iron, folic acid and other vitamins offers a number of strategic advantages because cereals flours are widely and regularly consumed, and mostly processed in centralized facilities with established distribution and marketing capacity. Cereal fortification has played a major role in improving the health of the world populations at large. Wheat is the most widely produced cereal in the world, most of which is destined for human consumption. The processing of whole wheat to flour is generally concentrated in a few large mills. The resulting flour is used to make bread, biscuits, pasta, and other products. In a population of school-age Filipino children, it was observed that the routine consumption of a wheat-flour bun fortified with only 33% of the RDA of vitamin A improved vitamin A status [9]. In January 1999, the Government of Indonesia, with support from UNICEF and through an initial premix donated by Mother Care/USAID, started a program for

Table 1. Linkages between micronutrient deficiencies and Millennium Development Goals

Goal	Impact of vitamin A deficiency	Impact of iron deficiency anemia	Impact of iodine deficiency disorders
Poverty and hunger impact (MDG1)	On countries: higher burden of death and disease to be managed	On countries: economic loss in affected countries = 1% of GDP	On countries: in iodine-deficient population mean IQ lowered by 10–15%
	On caregivers: care for the sick/dying On families: cost of funerals On families: loss of future earnings	On adults: reduces productivity On caregivers: care for the sick	On adults: negatively affects livelihoods On children: impairs learning On caregivers: care for the sick
Education and literacy impact (MDG2)	On children: decreased school attendance	On children: impaired mental development for 50% of 6- to 24-month-old children in the developing world: hard to learn and keep jobs	On children: impaired mental development for 18 million children globally: 60,000 severely mentally retarded
Gender equality impact (MDG3)	On women and girl children: caring for sick young children affects earning a livelihood	On adults: impaired productivity increases risks to livelihood Greater health impact on women	On women and girl children: caring for sick young children affects earning a livelihood and school attendance
Child mortality impact (MDG4)	On children: increased risk of death for >1 million young children yearly	On children: 15,000 infants at greater risk of death due to maternal anemia	On children: increased risk of stillbirths
Maternal health impact (MDG5)		On mothers: death of 50,000 women/year during pregnancy and childbirth	
Major infectious disease impact (MDG6)	On children: 40% of under-5s immunocompromised by vitamin A deficiency with reduced protection against diarrhea, measles, and other infections	On people: impact of malaria exacerbated by iron deficiency On children: anemia is linked to most malaria-related deaths in young children	

fortifying wheat flour with iron. This strategy is believed to have contributed substantially to the reduction of iron deficiency anemia in Indonesia [10].

Folic acid fortification of cereal flours is having remarkable impact in reducing women's risk of having a baby born with a birth defect of the spine or brain (spina bifida or anencephaly). Food fortification was determined to be the best strategy for increasing blood folate levels, as the critical period for adequate intake of folic acid is in the first weeks of pregnancy before most women know that they are pregnant and begin taking supplements. In the US, the fortification of enriched cereal grain products with folic acid began in 1996. By 1999 the National Health and Nutrition Examination Survey conducted by the Centers for Disease Control found that the average level of folic acid in the blood of US women had almost tripled in 5 years [11]. Fortification of flour, pasta and cornmeal has become mandatory in Canada since 1998, and a study in Ontario showed that the incidence of neural tube defects had fallen to 8.6 cases/10,000 pregnancies, down from 16.2 in 1995 [12].

Currently, nearly 40 countries fortify cereal flour. In Latin America flour fortification is implemented on a large scale. Fortification of wheat and maize flours with multiple nutrients has been made mandatory in South Africa and Nigeria. There is growing interest in wheat flour fortification in South and South East Asian countries like Nepal, Bangladesh, Pakistan, Afghanistan, India and China.

Fortification of Complementary Foods

In the first 6 months, the dietary requirements of infants can be fully met by breast milk, as specified in WHO guidelines. Thereafter, complementary foods need to be given to augment energy and nutrient intake. Although breastfeeding is common in most developing countries, children show growth faltering between 6 and 24 months of age due to inadequate complementary feeding. Most children are given a small portion of adult diet. The 'bulk' of the cereal-based diet does not allow the young child to consume sufficient quantities to meet their energy and protein requirements. Hence, from the food technology perspective, the challenge is to increase both the energy density of complementary foods and levels of micronutrients at an affordable price. From the public health perspective, we need a combination of proper regulation that protects infant health yet supports industrial innovation and strong public education on appropriate infant feeding practices and psychosocial care of the infant.

The fortification of commercially marketed staple foods such as cereal flours, cooking oils and dairy products could have a small but significant impact for preschool children. However infants and children under the age of 24 months consume a different dietary pattern than older individuals. Cereals are the first complementary foods to be introduced and are intended to accustom the infant to solid foods. Industrially produced fortified complementary foods are recommended by pediatricians worldwide as an essential part of a nutritionally adequate infant diet (beyond the age of 6 months) and as complementary to breast milk and home-prepared foods. This is essential in order to meet the micronutrient requirements of infants, especially for iron and zinc. Beyond the superior micronutrient content of industrially fortified complementary foods over home-prepared porridges and other traditional infant foods, they also have the advantages of delivering micronutrients of higher bioavailability, energy density and protein quality, and are safe and convenient.

Multiple fortification of infant cereals is common in developed countries. Since the 1950s, the National Supplementary Food Program administered by the Chilean Ministry of Health through primary care health centers, provided milk-based complementary foods free to children from birth to 5 years of age, along with other health and nutrition services. The milk is fortified with iron, ascorbic acid, zinc and copper. The program has helped reduce anemia in Chilean infants from 21 to approximately 1% today [13]. Similarly, data from the CDC pediatric nutrition surveillance system show a reduction in the prevalence of anemia among low income children in the US [14] which could be attributed to increased consumption of fortified ready-to-eat cereals [15]. In a survey in Canada it was observed that 96% of the children between 4 and 10 months received fortified cereals, which were the main source of iron in their diets [16].

Controlled trials in Chinese infants of 6–12 months of age revealed that feeding cereals fortified with iron resulted in a significant reduction in the prevalence of anemia [17]. Recent attention has been focused on the fortification of staple food with iron compounds which may have limited bioavailability and, hence, biological impact [18]. Plant foods high in protein (e.g., legumes) are often mixed with cereals in fortified complementary foods [19]. Both contain a large amount of phytic acid, a powerful inhibitor of trace element and mineral absorption. The influence of phytic acid on calcium, copper and magnesium absorption is of less concern than its effect on iron and zinc absorption [20]. Ascorbic acid is usually added in quantities that exceed the RDA to facilitate iron absorption in mixtures with high levels of phytate. Addition of ascorbic acid in iron-fortified chocolate flavored milk drink increased iron absorption in Jamaican children [21]. It has been observed in various studies that fortification of foods with iron does not have a negative effect on zinc absorption [22].

Given the severity of the problem, it is evident that the burden of micronutrient deficiency can be reduced through a holistic approach that includes promotion of healthy weaning practices, targeted micronutrient supplementation (e.g. high dose vitamin A supplementation every 6 months as recommended by WHO) and use of appropriate complementary foods along with improving the nutritional value of such foods [23].

Strategies to improve the availability of and accessibility to low cost complementary foods can play an important role in improving the nutritional status of infants and young children. It is possible to manage a large proportion of severely malnourished children at home using ready to use therapeutic foods or supplements or using a diet that combines home-based food with vitamin and mineral supplements.

Targeted Fortification Programs

Fortification of foods that are targeted to vulnerable and low-income groups needs high priority. There are several opportunities in developing countries which, if seized and applied, could make a vast difference to millions of people suffering from micronutrient deficiencies.

Fortified complementary foods provided through public feeding programs and commercially marketed foods have also had a good impact. In Ecuador, the Ministry of Public Health developed a complementary feeding program by targeting all eligible infants and young children between 6 and 24 months of age living in conditions of extreme poverty by providing coupons to redeem a micronutrient-fortified complementary food (Mi Papilla). At the final survey, the hemoglobin levels in children in the program group were significantly higher compared to children in the non-program group (27.6% prevalence of anemia in the program group versus 44.3% in the non-program group) [24]. In Mexico, the Progresa Program, a large incentive-based development program reaching children and pregnant and lactating women of 4.5 million families with fortified nutrition supplements was associated with better growth in height and hemoglobin values among the poorest and younger infants [25].

There is growing evidence for the impact of home-fortification of complementary foods using premixes in single-dose sachets containing micronutrients in a powder form that can be added to any homemade food for children at risk. These newer methods for addressing iron deficiency include micronutrient Sprinkles™, which were shown to be effective and efficacious in improving the hemoglobin status in anemic infants in several studies conducted in Ghana, Cambodia and many other countries with different levels of iron and various periods of time [26, 27].

The Government of Pakistan is planning to distribute Sprinkles™ through their ongoing Lady Health Worker Program, a large public sector primary health care program. In Bangladesh, BRAC, the largest national NGO in the country, is planning to distribute Sprinkles™ through their on-going Female Community Health Worker Program. In both these countries, Sprinkles™ would be produced locally through public-private partnerships, via a technology transfer agreement.

In India, several public programs such as the Integrated Child Development Services (ICDS), Mid Day Meal (MDM) and Targeted Public

Distribution System (TPDS) provide supplementary food to various age groups. Although ICDS has a life cycle approach reaching children 6 months to 6 years of age, as well as adolescent girls and pregnant and lactating mothers, they too often still only meet the macro level requirements of energy and protein and do not address micronutrient deficiencies sufficiently. However, recently with the efforts of the Government of India and several state governments and support from various international agencies, fortified supplementary foods are being distributed through these programs in states (fig. 2).

Distribution of fortified wheat flour through the TPDS to 0.6 million population living below the poverty line resulted in a significant reduction in the prevalence of anemia and vitamin A deficiency in the state of West Bengal.

The impact of fortified ready-to-eat food – a mix of wheat flour and chick pea flour distributed through ICDS in the state of Gujarat, reaching 0.35 million beneficiaries, revealed a significant reduction from 2 to 0.1% in the prevalence of night blindness amongst children in the intervention area.

In the state of West Bengal, *Khichdi* (rice, lentils and oil) is the supplementary food distributed through ICDS. A micronutrient premix popularized as *Vita ShaktiTM* consisting of vitamin A, iron and folic acid, which may be added to prepared *Khichdi* at the *Anganwadi* (village) center is also being used in ICDS. The feasibility and acceptability were proved by the high program compliance with both *Anganwadi* workers to implement and enroll children who consumed most of the *Khichdi* each time it was served to them. The study also demonstrated that fortified *Khichdi* was efficacious in improving iron status and reducing the prevalence of iron deficiency and iron deficiency anemia in children aged 3–6 years [28].

An indigenous multiple micronutrient dry powder sachet, meeting one full RDA per child under 2 years of age, has been developed and distributed in two Indian states. The operational feasibility and acceptability of this product tested on 70,000 children have shown high compliance by both mothers and children on parameters such as ease of administration, taste, compliance, etc., while distributing the products to the mothers who were trained in the usage of the sachets along with a single serving of the complementary food [unpublished data]. While the feasibility of distributing Sprinkles™ to over 15,000 children was also reported in Mongolia [29], high acceptability was reported in China because of the perceived benefits and ease of use [30].

Conclusion

The first 2 years of life is a critical window during which the optimal mental and physical development of the child needs to be enhanced. Adequate nutrition that combines energy density, proteins and adequate micronutrient levels is a critical component. This requires foods specially tailored and accessible either through commercial channels or through public programs. A number

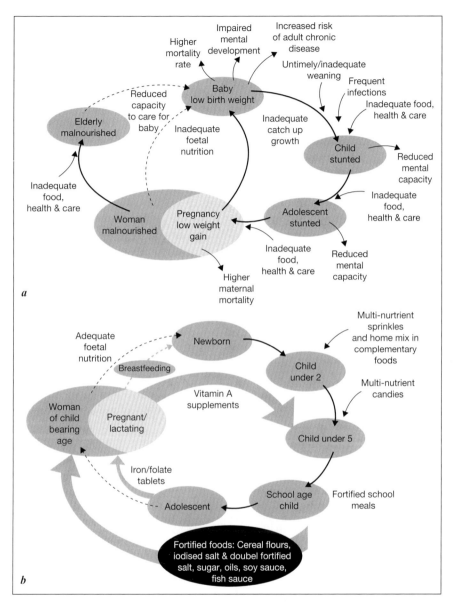

Fig. 2. a VMD risks at different stages of life. ***b*** Interventions tackling VMD at different ages. Source: United Nations Standing Committee on Nutrition.

of promising initiatives on cereal-based fortified foods have been proven effective and can be replicated and scaled-up. Given that most affected populations are extremely poor and that most governments have limited resources, cost limitations need to be borne in mind. Experiences from several countries have shown that affordable products can be produced and made accessible to the poorest segments of the population. However, much more work needs to be done to scale-up and sustain these efforts. Particularly in resource-poor settings, the sustainability of programs can be greatly enhanced through public-private-civil society partnerships. By improving the nutritional status of young infants we could make an enormous difference to the health and well-being of future generations around the world.

References

1 WHO, Administrative Committee on Coordination/Subcommittee on Nutrition: Forth Report on World Nutrition Situation. Geneva, WHO, 2000.
2 Underwood BA: Micronutrient malnutrition: is it being eliminated? Nutr Today 1998;33: 121–129.
3 Tomkins A: Malnutrition, morbidity and mortality in children and their mothers. Proc Nutr Soc 2000;59:135–146.
4 Cherian A, Seena S, Bullock RK, Antony AC: Incidence of neural tube defects in the least developed area of India: a population based study. Lancet 2005;366:930–931.
5 Bauernfeind JC, Arroyave G: Control of vitamin A deficiency by the nutrification of food approach; in Bauernfeind JC (ed): Vitamin A Deficiency and Its Control. Gainesville, Academic Press, 1986, pp 359–388.
6 Arroyave G, Mejia LA, Aguilar JR: The effect of vitamin A fortification of sugar on the serum vitamin A levels of preschool Guatemalan children: a longitudinal evaluation. Am J Clin Nutr 1981;34:41–49.
7 Arroyave G: Food fortification with emphasis on the addition of micronutrients to wheat flour. Arch Latinoam Nutr 1993;43:186–190.
8 Nestel P: Food Fortification in Developing Countries. Washington, US Agency for International Development, 1993.
9 Florentino SS, Rolf DW, Sanchez L, et al: Efficacy of a vitamin A-fortified wheat-flour bun on the vitamin A status of Filipino schoolchildren. Am J Clin Nutr 2000;72:738–744.
10 Canadian International Development Agency: A Report on 'Wheat Flour Fortification In Indonesia', Geneva, UNICEF, 2003.
11 Charatan F: Fortification of flour likely to halve neural tube defects, says CDC. BMJ 1999; 318:1506.
12 Gucciardi E, Pietrusiak M, Reynolds DL, Rouleau J: Incidence of neural tube defects in Ontario, 1986–1999. CMAJ 2002;167:237–240.
13 Walter T, Olivares M, Pizarro F, et al: Fortification; in Ramakrishnan U (ed): Nutritional Anemias. Boca Raton, CRC Press, 2001, pp 153–184.
14 Yip R, Binkin NJ, Fleshood L, Trowbridge FL: Declining prevalence of anemia among low-income children in the United States. JAMA 1987;258:1619–1623.
15 Whittaker P, Tufaro PR, Rader JI: Iron and folate in fortified cereals. J Am Coll Nutr 2001;20: 247–254.
16 Yeung DL, Pennell MD, Leung M, et al. Iron intake infants: the importance of infant cereals. Can Med Assoc J 1981;125:999–1002.
17 Li T, Wang WM, Yeung DL: Efficacy of iron-fortified infant cereals in the prevention of iron deficiency in infants in China. Nutr Rep Int 1998;37:695.
18 Lutter CK,Dewey KG: Nutrient composition for fortified complementary foods. J Nutr 2003;133:3011S–3020S.
19 Hurrell R: Influence of vegetable protein sources on trace element and mineral bioavailability. J Nutr 2003;133:2973S–2977S.
20 Dalton MA, Sargent JD, O'Connor GT, et al: Calcium and phosphorus supplementation of iron-fortified infant formula: no effect on iron status of healthy full-term infants. Am J Clin Nutr 1997;65:921–926.

21 Davidsson L, Walczyk T, Morris A, et al: Influence of ascorbic acid on iron absorption from an iron-fortified, chocolate-flavored milk drink in Jamaican children. Am J Clin Nutr 1998;67: 873–877.

22 Whittaker P: Iron and zinc interactions in humans. Am J Clin Nutr 1998;68:442S–446S.

23 United Nations System Standing Committee on Nutrition: 5th Report on the World Nutrition Situation: Nutrition for Improved Development Outcomes. New York, SCN, 2004, p 14.

24 Lutter C: Effectiveness of Ecuador's National Fortified Complementary Food Program for Children under 5 Years of Age (PANN 2000). Washington, Pan American Health Organization, 2004.

25 Torrejon CS, Castillo-Duran C, Hertrampf ED, Ruz M: Zinc and iron nutrition in Chilean children fed fortified milk provided by the Complementary National Food Program. Nutrition 2004;20:177–180.

26 Zlotkin S, Arthur P, Schauer C, et al: Home-fortification with iron and zinc sprinkles or iron sprinkles alone successfully treats anemia in infants and young children. J Nutr 2003;133: 1075–1080.

27 Giovannini M, Sala D, Usuelli M, et al: Double-blind, placebo-controlled trial comparing effects of supplementation with two different combinations of micronutrients delivered as sprinkles on growth, anemia, and iron deficiency in Cambodian infants. J Pediatr Gastroenterol Nutr 2006;42:306–312.

28 Varma JL, Das S, et al: Community-level micronutrient fortification of a food supplement in India: A controlled trial in preschool children aged 36–66 months. Am J Clin Nutr 2007;85:1127–1133.

29 Zlotkin SH, Schauer C, Christofides A, et al: Micronutrient sprinkles to control childhood anemia. PLoS Med 2005;2:24–28.

30 Yeung DL, Yap J, Cheng C: Consumer acceptance of a home food iron fortificant (abstract). International Nutritional Anemia Consultative Group Symposium, 2004. ILSI Research Foundation, 2004, p 18.

Discussion

Dr. Guno: We have moved from voluntary to mandatory fortifications. In the study by Florentino et al. [1] iron- and vitamin A-fortified wheat buns were given to school children and the efficacy trial showed that they were able to reduce the prevalence of iron deficiency anemia by as much as 92%. Our prevalence of iron deficiency anemia in infants is still at 66%. What do your long-term studies show? What happens to long-term outcomes such as school performance and productivity later in life?

Dr. Bulusu: As I showed in our study on wheat fortification in preschool children, at the end of 1 year of intervention we found that the decrease in the prevalence of anemia was up to 15–20% among the children, but we did not really look at cognitive development or school performance in these children. We do have qualitative results on these parameters collected through group discussions with the local community workers who are teachers in the Integrated Child Development Services (ICDS) as well as the Mid Day Meal (MDM) program, who say that the performance of these under-6-year-old children who come to the center (preschool education before they actually enter formal schools) has improved a lot, not only school performance in the sense of learning, but also their agility has improved. We just started the programs over the last 4–5 years and are still struggling with the form of iron compound to be used because often issues are raised about this.

Dr. Fisberg: In recent years we have seen that, in many developed countries, industries are privately fortifying various staple and industrial foods with iron. Many of these products, especially juices, yogurts and other products, are fortified with iron, usually 20–30% of the RDA. So if children eat all or the majority of these products, their iron levels might be above the upper limits. What do you believe would be the safety level for all these foods?

Dr. Bulusu: Until now in India, ever since Micronutrient Initiative (MI) started in 1998–1999, this question, which has been raised by several scientists in the country, has remained the same. Our target has mainly been through government programs, the MDM, the ICDS and the Targeted Public Distribution Scheme (TPDS) programs. Six to eight years ago there were no fortified products through government programs, except for the World Food Program which distributed their India Mix which was fortified with all the micronutrients at very high levels, 80% of the RDA. Today most of the multinational companies coming to India sell their fortified products over the shelf on the open market. I asked my president, who lives in Canada, to list the different fortified products consumed during the day in developed countries. Most of the people in developed countries cover the requirements of most of the micronutrients at breakfast itself. I do agree that there could be an issue of toxicity but in a developed country where people are consuming it and have been able to reduce most of the micronutrient deficiencies, I am sure that in a country like India, or any other developing country, it is safe and the only way to reach at least the poorest of the poor, who otherwise cannot afford fortified substances, through closely monitored government programs.

Dr. Brown: I don't know if this is something to worry about or not, but I would say that in the more affluent countries we have absolutely no control over the total nutrient intake from fortified products and I think this is something that we should be concerned about. Just one example, in the US 90% of infants are consuming more than the upper limit of zinc. In the same study where we looked at trends in zinc consumption over the 5 years for which we had CSFII dietary data, we found that just over those 5-year periods, from the mid to late 1990s, there was a significant increase in zinc intake among preschool children in the US, most of whom are already consuming above the upper limit [2]. When we brought that down by food source of zinc, there was absolutely no change in the zinc consumption from zinc endogenous or intrinsic to a food, but a significant year-by-year increase over that 5-year period in the amount of zinc consumed from fortified foods.

Dr. Bulusu: I would like to add one more point. In India we have a National Nutrition Monitoring Bureau that actually monitors the consumption profile of both the food intake as well as the nutrient intake. In most cases across the country it has been seen that the intake of micronutrients is less than 40–50% of the RDA [3]. So we still have another 40–50% if not 60% to be covered through micronutrient fortification of food.

Dr. Fisberg: I agree with you that in very developing countries it is important to have this kind of initiative. I really worry about some of the countries, especially those in the transitional phase, where we have to cope with the situation that 50% of small children have anemia, and at the same time the mothers are buying a lot of products from the supermarkets. We probably have to take some kind of control of it.

Dr. Solomons: The two stories that you began your talk with, one from Mexico and the other from Chile, are illustrative of two points. The point you made is related to their effectiveness to reduce micronutrient malnutrition. However, the authors from those nations today seem more concerned with a negative effect that both programs have had in provoking excess energy and macronutrient intakes along the way [4, 5]. The unintended consequence of both the Mexican and Chilean public health interventions was an increase in obesity rates in the children covered by the programs. India may or may not be in danger of that consequence. Your local sprinkles are basically calorie free and targeted to a very specific group. But, what I would add in the case of India is the unusual biological and epidemiological situation, the so-called 'Indian paradox', that is of the 'thin-fat' baby; this suggests that if you, Dr. Bulusu, also link your micronutrients to macronutrient-laden, sweet-tasting vehicles in government-sponsored programs, you may fall into the same problems the Chileans and Mexicans have experienced, with adverse consequences for metabolic health.

Dr. Bulusu: Thank you for that excellent point, but I would like to mention that in ICDS the supplementary nutrition components, whether anuka or nutri candy, are always provided along with the food. I would also like to add that though this program started way back in 1975 with the objective of providing 300 calories and 10 g of proteins, it still has not achieved its goal of controlling undernutrition, as is evident from the NFHS-II data. In most cases a substitution nutrition is used instead of supplementary nutrition, so the question of overfeeding may not arise in the near future.

Dr. Solomons: I would point out once again my concern for energy imbalance. India still has a vast number of rural poor with low access to dietary energy, but there is an increasing urbanization of the population. If your programs become general entitlements, without exquisite targeting to the neediest segments of the population, you run the risk of seeing the adverse outcomes and unintended consequences mentioned for Chile and Mexico [4, 5]. Chile and Mexico now openly admit it is the unintended consequence of an inspiration to do good; they did some good, they did some harm, but unfortunately they don't neutralize one each other; so they are rethinking the whole process to tailor to do good plus good.

Dr. Ibe: The costs of these programs, are they subsidized? Is there a move to make them attractive to industry so that they are marketed and made more accessible to the population?

Dr. Bulusu: The costs of the programs are not subsidized. The supplementary nutrition component was being given by the government, the micronutrient component was being supported by the MI to begin with. They are extremely cost-effective, for example 'Vita Shakti' costs just 3 Indian cents. As the cost is minuscule, today the government is bearing the cost in some states, which makes it sustainable.

Dr. Ibe: I am worried about the sustainability of the programs. If they are subsidized and paid by the government, is there any chance that at some point the government will refuse to pay, and then is it affordable?

Dr. Bulusu: There are 2 or 3 issues here. First of all 'fortification' was a forbidden word in India about 8 years back. Dr. Solomons was in India way back in 1999–2000, when we were having workshops on food fortification where questions about promoting multinational companies in the country were raised. To counteract this most of the products I am developing are within the country, that's one issue for sustainability. Secondly, there was no question of fortification for the poor, whereas that was the need. So these government programs, that are today bearing the cost of the supplementary nutrition component, have increased the budget several fold. Now the question is if they withdraw funding. First of all it won't happen because the government has just issued notification, after 9 years of struggle by the MI and World Food Program, that all food going to children in the country and pregnant and lactating mothers through the government-supported programs should be fortified with 9 micronutrients including iron, vitamin A, folic acid, vitamin C, iodine, the B complex group such as B_6, B_{12}, B_2, and others. We are also trying to target the open market which is going to take time due to the type of population in India where illiteracy is so high. For these people to come to a stage where they understand what are micronutrients, to take those micronutrients on a regular basis and to buy those fortified foods, the government needs to advocate micronutrient consumption. The government is presently promoting the concept of micronutrients in the country through government programs, but for the middle income and high income groups there is fortified flour on the market and today it is being bought by these groups. The poor income group is the beneficiary of these programs where it is supplied free of cost. But the time will come, perhaps in 10 or even 20 years, where, as in the richest countries such as the USA or Canada, every food is fortified and everybody has access to it.

Dr. Safavi: You have nicely shown the effect of supplementation, fortification and also education. My concern is that if we continue along one of these routes like supplementation or fortification or education alone, it won't be beneficial to the community. As long as fortification is being given, education should continue. I was also in India during the nutrition congress, and I have seen this gap between the communities in India as well as in other countries. The question is how can we solve this issue of fortifying all the products available, you mentioned chocolate and candies, to avoid problems such as toxicity that might rise during supplementation or the use of these products?

Dr. Bulusu: Part of the question on toxicity has already been answered. First of all, all three strategies need to work hand in hand until such time that we can alleviate the problem of micronutrient malnutrition. The second thing is the supplementation program, I don't know about Iran but in India it is very targeted. We have the biannual vitamin A supplementation program, but that is only for children from 9 to 36 months and today the government of India is planning to take it to 59 months. Pregnant and lactating mothers are supplemented with 100 tablets of iron and folic acid in the third trimester of pregnancy. In view of the increasing evidence of neural tube defect and spina bifida cases, with support from UNICEF and MI the government is presently supplementing particularly adolescent girls with iron and folic acid in some states because it has been realized that damage has already been done by the time an adolescent girl gets married and is supplemented in the third trimester of pregnancy. The other issue is that of compliance which today is only about 34% after 35 years of this program being in place, so it doesn't happen. I think it should take a minimum of another 25–30 years, if not more, in a country like India by the time fortification really gets to the stage that it becomes toxic. With dietary diversification over the last 50 years, we have not been able to eradicate even one single deficiency disorder in the country. I am not saying that we don't need to be careful because there is no toxicity, there could be toxicity. There was one incident in 2001 in the state of Assam where 23 children died during the biannual vitamin A campaign. Later a committee which investigated the whole issue said that it was not because of vitamin A per se but because of a change in the modus operandi of giving the vitamin A. So that was one case over the last 15–18 years in the country. I can at least talk about India, and of course we have offices in Nepal, Bangladesh, Pakistan, Sri Lanka and Indonesia, and to my knowledge also in these countries there has not been any case of hypertoxicity.

Dr. Agostoni: Maybe I have missed something; 23 children died, for what reason?

Dr. Bulusu: This was in 2001 during the biannual vitamin A supplementation campaign, and everybody wanted a push because coverage was so low. In the state of Assam, 23 children died, but it was basically due to the negligence of the local health workers in one particular area of the state where the spoon which was used to administer vitamin A was changed to a small container which was actually marked 500,000 and 200,000. Without proper training the local health worker was probably giving 500,000. But the doctors also said that it may not have been exclusively due to vitamin A alone, it could also have been because those children may also have had some other unknown physiological problems which may have been triggered off by the administration of 500,000 international units of vitamin A.

Dr. Agostoni: I am a little worried, 500,000 units of vitamin A could be the cause of these deaths?

Dr. Solomons: Calculating that given the under-5 mortality rate in the state of Assam the number of children who are eligible to be pulsed in that campaign would be 63 deaths of children on any given day of the year. Now how do you figure out which 23 of them died due to exposure to excess vitamin A? You could similarly argue that

Assam mothers kissed their children on any given day and 63 died. Hence, kissing children is hazardous.

Since Dr. Brown and I visited your country in 2000, the situation continues to evolve. It must be obvious that, through 59 years of Indian independence, the inability to eradicate even a single micronutrient deficiency means that the traditional dietary practices are ideal. The fact that Indian professional opinion now accepts a contribution of micronutrient fortification as a beneficial and necessary policy perhaps indicates some backing off from the former insistence that a strict vegetarian fare can provide all essential nutrients. There is a dialectic conflict. I think the concept of fortification in micronutrients has won in the ensuing debate over these 6 years, and that Dr. Bulusu and her persistence are a partial factor in that advance in the dialectical resolution.

Dr. Bulusu: Since then the government has changed the campaign mode and administration is not on a single day. Every state has been requested to conduct the vitamin A supplementation program over a period of time, e.g. a month, so in different districts supplementation is taken on different days, so that the local people and health workers are more vigilant on that issue.

References

1   Florentino SS, Rolf DW, Sanchez L, et al: Efficacy of a vitamin A-fortified wheat-flour bun on the vitamin A status of Filipino schoolchildren. Am J Clin Nutr 2000;72:738–744.
2   Arsenault JE, Brown KH: Zinc intake of US preschool children exceeds new dietary reference intakes. Am J Clin Nutr 2003;78:1011–1017.
3   NNMB Report 2003–04.
4   Rivera JA, Sotres-Alvarez D, Habicht JP, et al: Impact of the Mexican program for education, health, and nutrition (Progresa) on rates of growth and anemia in infants and young children: a randomized effectiveness study. JAMA 2004;291:2563–2570.
5   Torrejon CS, Castillo-Duran C, Hertrampf ED, Ruz M: Zinc and iron nutrition in Chilean children fed fortified milk provided by the Complementary National Food Program. Nutrition 2004;20:177–180.

Agostoni C, Brunser O (eds): Issues in Complementary Feeding.
Nestlé Nutr Workshop Ser Pediatr Program, vol 60, pp 107–121,
Nestec Ltd., Vevey/S. Karger AG, Basel, © 2007.

Processed Infant Cereals as Vehicles of Functional Components

Magnus Domellöf, Christina West

Department of Clinical Sciences, Pediatrics, Umeå University, Umeå, Sweden

Abstract

Cereals are the most common complementary foods all over the world and there is now a novel possibility to add functional components to target health problems that are not caused by a simple nutritional deficiency. So far there have been very few published trials on the addition of functional components to infant cereals. A single trial has suggested that infant cereals containing a combination of probiotics, prebiotics and zinc are an effective adjunct to oral rehydration solution in the treatment of acute gastroenteritis. Up to now there has been no evidence that infant cereals supplemented with probiotics or prebiotics have a preventive effect on diarrhea but a recent study has suggested that a milk fat globule membrane (MFGM) protein fraction added to an infant cereal reduces the risk of diarrhea in a developing country. There are some promising results suggesting that infant cereals supplemented with probiotics or prebiotics may prevent atopic eczema. The addition of prebiotic oligosaccharides to infant cereals may lead to softer stools, likely to benefit those infants who are suffering from constipation. More studies are needed to verify these results and to assess the effects of other functional components – especially probiotics, prebiotics, nucleotides, novel protein fractions and recombinant human milk proteins – added to infant cereals.

Copyright © 2007 Nestec Ltd., Vevey/S. Karger AG, Basel

Introduction

Exclusive breastfeeding ensures optimal nutrition for healthy infants during the first 6 months of life. Thereafter, the feeding of nutrient-dense complementary foods, along with continued breastfeeding, is critical to ensure optimal health, growth and development of infants and young children. The complementary feeding period (6–24 months of age) is therefore an especially important target for nutritional interventions.

Cereals are the most common complementary foods all over the world. Both traditional and industrially produced infant cereals are based on common grains such as rice, maize, wheat, oat or sorghum and are often combined with milk or legumes such as soy.

Traditional home-made or locally produced cereals in developing countries are often poorly adapted to the nutritional needs of infants, leading to malnutrition [1]. The fortification of infant cereals with micronutrients (iron, zinc, vitamin A, etc.) has been shown to be an effective tool to prevent basic nutritional deficiencies [2, 3]. However, there is now a novel possibility to add functional components in order to target important public health problems that are not caused by a simple nutritional deficiency. Examples of such health problems are infectious diarrhea in developing countries and allergies in industrialized countries.

Functional components of foods are usually defined as those having additional health effects beyond basic nutrition. In a European consensus document, a food product or component was regarded as functional if it was demonstrated to beneficially affect one or more target functions in the body, beyond adequate nutritional effects, in a way that is relevant to either improved health and/or reduction of risk of disease [4].

Functional components in infant food products include long chain polyunsaturated fatty acids (LCPUFAs), probiotics, prebiotics, nucleotides, protein fractions, amino acids, structured triglycerides, polyamines, recombinant proteins, hormones and growth factors. Several of these functional components are presently added to commercially available infant food products even though their health benefits are not clearly proven [5].

Most of the functional components added to infant foods are originally bioactive components of breast milk since the feeding of human milk has been shown to promote many health benefits, e.g. more favorable development of the brain, gut and immune system, less risk of infectious diseases, diabetes or cancer [6–8]. It is thus logical that most of these functional components have been tested primarily as supplements to infant formula and very few trials have so far been performed of functional components added to processed infant cereals (table 1).

Probiotics and Prebiotics

During the postnatal period, breastfed but not formula-fed infants establish an intestinal flora rich in lactic acid bacteria, e.g. bifidobacteria and lactobacilli [9]. Possible mechanisms for the protective effect of breast milk against infections include growth inhibition of pathogenic microorganisms through the production of lactic, acetic and other organic acids, with a consequent decrease of intraluminal pH that inhibits the growth of some bacterial pathogens. In contrast, formula feeding tends to favor a flora associated with

Table 1. Randomized, controlled trials of functional components in infant cereals

Author	Year	Component(s)	Main result
Moore et al. [40]	2003	FOS	Softer, more frequent stools
Duggan et al. [27]	2003	FOS	No prevention of diarrhea
Shamir et al. [22]	2005	*S. thermophilus, B. lactis, L. acidophilus,* FOS, zinc	Shorter duration of acute gastroenteritis (treatment)
Moro et al. [32]	2006	GOS, FOS	Prevention of atopic eczema
Zavaleta et al. [55]	2006	MFGM protein fraction	Prevention of diarrhea
West et al. (unpubl. study, 2007)	2006	LF19	Prevention of atopic eczema; no prevention of diarrhea

a near-neutral pH of the feces [10]. Furthermore, bifidobacteria and lacto-bacilli compete with potentially pathogenic bacteria for nutrients and epithelial adhesion sites. The gut microbiota also modulates the recovery of substrates through fermentation of nondigestible carbohydrates and nitrogen salvage, and affects mucosal growth and the absorption of water and nutrients [11]. Accumulating evidence also indicates that the gut flora modulates mucosal physiology, barrier function and systemic immunologic and inflammatory responses [12]. The realization that the intestinal flora modifies the function of the gut immune system has led to the concept of probiotic and prebiotic therapy as possible means to reduce the risk of infections and allergies [13]. Probiotics are live organisms which when administered in adequate amounts confer a health benefit on the host [14]. Prebiotics are non-digestible food ingredients that beneficially affect the host by selectively stimulating the growth and/or activity of a limited number of bacteria in the colon that have the potential to improve the host's health [15]. Commercially available prebiotics are galacto-oligosaccharides (GOS), fructo-oligosaccharides (FOS) and inulin-type fructans [16].

Treatment of Acute Gastroenteritis

Diarrheal diseases are a leading cause of mortality in infants and children worldwide, and continue to be a significant cause of morbidity in industrialized countries [17]. In recent years, the major advance in the treatment of acute gastroenteritis in children was the introduction of oral rehydration solution (ORS) in the early stages of illness [18]. In addition, rice-based ORS is superior to ORS alone in reducing the frequency and stool volume in acute gastroenteritis [19]. However, nutritional interventions during the diarrheal illness are usually not helpful in reducing the duration of diarrhea, and current recommendations suggest that the normal diet is continued during mild diarrhea [20].

Studies have clearly shown that probiotics is a useful adjunct to rehydration therapy in treating acute, infectious diarrhea in adults and children and this has also been supported by a Cochrane meta-analysis showing that the duration of diarrhea is shortened by about 1 day and that patients receiving probiotics had fewer stools on treatment day 2–3 [21].

There is one published randomized controlled trial (RCT) on the effects of probiotics and prebiotics in infant cereals in the treatment of acute gastroenteritis: Shamir et al. [22] randomized 65 infants at 6–12 months of age, suffering from acute gastroenteritis and mild to moderate dehydration, to receive either a lactose free soy protein-based rice cereal or the same cereal with added probiotics, prebiotics and zinc. The study was carried out in an ambulatory setting. The infants were first prescribed an ORS solution according to previously established guidelines. Thereafter, parents from both groups were instructed to feed 600 ml of cereals with or without supplements: *Streptococcus thermophilus, Bifidobacterium lactis* and *Lactobacillus acidophilus* (2×10^9 colony forming units each), FOS (0.3 g) and zinc (10 mg). The mean duration of diarrhea was 15 h shorter in the supplemented group compared to the control group (1.34 ± 0.71 vs. 1.97 ± 1.24 days, p = 0.017). There was no difference in time to resolution of fever or vomiting. On day 3, there was only one infant with watery stools in the supplemented group compared to 10 infants in the control group (p = 0.02). Unfortunately, due to the combined supplementation, it is not possible to know if this effect was due to the added probiotics, prebiotics or zinc. Zinc supplementation by itself has been shown in several trials to substantially reduce the duration and severity of symptoms in acute gastroenteritis [23].

Prevention of Diarrhea

Several RCTs have suggested that the addition of probiotics to infant formula may reduce the severity of diarrhea episodes. Recently, Weizman et al. [24] showed that a formula with *B. lactis* and a formula with *Lactobacillus reuteri* resulted in fewer and shorter episodes of diarrhea compared to standard formula. Thibault et al. [25] showed in a large trial (n = 971) that formula fermented with *Bifidobacterium breve* and *S. thermophilus* resulted in fewer cases of dehydration and fewer medical consultations but no difference in the incidence or duration of diarrhea episodes.

There are no published trials on the effect of infant cereals supplemented with probiotics on the prevention of diarrhea. However, preliminary results are available from an RCT by our group [West et al., unpubl. study] in which 179 mostly breastfed infants were assigned to cereals (rice and wheat porridge with milk proteins) with or without *Lactobacillus paracasei* strain F19 (LF19). The recommended intake was at least one serving of cereals daily from 4 to 13 months of age. In the LF19 group, one serving contained 1×10^8 colony forming units. Compliance was good in both groups: mean intake was 0.85 ($\pm$0.45) servings per day. There was no difference in the number of days with fever, respiratory illness or diarrhea between the groups. Infants in the LF19 group had fewer days with antibiotic prescriptions compared to placebo (1.6 vs. 2.2 days, p = 0.044).

The lack of effect on diarrhea morbidity cannot be explained by a low incidence or duration of gastroenteritis in the study of West et al. since the average number of days with diarrhea was 0.3 days/month compared to 0.2 days/month in the control group in the study of Weizman et al. The negative results of West et al. with regard to diarrhea support those of Thibault et al. (see above). However, in the study of Thibault et al., a more liberal definition of diarrhea was used resulting in a higher number of days with diarrhea (1.0 days/month). An alternative explanation for the lack of effect on diarrhea morbidity in the study of West et al. is that the preventive effect of probiotics on diarrhea is less pronounced in breastfed infants, as suggested by Oberhelman et al. [26] who found a decrease in the incidence of diarrhea in Peruvian 18- to 29-month-olds receiving a *Lactobacillus rhamnosus* GG supplement, an effect which was largely restricted to those toddlers who were not breastfed.

There is one published trial of prebiotic supplemented infant cereals assessing effects on diarrhea: Duggan et al. [27] randomized 282 breastfed Peruvian infants between the ages of 6 and 12 months to receive infant cereals (either rice- or oat-based at the choice of the family) with or without FOS supplementation (0.55/15 g serving) during 6 months. An identical study was performed in 349 infants with zinc added to both infant cereals. In both studies, FOS supplementation of formula was not associated with any difference in diarrhea prevalence or use of health care resources.

Prevention of Atopic Eczema

In a randomized study by Kalliomäki et al. [28, 29] in families at risk of allergy, capsules of *L. rhamnosus* GG given perinatally to mothers and infants resulted in a reduction in the prevalence of atopic eczema at 24 months of age (from 46 to 23%) without any effect on IgE concentrations at 24 months or skin prick tests at 4 years of age. Some studies have also suggested that probiotics may have a beneficial treatment effect on atopic eczema in children [30, 31].

There is only one published RCT on infant formula or cereals supplemented with probiotics or prebiotics, assessing the effect on atopic eczema: Moro et al. [32] randomized 259 term infants with a family history of atopy to infant formula with or without a mixture of 90% GOS and 10% FOS at a concentration of 8 g/l. A reduction was observed in the incidence of atopic

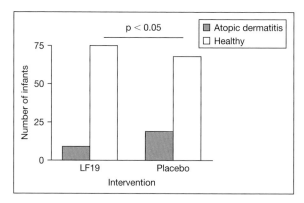

Fig. 1. Cumulative incidence of atopic eczema at 13 months.

eczema up to 6 months of age from 23% in the control group to 10% in the prebiotic group (p = 0.014). IgE or other measures of allergy were not presented in that study.

Preliminary data from the study by West et al. suggest that the incidence of atopic eczema up to 13 months of age was 50% lower in the LF19-supplemented group compared to controls (11 vs. 22%, fig. 1), suggesting that probiotics in infant cereals have a preventive effect against this disease [West, unpubl. study]. However, there was no difference in IgE concentrations.

The study by West et al. confirms the results of two previously published trials showing a preventive effect of prebiotics/probiotics on atopic eczema. Both the studies of West et al. and Kalliomäki et al. suggest that the preventive effect of prebiotics/probiotics on atopic eczema is mediated by an IgE-independent mechanism. Since atopic eczema has been associated with disruption of the intestinal mucosal barrier, one possible mechanism of probiotics is a reduction in intestinal permeability and thereby a reduction of antigen transfer across the intestinal mucosa [33].

Effect on Stool Consistency

Seven RCTs of prebiotic supplements to infant formulas have been published [32, 34–39]. All except one was performed in term infants. Five of the studies used a mixture of 90% GOS and 10% FOS at a concentration of 4–10 g/l. Two of the studies used FOS at a concentration of 1.5–3 g/l. Most of these studies showed that added oligosaccharides resulted in increased stool frequency and a softer stool consistency.

There is one published trial of prebiotic supplemented infant cereals assessing effects on stool quality: Moore et al. [40] randomized 56 infants to receive either a rice-based cereal with milk protein supplemented with FOS or the equivalent amount of maltodextrin (placebo) from 4 to 12 months of age.

Infants receiving FOS had significantly more stools per day (1.99 ± 0.62 vs. 1.58 ± 0.66, $p = 0.02$). For infants receiving FOS, stool consistency was less likely to be described as 'hard' and more likely to be described as 'soft' or 'loose'.

Other Effects of Probiotics and Prebiotics

Formulas and cereals supplemented with probiotics and prebiotics are generally well accepted and result in the same growth as standard formula. An increase in fecal bifidobacteria has been shown in several studies of oligosaccharide supplements to formula [34, 35, 37, 38], supporting their prebiotic effect. Except for effects on diarrhea and stool quality (see above), most studies show no effect on other gastrointestinal symptoms, e.g. regurgitation, vomiting, colics, etc.

Immunological effects of probiotics and prebiotics added to infant formulas or cereals (e.g. effects on immunoglobulin responses to childhood immunizations) have been suggested in some [West, unpubl. study; 41] but not all trials [27].

Other and Novel Functional Components

LCPUFAs are fundamental for central nervous system growth and development. Several studies have shown that LCPUFA supplementation of infant formula may lead to short-term effects on psychomotor development and visual acuity, but recent Cochrane meta-analyses of trials in preterm and term infants have concluded that there is still no evidence for long-term benefits [42, 43]. Since LCPUFA supplementation theoretically would have a better effect the earlier it is given during the first year of life [44], it has not primarily been considered for supplementation to infant cereals and there are no published studies of LCPUFA-supplemented infant cereals.

Compared to cow's milk, human milk has higher concentrations of nucleotides. Several RCTs of infant formulas supplemented with nucleotides have suggested beneficial effects on infant immune response but so far there is no evidence of a dose response or a consistency in the specificity of the response [45–49]. So far there have been no published trials of infant cereals supplemented with nucleotides.

Human recombinant lactoferrin and lysozyme have recently been expressed in rice [50, 51] and may have a protective effect against enteral infections [52], but as of yet, there are no clinical studies on these recombinant proteins added to infant formula, infant cereals or cereal-based ORS solutions.

However, novel protein components can also be found in bovine milk. A bovine milk protein fraction containing enriched milk fat globule membranes (MFGM) has recently become available. This fraction contains 120 proteins and other components, including several with possible antiviral and antibacterial activity (e.g. butyrophilin, MUC1, lactadherin, lactoferrin, sphingomyelin, gangliosides and sialic acid) as well as micronutrient binding proteins (e.g. lactoferrin, folic acid binding protein) [53]. Lönnerdal et al. [54] and Zavaleta et al. [55] recently presented results from an RCT, in which 6- to 11-month-old infants (n = 550) in periurban Lima, Peru, were fed a micronutrient-fortified, cereal- and milk-based meal (40 g/day) with (a) MFGM or (b) skim milk proteins twice daily for 6 months. The incidence of diarrhea was lower in the MFGM group (5.8 episodes/child/year vs. 6.3 in the control group; p < 0.05). S-Cu and vitamin B_{12} were significantly higher in the MFGM group than in the skim milk group but there was no difference in anemia prevalence, hemoglobin, serum ferritin, serum Zn, serum folate or growth between groups.

Effect Modifiers

It is not always possible to extrapolate the results from trials of bioactive components given as a separate supplement (e.g. drops, capsules) to the same bioactive component added to infant cereals. As an example, we have shown that iron given as a separate supplement has different effects on hemoglobin and serum ferritin compared to the same dose of iron given as iron-fortified foods [56]. Similarly, it is not recommended to extrapolate the results from trials of a functional component in infant formula to the same functional component added to infant cereals. Infants receiving infant cereals are commonly also breastfed, in contrast to formula-fed infants who are usually not breastfed, and the functional components may have different effects depending on whether the infant is breastfed or not [26]. It is also important to consider which liquid is used to reconstitute infant cereals. In the Peruvian study by Duggan et al. [27], the infant cereal powder was mixed with milk, breast milk or water. It is likely that these liquids will influence the effect of the functional components differently. Furthermore, it is important not to generalize effects of probiotics and prebiotics since different strains of bacteria in different doses as well as different combinations of oligosaccharides in different doses may have different clinical effects [10, 57]. Even though most tested functional components are well tolerated, safety aspects and long-term outcomes should be included in all clinical trials.

Conclusion

Even though several randomized trials have been published on the addition of functional components to infant formulas, there are very few published trials on the addition of functional components to infant cereals (table 1).

Probiotics have been shown to be an effective adjunct to ORS therapy in the treatment of acute gastroenteritis and a single trial has suggested that this is also true for infant cereals containing a combination of probiotics, prebiotics and zinc. As of yet there is no evidence that infant cereals supplemented with probiotics or prebiotics have a preventive effect on diarrhea but a recent study has suggested that an MFGM protein fraction added to an infant cereal reduces the risk of diarrhea in a developing country. There are some promising results suggesting that infant cereals supplemented with probiotics or prebiotics may reduce the incidence of atopic eczema. It is also possible that the addition of prebiotic oligosaccharides to infant cereals increases stool frequency and leads to a softer stool consistency, likely to benefit those infants who are suffering from constipation.

Since the number of studies is very small, all of the above results need to be verified in further studies. The promising initial results showing clinical effects of infant cereals with added functional components on treatment and prevention of acute gastroenteritis and prevention of atopic eczema are especially interesting. More studies are needed to assess the effects of functional components – especially probiotics, prebiotics, nucleotides, novel protein fractions and recombinant human milk proteins – added to infant cereals and cereal-based ORS solutions.

References

1 Lutter CK, Rivera JA: Nutritional status of infants and young children and characteristics of their diets. J Nutr 2003;133:2941S–2949S.
2 Lartey A, Manu A, Brown KH, et al: A randomized, community-based trial of the effects of improved, centrally processed complementary foods on growth and micronutrient status of Ghanaian infants from 6 to 12 mo of age. Am J Clin Nutr 1999;70:391–404.
3 Faber M, Kvalsvig JD, Lombard CJ, et al: Effect of a fortified maize-meal porridge on anemia, micronutrient status, and motor development of infants. Am J Clin Nutr 2005;82:1032–1039.
4 Diplock AT, Aggett PJ, Ashwell M, et al: Scientific concepts of functional foods in Europe. Consensus document. Br J Nutr 1999;81(suppl 1):S1–S27.
5 Agostoni C, Domellof M: Infant formulae: from ESPGAN recommendations towards ESPGHAN-coordinated global standards. J Pediatr Gastroenterol Nutr 2005;41:580–583.
6 Lucas A, Morley R, Isaacs E: Nutrition and mental development. Nutr Rev 2001;59:S24–S33.
7 Walker WA: The dynamic effects of breastfeeding on intestinal development and host defense. Adv Exp Med Biol 2004;554:155–170.
8 Schack-Nielsen L, Larnkjaer A, Michaelsen KF: Long term effects of breastfeeding on the infant and mother. Adv Exp Med Biol 2005;569:16–23.
9 Fanaro S, Chierici R, Guerrini P, et al: Intestinal microflora in early infancy: composition and development. Acta Paediatr Suppl 2003;91:48–55.
10 Agostoni C, Axelsson I, Goulet O, et al: Prebiotic oligosaccharides in dietetic products for infants: a commentary by the ESPGHAN Committee on Nutrition. J Pediatr Gastroenterol Nutr 2004;39:465–473.
11 Kelleher SL, Casas I, Carbajal N, et al: Supplementation of infant formula with the probiotic Lactobacillus reuteri and zinc: impact on enteric infection and nutrition in infant rhesus monkeys. J Pediatr Gastroenterol Nutr 2002;35:162–168.
12 Sudo N, Sawamura S, Tanaka K, et al: The requirement of intestinal bacterial flora for the development of an IgE production system fully susceptible to oral tolerance induction. J Immunol 1997;159:1739–1745.
13 Isolauri E, Sutas Y, Kankaanpaa P, et al: Probiotics: effects on immunity. Am J Clin Nutr 2001;73:444S–450S.

14 Joint FAO/WHO expert consultation: Health and nutritional properties of probiotics in food including powder milk with live lactic acid bacteria, Cordoba, 2001.

15 Roberfroid MB: Prebiotics: preferential substrates for specific germs? Am J Clin Nutr 2001;73:406S–409S.

16 Veereman-Wauters G: Application of prebiotics in infant foods. Br J Nutr 2005;93(suppl 1): S57–S60.

17 Cheng AC, McDonald JR, Thielman NM: Infectious diarrhea in developed and developing countries. J Clin Gastroenterol 2005;39:757–773.

18 Walker-Smith JA, Sandhu BK, Isolauri E, et al: Guidelines prepared by the ESPGAN Working Group on Acute Diarrhoea. Recommendations for feeding in childhood gastroenteritis. European Society of Pediatric Gastroenterology and Nutrition. J Pediatr Gastroenterol Nutr 1997;24:619–620.

19 Wall CR, Swanson CE, Cleghorn GJ: A controlled trial comparing the efficacy of rice-based and hypotonic glucose oral rehydration solutions in infants and young children with gastroenteritis. J Gastroenterol Hepatol 1997;12:24–28.

20 Practice parameter: the management of acute gastroenteritis in young children. American Academy of Pediatrics, Provisional Committee on Quality Improvement, Subcommittee on Acute Gastroenteritis. Pediatrics 1996;97:424–435.

21 Allen SJ, Okoko B, Martinez E, et al: Probiotics for treating infectious diarrhoea. Cochrane Database Syst Rev 2004;2:CD003048.

22 Shamir R, Makhoul IR, Etzioni A, et al: Evaluation of a diet containing probiotics and zinc for the treatment of mild diarrheal illness in children younger than one year of age. J Am Coll Nutr 2005;24:370–375.

23 Strand TA, Chandyo RK, Bahl R, et al: Effectiveness and efficacy of zinc for the treatment of acute diarrhea in young children. Pediatrics 2002;109:898–903.

24 Weizman Z, Asli G, Alsheikh A: Effect of a probiotic infant formula on infections in child care centers: comparison of two probiotic agents. Pediatrics 2005;115:5–9.

25 Thibault H, Aubert-Jacquin C, Goulet O: Effects of long-term consumption of a fermented infant formula (with *Bifidobacterium breve* c50 and *Streptococcus thermophilus* 065) on acute diarrhea in healthy infants. J Pediatr Gastroenterol Nutr 2004;39:147–152.

26 Oberhelman RA, Gilman RH, Sheen P, et al: A placebo-controlled trial of *Lactobacillus* GG to prevent diarrhea in undernourished Peruvian children. J Pediatr 1999;134:15–20.

27 Duggan C, Penny ME, Hibberd P, et al: Oligofructose-supplemented infant cereal: 2 randomized, blinded, community-based trials in Peruvian infants. Am J Clin Nutr 2003;77:937–942.

28 Kalliomaki M, Salminen S, Arvilommi H, et al: Probiotics in primary prevention of atopic disease: a randomised placebo-controlled trial. Lancet 2001;357:1076–1079.

29 Kalliomaki M, Salminen S, Poussa T, et al: Probiotics and prevention of atopic disease: 4-year follow-up of a randomised placebo-controlled trial. Lancet 2003;361:1869–1871.

30 Weston S, Halbert A, Richmond P, et al: Effects of probiotics on atopic dermatitis: a randomised controlled trial. Arch Dis Child 2005;90:892–897.

31 Rosenfeldt V, Benfeldt E, Nielsen SD, et al: Effect of probiotic *Lactobacillus* strains in children with atopic dermatitis. J Allergy Clin Immunol 2003;111:389–395.

32 Moro G, Arslanoglu S, Stahl B, et al: A mixture of prebiotic oligosaccharides reduces the incidence of atopic dermatitis during the first six months of age. Arch Dis Child 2006;91:814–819.

33 Rosenfeldt V, Benfeldt E, Valerius NH, et al: Effect of probiotics on gastrointestinal symptoms and small intestinal permeability in children with atopic dermatitis. J Pediatr 2004;145:612–616.

34 Boehm G, Lidestri M, Casetta P, et al: Supplementation of a bovine milk formula with an oligosaccharide mixture increases counts of faecal bifidobacteria in preterm infants. Arch Dis Child Fetal Neonatal Ed 2002;86:F178–F181.

35 Moro G, Minoli I, Mosca M, et al: Dosage-related bifidogenic effects of galacto- and fructooligosaccharides in formula-fed term infants. J Pediatr Gastroenterol Nutr 2002;34:291–295.

36 Schmelzle H, Wirth S, Skopnik H, et al: Randomized double-blind study of the nutritional efficacy and bifidogenicity of a new infant formula containing partially hydrolyzed protein, a high beta-palmitic acid level, and nondigestible oligosaccharides. J Pediatr Gastroenterol Nutr 2003;36:343–351.

37 Fanaro S, Jelinek J, Stahl B, et al: Acidic oligosaccharides from pectin hydrolysate as new component for infant formulae: effect on intestinal flora, stool characteristics, and pH. J Pediatr Gastroenterol Nutr 2005;41:186–190.

38 Euler AR, Mitchell DK, Kline R, et al: Prebiotic effect of fructo-oligosaccharide supplemented term infant formula at two concentrations compared with unsupplemented formula and human milk. J Pediatr Gastroenterol Nutr 2005;40:157–164.
39 Bettler J, Euler AR: An evaluation of the growth of term infants fed formula supplemented with fructo-oligosaccharide. Int J Probiotics Prebiotics 2006;1:19–26.
40 Moore N, Chao C, Yang LP, et al: Effects of fructo-oligosaccharide-supplemented infant cereal: a double-blind, randomized trial. Br J Nutr 2003;90:581–587.
41 Saavedra JM, Tschernia A: Human studies with probiotics and prebiotics: clinical implications. Br J Nutr 2002;87(suppl 2):S241–S246.
42 Simmer K, Patole S: Longchain polyunsaturated fatty acid supplementation in preterm infants. Cochrane Database Syst Rev 2004;1:CD000375.
43 Simmer K: Longchain polyunsaturated fatty acid supplementation in infants born at term. Cochrane Database Syst Rev 2001;4:CD000376.
44 Cheatham CL, Colombo J, Carlson SE: N-3 fatty acids and cognitive and visual acuity development: methodologic and conceptual considerations. Am J Clin Nutr 2006;83:1458S–1466S.
45 Pickering LK, Granoff DM, Erickson JR, et al: Modulation of the immune system by human milk and infant formula containing nucleotides. Pediatrics 1998;101:242–249.
46 Hawkes JS, Gibson RA, Roberton D, et al: Effect of dietary nucleotide supplementation on growth and immune function in term infants: a randomized controlled trial. Eur J Clin Nutr 2006;60:254–264.
47 Buck RH, Thomas DL, Winship TR, et al: Effect of dietary ribonucleotides on infant immune status. 2. Immune cell development. Pediatr Res 2004;56:891–900.
48 Yau KI, Huang CB, Chen W, et al: Effect of nucleotides on diarrhea and immune responses in healthy term infants in Taiwan. J Pediatr Gastroenterol Nutr 2003;36:37–43.
49 Ostrom KM, Cordle CT, Schaller JP, et al: Immune status of infants fed soy-based formulas with or without added nucleotides for 1 year. Part 1. Vaccine responses, and morbidity. J Pediatr Gastroenterol Nutr 2002;34:137–144.
50 Suzuki YA, Kelleher SL, Yalda D, et al: Expression, characterization, and biologic activity of recombinant human lactoferrin in rice. J Pediatr Gastroenterol Nutr 2003;36:190–199.
51 Huang J, Wu L, Yalda D, et al: Expression of functional recombinant human lysozyme in transgenic rice cell culture. Transgenic Res 2002;11:229–239.
52 Bethell DR, Huang J: Recombinant human lactoferrin treatment for global health issues: iron deficiency and acute diarrhea. Biometals 2004;17:337–342.
53 Reinhardt TA, Lippolis JD: Bovine milk fat globule membrane proteome. J Dairy Res 2006;73: 406–416.
54 Lönnerdal B, Valencia N, Graverholt G, et al: Effect of fortifying complementary food with a bioactive milk protein fraction with micronutrients on growth and micronutrient status of Peruvian infants (abstract). J Pediatr Gastroenterol Nutr 2006;42:E88.
55 Zavaleta N, Valencia N, Graverholt G, et al: Incidence and duration of diarrhea in Peruvian infants consuming complementary food with bioactive milk fat globule membrane proteins (abstract). J Pediatr Gastroenterol Nutr 2006;42:E39.
56 Domellöf M, Lind T, Lönnerdal B, et al: Effects of the mode of oral iron administration on serum ferritin and hemoglobin in infants. Am J Clin Nutr, submitted.
57 Agostoni C, Axelsson I, Braegger C, et al: Probiotic bacteria in dietetic products for infants: a commentary by the ESPGHAN Committee on Nutrition. J Pediatr Gastroenterol Nutr 2004;38: 365–374.

Discussion

Dr. Pazvakavambwa: Would the etiology of the diarrhea, viral diarrhea versus non-viral, make a difference? When these probiotics are added to the cereal, is it after cooking, is the cereal warm, heated, or at what stage is it added?

Dr. Domellöf: In a recent meta-analysis, there was a significant effect on viral gastroenteritis [1]. Regarding the second question, most of these cereals are manufactured with probiotics already added. Since they are living organisms, the product should not be heated to more than serving temperature in the home.

Dr. Simell: Why have none of the studies characterized the infectious agent causing the diarrhea? The other question I have regards the zonulin. Many of you are familiar with the recent data from Sapone et al. [2] looking at the function of zonulin as a gut permeability regulator, where gluten especially seems to be a very important contributor to the permeability of the gut. Have you or others looked at the possible negative effects of the cereals on the effect of probiotics? As suggested in your studies, there may be some negative effects as well. Has the zonulin concentration changed in any of these cases?

Dr. Domellöf: We did not observe any negative interaction between the cereals themselves and the effects of the probiotics, even though the trial was not designed to study that. Regarding intestinal permeability, this has been suggested to be a mechanism for the effect of probiotics on atopic eczema [3]. We have not specifically looked at zonulin. With regard to pathogenic agents, we did not investigate them in this study. However, in Sweden, bacterial diarrhea is very rare and the most common cause of viral diarrhea is rotavirus.

Dr. Guandalini: Thank you, a very interesting presentation and also very promising in terms of future studies. I want also to go along the same line of questions by adding some comments and also try to answer the questions that were raised. You are right, the effect of probiotics is evident mainly if not exclusively on diarrhea of viral origin, specifically rotavirus. There are a few studies in children with acute diarrhea, including our own [4] which remains the largest published in terms of the number of children studied, that looked at etiology with a rather comprehensive approach. We found something which other studies have since confirmed, including subsequent meta-analyses: that probiotics, or more precisely lactobacilli such as the *Lactobacillus* GG we utilized, are only active in the context of viral, not bacterial, diarrheas. Of course, it is conceivable that other probiotics may have different mechanisms of action and thus different efficacy. We really know close to nothing about the pharmacodynamics, pharmacokinetics of these products. I think we are just beginning to understand how these microorganisms work. Furthermore, I would like to add that probiotics have been found to be effective for instance in preventing antibiotic-associated diarrhea, obviously a very common problem. And then there is the issue of nosocomial diarrhea which is also of utmost importance. Already in 1994 in Baltimore Saavedra et al. [5] documented the efficacy of *Bifidobacterium bifidum* and the *Streptococcus thermophilus* in preventing the spread of rotaviral diarrhea in the wards. Subsequently there were two more studies, one by Szajewska et al. [6] which also showed the protective efficacy of *Lactobacillus* GG in a hospital ward, particularly in terms of preventing the spread of rotavirus-associated severe diarrhea. A subsequent study from Italy, however in conflict with these observations, failed to show a protective effect by *Lactobacillus* GG in hospitalized children [7]. So in essence and as Dr. Morelli delineated yesterday, I really think probiotics represent an exciting area, definitely worth pursuing. Chances are within 10 years, in the next Nestlé workshops, we will be discussing much more about their efficacy. Finally, on the question of permeability, it is clear to me that probiotics do have an effect in regulating intestinal permeability, as shown by several in vitro and in vivo studies. There was a pilot study in a few Crohn's patients [8], where the double-sugar technique was used to investigate the effect of *Lactobacillus* GG on the permeability of the intestine, and it was very clear in all patients that there was a striking improvement, albeit transient, as it regressed in approximately 4 months in spite of ongoing intake.

Dr. Haschke: Three short comments. The first refers to the study by Moran [9], where he found a reduction in atopic manifestations by feeding infants a hydrolyzed formula, as we saw without prebiotics. In the group without prebiotics he found that 25% of the infants had atopic eczema. This is far beyond any of the other studies which show that with hydrolyzed formulas the prevalence of atopic eczema is 10–11%. This is exactly what he achieved in this group. So it is not clear, especially as this was a hydrolyzed formula, whether this was an effect of the prebiotics or of the particular protein composition together with the prebiotics. It is very difficult to extrapolate to non-hydrolyzed formulas and to cereals. The second comment is related to the Isolauri study on the supplementation of lactating mothers and their infants with *Lactobacillus* GG during the perinatal period and thereafter. You showed the results until 2 years. Two weeks ago Dr. Isolauri presented the results until 7 years; the clinical results, and the preventive effect of *Lactobacillus* GG is still evident until 7 years of age; these are clinical data for atopic eczema. The third comment refers to whether probiotics or certain strains of probiotics are effective in bacterial or viral diarrhea, which is not clear. It depends very probably on which strain we are using. There is a study which was recently conducted at the ICDDR in Dacca where the *Lactobacillus* ST11 strain was tested; this strain had a clear effect on bacterial diarrhea but not on viral diarrhea. So we still have to learn a lot about the efficacy of individual strains in different situations before we can really make a general recommendation. I think it is very important to look at the cause of diarrhea.

Dr. Ribeiro: I have a different concept about this and the real results that have been presented in the literature to date. We have done three trials now with *Lactobacillus* GG and when we compared the data published so far on so-called diarrhea with our cases, e.g. 5 ml/kg/h of stool output, we could not see a difference over time in our area. At one time rotavirus was around 40% of the etiology and now more recently it is around 70–75%. There was no difference in terms of diarrhea duration and also in stool output. But what is promising is when you look at the prevention studies in daycare centers we see fewer longer cases of diarrhea; so we could observe a decrease in the duration in less persistent cases. I don't know what your idea is when faced with severe diarrhea regardless of the etiology as seen in our setting. A point that I am very concerned about is that we keep talking about probiotics as something that could be extrapolated everywhere in the world, and we have to be concerned about the microbiota we are dealing with; I don't think we can compare Swedish and north European microbiota. What is the environment, what is the colonization of the intestine in another part of the world compared to here in Brazil where we have a completely different intestinal colonization?

Dr. Domellöf: I agree with you that it is very important to conduct studies on prevention of diarrhea in low income regions.

Dr. Brunser: I agree with Dr. Haschke in the sense that we don't have a clear understanding of the way in which prebiotics and probiotics work. Many years ago we did a study in which we provided nucleotides to children and studied the incidence of diarrhea. We discovered that the nucleotides indeed prevented the first episodes of diarrhea, and we were happy because it was known that nucleotides improve T-cell immunity and to this we attributed the effect [10]. However, about 4 years ago an article appeared showing that nucleotides increase the growth of bifidobacteria in the gut; thus when studying the effects of a probiotic or a prebiotic one has to be very careful because they may act simultaneously through different mechanisms in the chain of events that prevent diarrhea. The other point is that one of the effects of prebiotics is that they enhance the recovery of the normal flora. We recently published an article in *Pediatric Research* [11] demonstrating that after children had been treated with amoxicillin for a week, the administration of a mixture of inulin and fructo-oligosaccharides resulted in the recovery of normal bifidobacteria counts. It took about 3 or 4 weeks for the controls to obtain normal bifidobacteria counts [11]. One minor point, in a study of gastric permeability in young adults, medical students who acutely drank alcohol or smoked were fed yogurt with *Lactobacillus johnsonii* (La1). Measurement of gastric mucosal permeability demonstrated that La1 and also smoking, surprisingly, decreased the urinary excretion of sucrose [12]. The effect of smoking is probably due to nicotine that induces vasoconstriction in the mucosa and this decreases excretion. But it was felt that La1 induced improvement in permeability [13]. So the problem is that more than one mechanism may operate simultaneously many times, and one has to look for effects in unexpected areas.

Dr. Solomons: Looking at your final slide on cereal, it is impressive that the treatment is a major constraint to the preservation of certain organisms in their living state; but it also supports the notion that perhaps some of the chemical compounds are sensitive. So the challenge to the cereal industry, in their manufacture of complementary feeding, is to make products that never get heated and in which the water is safe. So I would like to see the industry go in that direction – an innovative new idea, in my way of thinking. As a second point would be maternal education to give the mothers confidence to prepare foods without the terminal heating, which would destroy what we hope to be 'bioactive' at the moment of consumption by the infant.

Dr. Haschke: Just to reply to Dr. Solomons' comment. The solution exists; it is the single packaging of cereals, because cereals are given to infants beyond 6 months of age so they are not as susceptible to certain bacteria as very small infants during the first few weeks of life. The problem of contamination is almost always due to inadequate storage of the product or use of contaminated water, so heating of water and cooling it down before mixing it with the cereal and single bag sachets is possible, but this unfortunately increases the cost. This is a solution which is not the first choice for developing countries.

Dr. Giovannini: What is your personal opinion: is it better to add probiotics to the food by sachet or should it be in the food? There are two points: (1) how long is the efficacy because storage and transport are sometimes problematic, and (2) stability, in the case of probiotics in food cold is needed.

Dr. Domellöf: I think both of these options have to be explored and the recommendation might be different in different settings and different cultures. Probably the addition of probiotics as a component of the complementary food would improve compliance because, as we heard yesterday, taking a separate supplement is more demanding for the parents, but on the other hand you have the stability issues that were mentioned.

Dr. Cardoso: The bifidogenic effect of breast milk or formula with probiotics is easy to understand. But infants more than 6 months old who receive other types of foods in different countries are eating a lot of potentially functional ingredients at meals that can have a bifidogenic effect. How can you separate this when you give a fructo-oligosaccharide or galacto-oligosaccharide to these infants with cereals? You noted some differences in terms of intestinal transit, soft feces or recuperation of tissue, etc. How can you separate this?

Dr. Domellöf: The softening of stools is not a bifidogenic effect, it is an effect of the oligosaccharides themselves. There are several studies that have documented an increase in bifidobacteria after giving infant formula with probiotics [14]. Stool cultures have not usually been performed in the published trials on probiotics in infant cereals, but it would be interesting to verify the bifidogenic effect also in infants with a mixed diet.

Dr. Jongpiputvanich: You mentioned that there is no consistent beneficial effect of some functional components such as LCPUFA nucleotides even in full-term babies. Why do we have to add these nutrients to supplementary feeding for older babies? It seems to me that if one nutrient is added, the price will increase. It looks like a cosmetic change, not a beneficial effect.

Dr. Domellöf: Most of these components have been tested primarily in infant formula but several studies now suggest that they actually may have positive health effects during the weaning period. On the other hand, I agree with you that it is important to consider cost-effectiveness and that possible health benefits must be verified in properly powered clinical studies before bringing these products to the market.

References

1 Szajewska H, Setty M, Mrukowicz J, Guandalini S: Probiotics in gastrointestinal diseases in children: hard and not-so-hard evidence of efficacy. J Pediatr Gastroenterol Nutr 2006;42: 454–475.
2 Sapone A, de Magistris L, Pietzak M, et al: Zonulin upregulation is associated with increased gut permeability in subjects with type 1 diabetes and their relatives. Diabetes 2006;55: 1443–1449.
3 Isolauri E, Sutas Y, Kankaanpaa P, et al: Probiotics: effects on immunity. Am J Clin Nutr 2001;73(suppl):444S–450S.
4 Guandalini S, Pensabene L, Zikri MA, et al: *Lactobacillus* GG administered in oral rehydration solution to children with acute diarrhea: a multicenter European trial. J Pediatr Gastroenterol Nutr 2000;30:54–60.
5 Saavedra JM, Bauman NA, Oung I, et al: Feeding of *Bifidobacterium bifidum* and *Streptococcus thermophilus* to infants in hospital for prevention of diarrhoea and shedding of rotavirus. Lancet 1994;344:1046–1049.
6 Szajewska H, Kotowska M, Mrukowicz JZ, et al: Efficacy of *Lactobacillus* GG in prevention of nosocomial diarrhea in infants. J Pediatr 2001;138:361–365.
7 Mastretta E, Longo P, Laccisaglia A, et al: Effect of *Lactobacillus* GG and breast-feeding in the prevention of rotavirus nosocomial infection. J Pediatr Gastroenterol Nutr 2002;35: 527–531.
8 Gupta P, Andrew H, Kirschner BS, Guandalini S: Is *Lactobacillus* GG helpful in children with Crohn's disease? Results of a preliminary, open-label study. J Pediatr Gastroenterol Nutr 2000;31:453–457.
9 Moran JR: Effects of prolonged exposure to partially hydrolyzed milk protein. J Pediatr 1992;121: S90–S94.
10 Brunser O, Espinoza J, Araya M, et al: Effect of dietary nucleotide supplementation on diarrhoeal disease in infants. Acta Paediatr 1994;83:188–191.
11 Brunser O, Gotteland M, Cruchet S, et al: Effect of a milk formula with prebiotics on the intestinal microbiota of infants after an antibiotic treatment. Pediatr Res 2006;59:451–456.
12 Gotteland M, Cruchet S, Frau V, et al: Effect of acute cigarette smoking, alone or with alcohol, on gastric barrier function in healthy volunteers. Dig Liver Dis 2002;34:702–706.
13 Gotteland M, Cruchet S, Verbeke S: Effect of *Lactobacillus* ingestion on the gastrointestinal mucosal barrier alterations induced by indometacin in humans. Aliment Pharmacol Ther 2001;15:11–17.
14 Fanaro S, Boehm G, Garssen J, et al: Galacto-oligosaccharides and long-chain fructo-oligosaccharides as prebiotics in infant formulas: a review. Acta Paediatr Suppl 2005;94: 22–26.

Agostoni C, Brunser O (eds): Issues in Complementary Feeding.
Nestlé Nutr Workshop Ser Pediatr Program, vol 60, pp 123–138,
Nestec Ltd., Vevey/S. Karger AG, Basel, © 2007.

Functional Ingredients in the Complementary Feeding Period and Long-Term Effects

Carlo Agostoni, Enrica Riva, Marcello Giovannini

Department of Pediatrics, San Paolo Hospital, University of Milan, Milan, Italy

Abstract

The complementary feeding period is a critical stage for growth and development. Infants in developing countries and selected individuals in developed countries may benefit from micronutrient supplementation, but long-term effects are still poorly explored. We have some evidence, coming from observational studies, of the role of iron in the second semester of life for optimal brain development and functioning through early adulthood, but the advantage seems to be restricted to those infants who are effectively iron-deficient. For long-chain polyunsaturated fatty acids we have limited observations from randomized trials that they could promote the maturation of visual acuity in the short-term, without direct evidence linking supplementation during the complementary feeding period to later functional measurements. Probiotics and prebiotics, as well as other micronutrients, such as zinc, represent new promising areas of investigating effects on the immune system. The medium- and long-term effects need to be extensively explored, and any type of association recorded to check the safety of dietary supplements, considering their overconsumption, starting at early ages, in western countries.

Introduction

Nutritional factors during early development might have not only short-term effects on growth, body composition and body functions but also long-term effects on health, disease and mortality risks in adulthood, as well as development of neural functions and behavior, a phenomenon called 'metabolic programming'. The interactions of nutrients and gene expression form the basis of many of these programming effects [1]. Therefore, interest in functional ingredients for the enhancement of the genetic and environmental potentials for health, growth and development is emerging within the pediatric community.

During the intrauterine life and the early phases of the extrauterine life nutrients that have been demonstrated (in either animal or human studies) to have the potential for later functional advantages (from growth and neurodevelopment to the efficiency of the immune system) include minerals and trace elements (iron, zinc, iodine, copper and selenium), vitamins (vitamin A, folic acid, vitamin B_6, vitamin B_{12}, vitamin C, vitamin D, vitamin E), the essential fatty acid linoleic acid, and long-chain polyunsaturated fatty acids [LCP-UFA; including arachidonic acid (ARA) and docosahexaenoic acid (DHA)] [1]. Recently, also probiotics and prebiotics have been added to the concepts of functional nutrients, that is compounds having positive effects on biological processes and functional mechanisms, leading to a general advantage for the individual in terms of health and quality of life.

Now, new questions arise as to whether also the complementary feeding period may represent a further 'sensitive' period, in which selected nutrients might advantageously program the growing organisms, in both developing and well-developed countries. For the purposes of our discussion we will consider as 'complementary feeding period' the interval included between 4–6 and 18–24 months of age.

Clearly, different approaches are required according to the environmental background:

- Developing countries show primary needs to improve general health conditions, first of all growth, development and incidence of disease, closely connected to the nutritional status of young infants. Within this context, micronutrient supplementation has gained considerable attention, for a relatively low cost-benefit ratio, and the possibility to prevent conditions (such as iron deficiency anemia) that could impact later developmental abilities.
- Well-developed countries as well as countries in rapid transition offer opportunities to enrich diets with functional ingredients to maximize the individual genetic potential for growth, while decreasing the risk for the early appearance of unfavorable markers of the metabolic syndrome. The LCPUFA as well as bioactive intestinal agents are two examples. Since the primary goal of a health intervention is the avoidance of any damage, we must take care that dietary supplements are not associated with untoward effects, and also assess their effective utility.

Functional Ingredients and Complementary Feeding in Developing Countries

In most developing countries the main (or even only) available weaning foods are represented by local staple cereal foods such as maize, rice or cassava.

In these communities, where energy-protein malnutrition is endemic, the 6- to 24-month period is the most critical for nutritional interventions and the introduction of specifically designed supplements can prevent the onset of wasting in a large proportion of children [2]. Malnutrition at an early age may have long-term effects on growth achievement as well as the incidence of disease and brain development (with identifiable anatomic changes), leading to lower levels of intellectual achievement in school-age children and final intelligence quotient scores [3]. As a matter of fact, while the minimal requirements for energy and protein intakes intake are seldom met and represent a primary health determinant, interventions based on micronutrient supplements are planned in order to improve health conditions, growth and developmental outcomes. Several studies have been conducted in developing countries by supplementing from 6- up to 12- to 24-month (or even longer) infants at high risk of malnutrition. In these settings micronutrients (mostly iron, less often zinc, sometimes mixed with other micronutrients) have been introduced at the starting of the complementary feeding period to look at short-term effects on biological markers and health outcomes while no information is available on later effects [4].

To specifically assess the effects of iron supplements, anthropometric measurements, developmental indices, blood indicators of iron status (blood levels of hemoglobin, iron, ferritin), incidence of disease together with adverse reactions have commonly been considered. The assessment of other biological markers as well as later effects, such as growth and intellectual (educational) achievement, and markers of disease, including the early indicators of metabolic impairment are clearly necessary to optimize interventions. A rapid transition towards affluent conditions puts infants from developing countries at particular risk of growth acceleration and related unfavorable biological and anthropometric parameters [5, 6]. In general, growth progression is not influenced by micronutrient supplementation in the complementary feeding period (except in a few reports) since the energy and protein deficiencies represent the major limiting factors. Developmental progresses with supplements are more easily found at short-term assessments [7, 8], but many reports indicate that there is no convincing evidence that iron treatment has an effect on mental development in children aged less than 2 years [9]. Future studies from developing countries should supply data on the medium- and long-term outcomes of dietary supplements in the period of dietary diversification, to define the cost/benefit ratio of nutritional interventions.

Functional Ingredients and Complementary Feeding in Developed and Rapidly Progressing ('Transition') Countries

Even if surveys on several dietary supplements are available in more advantaged settings, very few studies have been published concerning nutrients

Table 1. Structural correlates from experimental models (mostly animals) of long-term functional effects of early iron deficiency in humans [as reviewed in 4]

Reduced brain iron
    → Great variability by brain region
    → Areas and functions differently involved
Alterations of brain metabolism
    → Failure of iron incorporation into protein structures
    → Altered dendritic structure, mainly in hippocampal areas
    → Poorer recognition memory
Alterations of myelination
    → Decrease in myelin lipids and proteins
    → Decreased proliferation of oligodendrocytes (fewer?, less functional?)
    → Slower conduction in the auditory and visual systems
    → Other poorer outcomes?
Alterations of neurotransmission
    → Deranged metabolism of enzymes involved in neurotransmitter synthesis (serotonin, norepinephrine, dopamine)
    → Alterations of dopamine receptors and transporters connected to the extent of iron loss
    → Social/emotional alterations, affective changes
    → Altered experience-dependent processes
    → Altered interactions with the environment
Altered gene and protein profiles

supplemented during the complementary feeding period and assessment of functional effects at medium-term (18–24 months of age) and long-term (at preschool age at least).

Only for iron do we have some evidence from observational studies, while for LCPUFA we are merely able to collect partial observations from randomized controlled trials (RCT). For other functional nutrients (such as probiotics, prebiotics, zinc and some minerals/vitamins) we have still more partial and indirect evidence, and it is, therefore, mostly speculation.

Iron

Iron deficiency in the 6- to 24-month period represents a challenging question even in affluent environments, and its effects may be more easily isolated, since energy and protein intakes are generally more than adequate. This time period is characterized by the peak hippocampal and cortical regional development, as well as myelinogenesis, dendritogenesis and synaptogenesis in the brain [4], all critical processes that, if early deranged, may justify the bases for later anatomofunctional consequences (table 1). Case-controlled studies usually include assessment before and immediately after iron supplementation and/or therapy [4]. Therefore, the issue of the medium- and long-term functional value of iron supplements in the complementary feeding period may be summarized in some fundamental points from observational studies in humans:

- The mean cell hemoglobin levels during infancy, and more markedly during the 6- to 12-month period, have been associated with neurodevelopmental indices at either preschool age [10–15] or school age [16–18].
- Lozoff et al. [19] found that early iron deficiency is still associated with lower performance in arithmetic and writing achievement and motor function, together with affective and social/emotional differences, during early adolescence (11–14 years of age). A widening gap for mental scores through 19 years of age has also been observed, which was particularly marked for children from more disadvantaged families [20].
- A recent, more sophisticated investigation showed longer wave latencies using auditory brainstem response and visual evoked potentials in 4-year-old children identified as having iron deficiency anemia at 6, 12 and 18 months [21].

Since no study included original RCT, observations generally result from the follow-up of infants who had formerly been anemics compared to those who had higher hemoglobin levels. On the whole, it seems that the prevention of iron deficiency anemia is critical to prevent later neurodevelopmental impairments (fig. 1). The hypotheses on the structural and biochemical correlates for the long-term effects are summarized in table 1.

The question then arises whether an indiscriminate supply of dietary iron as a supplement should be planned at 6–12 months of age or whether a screening procedure would be preferable in order to identify effectively iron-deficient infants requiring a dietary supplementation. To plan an indiscriminate supply, one should make sure that no untoward effects will follow for those who are already iron sufficient. There are reports of untoward effects of iron supplements on the incidence of disease [22] and weight and/or length progression [23] for previously iron-replete infants. On the other hand, if infants are going to be screened for iron status to individualize the intervention, we need to consider the ethical problem of an invasive procedure for blood sampling. We also need to consider a nutritional paradox: infants breastfed for an extended period are prone to have a low iron status [24], but breastfeeding itself has been associated in a duration-dependent fashion with higher intelligence quotient scores in adults [25].

An alternative way to solve the question could be represented by the early introduction of a natural food, such as meat, in subjects more exposed to iron deficiency (breastfed infants). Two recent studies (the first, an observational follow-up survey and the second, an RCT) have shown associations between meat intake at 4–16 months [26] and at 5–7 months [27] with more favorable psychomotor developmental indices at 22 months and behavioral indices at 12 months, respectively. Accordingly, the development of cereal iron fortification [28] might improve the mineral bioavailability from vegetables, adding a

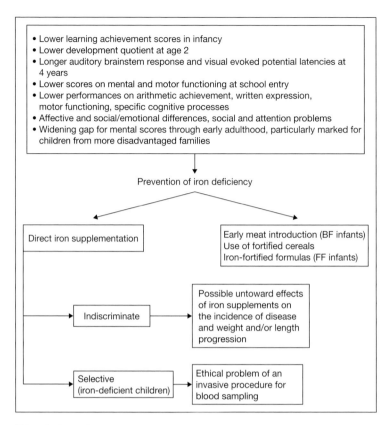

• Lower learning achievement scores in infancy
• Lower development quotient at age 2
• Longer auditory brainstem response and visual evoked potential latencies at 4 years
• Lower scores on mental and motor functioning at school entry
• Lower performances on arithmetic achievement, written expression, motor functioning, specific cognitive processes
• Affective and social/emotional differences, social and attention problems
• Widening gap for mental scores through early adulthood, particularly marked for children from more disadvantaged families

Prevention of iron deficiency

Direct iron supplementation

Early meat introduction (BF infants)
Use of fortified cereals
Iron-fortified formulas (FF infants)

Indiscriminate

Possible untoward effects of iron supplements on the incidence of disease and weight and/or length progression

Selective (iron-deficient children)

Ethical problem of an invasive procedure for blood sampling

Fig. 1. Iron deficiency in the complementary feeding period: long-term effects of observational studies and preventive strategies. BF = Breastfed; FF = formula-fed.

new relevant dietary source of the mineral for infants in the complementary feeding period.

Long-Chain Polyunsaturated Fatty Acids

The issue of LCPUFA as functional nutrients in childhood nutrition is relatively more recent than the iron issue. Since also the concept of RCT in nutrition as gold standard for the scientific evidence is relatively recent, more RCTs are available for LCPUFA, but only some performed in the first semester of life have been assessed in the long-term, while the few conducted in the second semester have been limited to observations in the short-term.

The biochemical and structural changes attributable to the dietary enrichment with LCPUFA at the possible origin of neural functional effects are summarized in table 2. Since the accretion of LCPUFA in the human brain goes on during the postnatal period up to at least 2 years of age [29], particularly in the case of DHA [30], we could infer that LCPUFA supplied through this

Table 2. Structural correlates from experimental models (mostly cultured cells) of functional effects of early dietary LCPUFA supply in humans [as reviewed in 37]

Altered membrane fluidity, volume and packing
Changed lipid phase properties
Modified membrane lipid-protein interactions within specific microdomains
→ Changed physical properties and membrane excitability
→ Modified ability of membrane proteins to bind ligands and activate enzymes
→ Altered receptor activity, antigenic recognition, signal transduction
→ Modified electrical properties of membranes
 → Development of synaptic processes (ARA)
 → Modulation of neurotransmitter uptake and release (DHA)
 → Direct effect on the expression of genes regulating cell differentiation and growth
  → Growth stimulation on retinal neurons, higher rhodopsin concentrations (DHA)
  → Overexpression of retinal genes (DHA)
  → Overexpression of ion channels involved in retinal synaptogenesis (DHA)
   → Overall contribution to the development and maturation of retina (other brain regions?)
Modification of eicosanoid function
 → Decreased inflammatory processes and platelet aggregation
 → Influence on arterial wall compliance and blood pressure

---

entire period of the rapid development of the brain and membranes might influence the neurodevelopmental outcome and also some more general adaptive functions of membranes and tissues. Unfortunately, a direct association of LCPUFA supplementation in the 4- to 6- to 12- to 24-month period and functional measurements in the long-term is lacking. The major points are summarized as follows (fig. 2):

- Most studies on LCPUFA effects consider the exclusive milk feeding period (in either preterm or term infants) with assessment in the short-term, that is at the end of the supplementation period. A few studies have investigated the effects of LCPUFA-enriched formula feeding in the first 4–6 months of life beyond the supplementation period, that is at 10 months of age and at medium-term (18–24 months), with either positive effects [31, 32] or no effects [33, 34], respectively.
- One study considered the effects at 5 years on blood pressure values, who were lower in a group fed an LCPUFA-enriched formula in the first 4 months of life [35]. The neurodevelopmental performance of the same infants was evaluated at 5 years, but the results have not yet been published.
- One RCT showed that a dietary LCPUFA enrichment of human milk through the maternal diet is associated with higher intelligence quotient scores at 4 years of age [36].

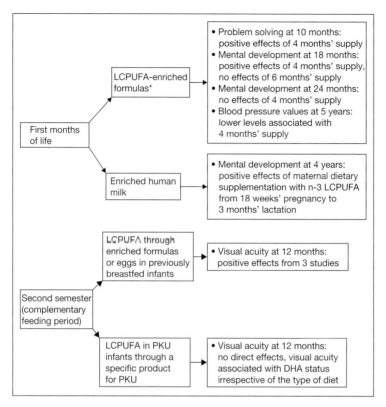

Fig. 2. LCPUFA supply: medium- and long-term effects from trials in the first semester and short-term effects from trials in the complementary feeding period. *Differing regarding sources and biochemical forms (phospholipds vs. triglycerides) and internal ratios (ARA:DHA ranging from 1:1 to 2:1) and absolute content of LCPUFA. PKU = Phenylketonuria.

- Three trials showed favorable functional effects of the dietary enrichment of LCPUFA through a formula [37, 38] or eggs [39] during the complementary feeding period with neurophysiological tests exploring visual acuity at 12 months, that is there was only short-term assessment. There have been similar findings in infants affected by phenylketonuria and followed up for 12 months in an LCPUFA supplementation trial, in which an association between plasma DHA levels and better visual acuity measured with visual evoked potentials was found in the course of 1 year [40].

Hopefully more long-term assessments of early LCPUFA dietary supplementation could become available in the near future, but a lack of a consistent pattern of the results has already been anticipated due to the 'differences in the levels, nature and duration of supplementations, the use of tools that are insufficiently sensitive to measure small changes in performance, and the complexities caused by the longevity and reversibility of diet-induced changes in developmental outcomes' [41, 42].

Other Micronutrients, Probiotics and Prebiotics

Zinc and other micronutrients have been considered for trials in both developing and developed countries, closely associated with the issue of iron supplementation, and, accordingly, no observations in either the medium- and long-term are available. Some contrasting observations might be explained on the basis of the co-presence of subjects with adequate zinc status and others with poorer stores who probably benefited most from the supplementation. A marginal zinc status in breastfed groups at the beginning of the complementary feeding period could represent an additional explanation for the observations linking the amount of meat eaten in the complementary feeding period to later developmental indices [26, 27] and suggests the need for further research.

An increasing interest in the potential effects of probiotcs and prebiotics administered at early ages is developing today. It is speculated that the manipulation of the infants' intestinal flora, either directly, with specific probiotic strains, or indirectly, by administering prebiotics, could develop patterns more favorably connected with less allergic reactions, fewer infective episodes (gastrointestinal, but also respiratory), and less gastrointestinal disturbances (constipation, colic episodes). The model is the breastfed, compared to the formula-fed, infant. While some RCTs with prebiotic- and/or probiotic-enriched formulas are available for the first months of life, there are fewer trials regarding the complementary feeding period, concerning oligofructose-enriched cereals [43, 44]; other studies, however, have considered the effects of administering probiotic strains within a formula [45, 46]. Available results are limited to the period of the supplementation trial, and are suggestive of possible preventive effects on the expression of allergy and the incidence of fever and diarrhea, particularly for probiotics. In any case, no studies are available on medium- and long-term effects.

Dietary Supplementation: Useful or Useless?

It is a well-known, common dietary practice to give children dietary supplements in the 4- to 24-month period of age. Inadequate iron and zinc intakes are highly prevalent in developing countries, especially during the period of complementary feeding when micronutrient requirements are high and breast milk contributes little. Severe diarrheal episodes, especially in case of persistent symptoms, represent a further condition requiring supplementation of dietary zinc [47]. More data are needed on the routine inclusion of zinc in iron supplements given to children with the simultaneous inclusion of other micronutrients, to prevent negative interactions [48]. Once more, we need to expand our knowledge on the effects in the medium (preschool age) and long (school age) term.

In well-developed, rich countries it is a relatively common practice to add dietary supplements to infants' nutrition, starting at 4–6 months of age. More than half of the US preschool children take vitamin and mineral supplements [49]. Children who are given supplements tend to have mothers who are older, more educated, married, insured, and receiving care from a private health care provider, have a greater household income, and took in turn supplements during pregnancy. Child health characteristics associated with supplement use included first birth order and having eating problems or poor appetite. The sociodemographic and health predictors identified for supplement use therefore suggest that groups at risk for nonuse are likely the same groups whose circumstances might suggest the need for supplementation.

According to a recent survey from the US [50], 8% of infants aged 4–5 months received some type of dietary supplements, and the prevalence of supplement use increased with age to 19% among infants aged 6–11 months and 31% among toddlers aged 12–24 months. The vast majority of supplement users (97%) received only one type of supplement, most commonly a multivitamin and/or mineral supplement. Vitamin/mineral supplement use among infants and toddlers was associated with being a first-born child, particularly if reported as being a 'picky eater'. Accordingly, healthy infants and toddlers can achieve recommended levels of intake from food alone, and dietetics professionals should encourage caregivers to use foods rather than supplements as the primary source of nutrients in children's diets. Since vitamin and mineral supplements could help infants and toddlers with special nutrient needs or marginal supply to achieve adequate intakes, care must be taken to ensure that supplements do not lead to an excessive intake, especially for nutrients that are widely used as food fortificants, including vitamin A, zinc, and folate. Another recent survey from the US has reached quite similar results and conclusions [51]. Among micronutrients, zinc intake is becoming excessive in preschool American children [52]. Paradoxically, early vitamin supplementation (within the first 6 months) has been associated with an increased risk of asthma in black children and food allergies in exclusively formula-fed children [53].

Conclusions

The complementary feeding period is a critical stage for growth and development. Infants in developing countries and selected individuals in developed countries may benefit from micronutrient supplementation, but long-term effects are still poorly explored, except for iron. Supplemented LCPUFA of the n-3 series (DHA) might promote visual acuity maturation up to 12 months with potential long-lasting effects. Probiotics, prebiotics and zinc represent new promising areas of investigation. Not only the medium- and long-term effects need to be explored, but also any type of association recorded to check the safety of dietary supplementation, considering their overconsumption from early ages in affluent countries.

References

1 Koletzko B, Aggett PJ, Bindels JG, et al: Growth, development and differentiation: a functional food science approach. Br J Nutr 1998;80(suppl 1):S5–S45.
2 Rivera JA, Habicht JP: Effect of supplementary feeding on the prevention of mild-to-moderate wasting in conditions of endemic malnutrition in Guatemala. Bull World Health Organ 2002;80: 926–932.
3 Ivanovic DM, Leiva BP, Perez HT, et al: Long-term effects of severe undernutrition during the first year of life on brain development and learning in Chilean high-school graduates. Nutrition 2000;16:1056–1063.
4 Lozoff B, Beard J, Connor J, et al: Long-lasting neural and behavioural effects on iron deficiency in infancy. Nutr Rev 2006;64:S34–S43.
5 Gonzalez-Barranco J, Rios-Torres JM, Castillo-Martinez L, et al: Effect of malnutrition during the first year of life on adult plasma insulin and glucose tolerance. Metabolism 2003;52: 1005–1011.
6 Monteiro PO, Victora CG: Rapid growth in infancy and childhood and obesity in later life – a systematic review. Obes Rev 2005;6:143–154.
7 Lind T, Lonnerdal B, Stenlund H, et al: A community-based randomized controlled trial of iron and zinc supplementation in Indonesian infants: effects on growth and development. Am J Clin Nutr 2004;80:729–736.
8 Black MM, Baqui AH, Zaman K, et al: Iron and zinc supplementation promote motor development and exploratory behavior among Bangladeshi infants. Am J Clin Nutr 2004;80:903–910.
9 Sachdev H, Gera T, Nestel P: Effect of iron supplementation on mental and motor development in children: systematic review of randomised controlled trials. Public Health Nutr 2005;8:117–132.
10 Palti H, Pevsner B, Adler B: Does anemia in infancy affect achievement on developmental and intelligence tests? Hum Biol 1983;55:189–194.
11 Dommergues JP, Archambeaud B, Ducot Y, et al: Iron deficiency and psychomotor development scores: a longitudinal study between ages 10 months and 4 years. Arch Fr Pediatr 1989;46:487–490.
12 Wasserman G, Graziano JH, Factor-Litvak P, et al: Independent effects of lead exposure and iron deficiency anemia on developmental outcome at age 2 years. J Pediatr 1992;121: 695–703.
13 Lozoff B, Jimenez E, Wolf AW: Long-term developmental outcome of infants with iron deficiency. N Engl J Med 1991;325:687–694.
14 Corapci F, Radan AE, Lozoff B: Iron deficiency in infancy and mother-child interaction at 5 years. J Dev Behav Pediatr 2006;27:371–378.
15 De Andraca I, Walter T, Castillo M, et al: Iron Deficiency Anemia and Its Effects upon Psychological Development at Preschool Age: A Longitudinal Study. Nestlé Foundation Nutrition Annual Report (1990). Vevey, Nestec, 1991, pp 53–62.
16 Cantwell RJ: The long term neurological sequelae of anemia in infancy. (abstract). Pediatr Res 1974;342:68.
17 Palti H, Meijer A, Adler B: Learning achievement and behavior at school of anemic and non-anemic infants. Early Hum Dev 1985;10:217–223.
18 Hurtado EK, Claussen AH, Scott KG: Early childhood anemia and mild or moderate mental retardation. Am J Clin Nutr 1999;69:115–119.
19 Lozoff B, Jimenez E, Hagen J, et al: Poorer behavioral and developmental outcome more than 10 years after treatment for iron deficiency in infancy. Pediatrics 2000;105:E51.

20 Lozoff B, Jimenez E, Walter T: Double burden of iron deficiency and low socio-economic status: a growth curve analysis of cognitive test scores to 19 years. Arch Pediatr Adolesc Med, in press.

21 Algarin C, Peirano P, Garrido M, et al: Iron deficiency anemia in infancy: Long-lasting effects on auditory and visual system functioning. Pediatr Res 2003;53:217–223.

22 Dewey KG, Domellof M, Cohen RJ, et al: Iron supplementation affects growth and morbidity of breast-fed infants: results of a randomized trial in Sweden and Honduras. J Nutr 2002;132:3249–3255.

23 Majumdar I, Paul P, Talib VH, Ranga S: The effect of iron therapy on the growth of iron-replete and iron-deplete children. J Trop Pediatr 2003;49:84–88.

24 Domellof M, Lonnerdal B, Abrams SA, Hernell O: Iron absorption in breast-fed infants: effects of age, iron status, iron supplements, and complementary foods. Am J Clin Nutr 2002;76: 198–204.

25 Mortensen EL, Michaelsen KF, Sanders SA, Reinisch JM: The association between duration of breastfeeding and adult intelligence. JAMA 2002;287:2365–2371.

26 Morgan J, Taylor A, Fewtrell M: Meat consumption is positively associated with psychomotor outcome in children up to 24 months of age. J Pediatr Gastroenterol Nutr 2004;39:493–498.

27 Krebs NF, Westcott JE, Butler N, et al: Meat as a first complementary food for breastfed infants: feasibility and impact on zinc intake and status. J Pediatr Gastroenterol Nutr 2006;42: 207–214.

28 Davidsson L, Kastenmayer P, Szajewska H, et al: Iron bioavailability in infants from an infant cereal fortified with ferric pyrophosphate or ferrous fumarate. Am J Clin Nutr 2000;71: 1597–1602.

29 Martinez M: Tissue levels of polyunsaturated fatty acids during early human development. J Pediatr 1992;120:129–138.

30 Martinez M, Mougan I: Fatty acid composition of human brain phospholipids during normal development. J Neurochem 1998;71:2528–2533.

31 Willatts P, Forsyth JS, Di Modugno MK, et al: Effect of long-chain polyunsaturated fatty acids in infant formula on problem solving at 10 months of age. Lancet 1998;352:688–691.

32 Birch EE, Garfield S, Hoffman DR, et al: A randomized controlled trial of early dietary supply of long-chain polyunsaturated fatty acids and mental development in term infants. Dev Med Child Neurol 2000;42:174–181.

33 Agostoni C, Trojan S, Bellù R, et al: Developmental quotient at 24 months and fatty acid composition of diet in early infancy: a follow-up study. Arch Dis Child 1997;76:421–424.

34 Lucas A, Stafford M, Morley R, et al: Efficacy and safety of long-chain polyunsaturated fatty acid supplementation of infant-formula milk: a randomised trial. Lancet 1999;354:1948–1954.

35 Forsyth JS, Willatts P, Agostoni C, et al: Long chain polyunsaturated fatty acid supplementation in infant formula and blood pressure in later childhood: follow up of a randomised controlled trial. BMJ 2003;326:953–957.

36 Helland IB, Smith L, Saarem K, et al: Maternal supplementation with very-long-chain n-3 fatty acids during pregnancy and lactation augments children's IQ at 4 years of age. Pediatrics 2003;111:e39–e44.

37 Birch EE, Hoffman DR, Castaneda YS, et al: A randomized controlled trial of long-chain polyunsaturated fatty acid supplementation of formula in term infants after weaning at 6 wk of age. Am J Clin Nutr 2002;75:570–580.

38 Hoffman DR, Birch EE, Castaneda YS, et al: Visual function in breast-fed term infants weaned to formula with or without long-chain polyunsaturates at 4 to 6 months: a randomized clinical trial. J Pediatr 2003;142:669–677.

39 Hoffman DR, Theuer RC, Castaneda YS, et al: Maturation of visual acuity is accelerated in breast-fed term infants fed baby food containing DHA-enriched egg yolk. J Nutr 2004;134: 2307–2313.

40 Agostoni C, Harvie A, McCulloch DL, et al: A randomized trial of long-chain polyunsaturated fatty acid supplementation in infants with phenylketonuria. Dev Med Child Neurol 2006;48: 207–212.

41 Lauritzen L, Hansen HS, Jorgensen MH, Michaelsen KF: The essentiality of long chain n-3 fatty acids in relation to development and function of the brain and retina. Prog Lipid Res 2001;40:1–94.

42 Uauy R, Dangour AD: Nutrition in brain development and aging: role of essential fatty acids. Nutr Rev 2006;64:S24–S33.
43 Duggan C, Penny ME, Hibberd P, et al: Oligofructose-supplemented infant cereal: 2 randomized, blinded, community-based trials in Peruvian infants. Am J Clin Nutr 2003;77:937–942.
44 Moore N, Chao C, Yang LP, et al: Effects of fructo-oligosaccharide-supplemented infant cereal: a double-blind, randomized trial. Br J Nutr 2003;90:581–587.
45 Weizman Z, Asli G, Alsheikh A: Effect of a probiotic infant formula on infections in child care centers: comparison of two probiotic agents. Pediatrics 2005;115:5–9.
46 Shamir R, Makhoul IR, Etzioni A, Shehadeh N: Evaluation of a diet containing probiotics and zinc for the treatment of mild diarrheal illness in children younger than one year of age. J Am Coll Nutr 2005;24:370–375.
47 Allen LH: Zinc and micronutrient supplements for children. Am J Clin Nutr 1998;68 (suppl):495S–498S.
48 Lind T, Lonnerdal B, Stenlund H, et al: A community-based randomized controlled trial of iron and zinc supplementation in Indonesian infants: interactions between iron and zinc. Am J Clin Nutr 2003;77:883–890.
49 Yu SM, Kogan MD, Gergen P: Vitamin-mineral supplement use among preschool children in the United States. Pediatrics 1997;100:E4.
50 Briefel R, Hanson C, Fox MK, et al: Feeding Infants and Toddlers Study: do vitamin and mineral supplements contribute to nutrient adequacy or excess among US infants and toddlers? J Am Diet Assoc 2006;106(suppl 1):S52–S65.
51 Eichenberger Gilmore JM, Hong L, Broffitt B, Levy SM: Longitudinal patterns of vitamin and mineral supplement use in young white children. J Am Diet Assoc 2005;105:763–772.
52 Arsenault JE, Brown KH: Zinc intake of US preschool children exceeds new dietary reference intakes. Am J Clin Nutr 2003;78:1011–1017.
53 Milner JD, Stein DM, McCarter R, Moon RY: Early infant multivitamin supplementation is associated with increased risk for food allergy and asthma. Pediatrics 2004;114:27–32.

Discussion

Dr. Calçado: Do you think there is enough evidence nowadays to put lactating mothers on n-3 supplementation, to increase DHA in breast milk in order to improve cortex and retinal chemical composition?

Dr. Agostoni: The question is: if I supplement lactating mothers, would I supplement the pregnant mothers? I would follow the suggestion from the literature showing an effect starting with 200 mg DHA/day from 18–20 weeks of gestation. The data suggest that during intrauterine life the growing fetus in the third trimester of life accumulates 40–60 mg/day of n-3 LCP and this could be roughly translated into 200 mg DHA to the mothers starting before the third trimester of life.

Dr. Biasucci: I have two considerations for you. The first one concerns the possibility of supplementing pregnant mothers, and the second one is related to the crucial and critical period of complementary feeding. What is your opinion regarding a natural approach, which would also be acceptable in developing countries, such as educating mothers to use fish in their babies' diets, more than artificial or pharmacological supplementation?

Dr. Agostoni: Certainly I agree. In our Cambodian study, the main solid food during the complementary feeding period was made up of a soup with cereals in which some fish is added. Indeed they have 3-fold the DHA levels of an Italian reference population [1]. The second point is not just fish but egg yolk. Egg yolk is an excellent source of phospholipids with DHA and arachidonic acid. I remember a paper in the *American Journal of Clinical Nutrition* 15 years ago when I started as a nutritionist showing that in several areas in China egg yolk is started at 3 months [2]. Even if both fish and egg are not the best preferred indications of immune allergologists, I underline that there is no evidence from a normal healthy population.

Dr. Domellöf: I would like to expand on the iron issue. As was mentioned, several studies suggest that iron supplementation is beneficial for neural development but, on the other hand, excessive iron supplementation of infants who are already iron-sufficient might lead to poor growth and may also increase the risk for infections, especially in endemic malaria regions. So how do you suggest that we determine which children should receive extra iron supplements?

Dr. Agostoni: You mean our experience with sprinkles [3]. What am I suggesting? I like the term 'holistic approach', first of all to support breastfeeding because it is the main source of available iron and it does no harm; at the point that when you take the supply of iron from human milk into consideration you are getting some contradictions looking at intake recommendations. As a second suggestion I would say meat because meat is also an excellent source of many functional components such as zinc, iron and the LCP supplied even in minimal amounts. In very good work you have nicely shown that there is a strict regulation of iron absorption according to individual status and to the dietary source utilized. To optimize absorption, vitamin C must also be considered to improve the ratio in special preparations, and zinc with copper to prevent negative interactions. I think that it is possible even using internal resources in developing or transition countries; hopefully this will be a policy of the future.

Dr. Solomons: I don't have an answer but I have several questions. One has to do with the philosophical question of why is the more rapid development of infants beneficial. I guess when humans were also prey as well as hunters and when other animals such as birds of prey or anacondas in the Amazon were looking around for young infants to eat it would seem to me that the infant who was more quite, less exploratory, had less visual acuity so it wasn't fascinated by what he was seeing, would have been the less likely to be eaten. On the other hand, the advanced infant, looking around, crawling at the edge of his cliff, would have been the suitable prey. So it may be that at that time nature wanted babies to be more quiet. Now we are rethinking the issue of whether fast or slow is better. I would say that developmental mind landmarks have a similar kind of philosophical question. The second has to do with the ethics of screening for iron status versus the ethics of giving iron without screening, and it is a very interesting question. Dr. Haschke mentioned that there are technological solutions, I would suggest that there are technological solutions to iron screening, and Dr. Rainer Gross, who passed away a month ago, was working in Indonesia on a transducer, a skin Doppler, which could look at the underlying capillaries with energy and photons [4]. This essentially could do a hematocrit in a flowing capillary, so this kind of technological solution would eliminate any invasion, if you will, to the screening. I am convinced that between the two options that screening is preferable to indiscriminate iron supplementation.

Dr. Agostoni: Thank you for the second point, it is quite interesting indeed to develop a noninvasive method for assessing hematocrit. As to the first question about evolution, it could perhaps be advantageous to have fast adaptation to technologies, internet and e-mails and so on.

Dr. Brown: I want to speak on the second point that Dr. Solomons raised. I was going to speak about the iron issue more from a perspective of the methodologic dilemma that we face, namely that the beneficial effects of iron seem not surprisingly to occur in iron-deficient infants and young children, and the adverse effects occur in those who initially are iron replete. So if we are looking for either beneficial or adverse effects of an intervention, we can only interpret the results of those studies if we interpret them in light of initial status. In a study that does not do that, the beneficial and adverse effects may cancel each other out, and so we can get any result without looking at the modifying effect of initial status. That then has implications on sample size and whether we have statistical power in these studies to actually detect these effects. I would argue that the adverse effects of iron in iron-replete children may occur not only in malaria endemic zones but in other parts of the world like Chile, Honduras, Sweden and Indonesia. We won't see those effects if we are not looking at iron in relation to initial status.

Dr. Agostoni: Yes, I agree. It is perhaps easier to define an optimal dosage for LCP and the dose-related effects, also taking the initial status into consideration.

Dr. Brunser: I want to raise a point about genetic polymorphism, which is important because in the same locus there may be alleles that are not exactly similar, and this generates dispersion of values. Nobody is entirely equal to his neighbor and this has advantages because these slight differences represent different adaptation possibilities. From our point of view, this creates problems because we have to increase the number of individuals incorporated into our studies to obtain significant differences: it is this background 'noise' that has to be kept in mind when analyzing results. This is complicated for us because larger numbers of individuals have to be studied to demonstrate significant differences.

Dr. Turck: I am not sure that I quite understood your answer to the following question: should we supplement lactating mothers with DHA? Did you say yes?

Dr. Agostoni: I said that if we decide to supplement, we should start at 18–22 weeks of gestation because we have to ensure an adequate supply of LCP to the fetus that, from this time onwards to the end of pregnancy, receives progressively increasing levels of LCP. It is like giving folic acid after the periconceptional period; its preventive effects are clearly reduced. If we give DHA during lactation, the mother may benefit, but I am not sure if the infant will benefit. If we give DHA in the last trimester of pregnancy we benefit the mother and probably also the infant, so I would supplement the mother.

Dr. Turck: To me supplementation is needed when an individual cannot fulfill his/her requirements from the regular diet. There may be problems, financial or sociocultural or even technical problems to obtaining DHA from the diet, but I think that we are not only raising a scientific issue but also an ethical issue. If we start to advise that lactating mothers be supplemented with DHA then the idea emerges that, in a sense, lactation becomes a sickness because we may need supplementation in several specific nutrients. So the question is difficult to answer and I think we have to be very cautious in the type of advice that we give to lactating mothers, at least for this issue with DHA.

Dr. Agostoni: I would say there are two categories mostly exposed to a poor transfer of DHA to the fetus. The first are mothers with intrauterine growth retardation who have very low DHA transfer [5]. The second category is smokers. It has been shown that infants born to smoking mothers have a poor DHA status [6]; smokers transfer lower DHA levels to the fetus. But the effects of maternal dietary supplementation have still to be investigated.

Dr. Haschke: All these discussions on the 2:1 ratio of arachidonic acid versus DHA is related to the American population because they are meat eaters. If you look at Japan, the ratio in breast milk of arachidonic acid to DHA is quite different, it is 1:1 or even less. So I think we should pay more attention to what people are eating in different regions. To follow up on the study which I mentioned yesterday by Dr. Bergmann which was presented at ESPGHAN this year, they started to supplement mothers with DHA at 30 weeks of gestation, and it was clearly shown that the DHA status of the mother was related to the DHA content in breast milk. And finally at birth and at 3 month of age, a clear effect of the supplementation was seen in the offspring. Again the ratio of arachidonic acid to DHA in breast milk was 1:1 or even below. So we have to learn more about supplementation, but it has an effect in certain populations.

References

1 Agostoni C, Giovannini M, Sala D, et al: Double-blind, placebo-controlled trial comparing effects of supplementation of two micronutrient sprinkles on fatty acid status in Cambodian infants. J Pediatr Gastroenterol Nutr 2007;44:136–142.
2 Simopoulos AP, Salem N Jr: Egg yolk as a source of long-chain polyunsaturated fatty acids in infant feeding. Am J Clin Nutr 1992;55:411–414.
3 Giovannini M, Sala D, Usuelli M, et al: Double-blind, placebo-controlled trial comparing effects of supplementation with two different combinations of micronutrients delivered as sprinkles on growth, anemia, and iron deficiency in cambodian infants. J Pediatr Gastroenterol Nutr 2006;42:306–312.
4 Gross R, Glivitski M, Gross P, Frank K: Anemia and hemoglobin status. A new concept and new method of assessment. Food Nutr Bull 1996;17:160–168.
5 Cetin I, Giovannini N, Alvino G, et al: Intrauterine growth restriction is associated with changes in polyunsaturated fatty acid fetal-maternal relationships. Pediatr Res 2002;52:750–755.
6 Agostoni C, Galli C, Riva E, et al: Reduced docosahexaenoic acid synthesis may contribute to growth restriction in infants born to mothers who smoke. J Pediatr 2005;147:854–856.

Agostoni C, Brunser O (eds): Issues in Complementary Feeding.
Nestlé Nutr Workshop Ser Pediatr Program, vol 60, pp 139–155,
Nestec Ltd., Vevey/S. Karger AG, Basel, © 2007.

The Influence of Gluten: Weaning Recommendations for Healthy Children and Children at Risk for Celiac Disease

Stefano Guandalini

Section of Pediatric Gastroenterology, Hepatology and Nutrition, Department of Pediatrics,
University of Chicago, Chicago, IL, USA

Abstract

In most developed countries, gluten is currently most commonly introduced between 4 and 6 months of age, in spite of little evidence to support this practice. As for infants at risk of developing food allergies, there is clear evidence that introducing solid foods before the end of the 3rd month is detrimental and should be avoided. A recent growing body of evidence however challenges the notion that solids (and among them, gluten-containing foods) should be introduced beyond the 6th month of life. Another important aspect of gluten introduction into the diet has to do with its possible role in causing type-1 diabetes (IDDM). Recently, a large epidemiological investigation in a cohort of children at risk for IDDM found that exposure to cereals (rice, wheat, oats, barley, rye) that occurred early (≤ 3 months) as well as late (≥ 7 months) resulted in a significantly higher risk of the appearance of islet cell autoimmunity compared to the introduction between 4 and 6 months. As for celiac disease, the protective role of breastfeeding can be considered ascertained, especially the protection offered by having gluten introduced while breastfeeding is continued. Evidence is emerging that early (≤ 3 months) and perhaps even late (7 months or after) first exposure to gluten may favor the onset of celiac disease in predisposed individuals. Additionally, large amounts of gluten at weaning are associated with an increased risk of developing celiac disease, as documented in studies from Scandinavian countries. In celiac children observed in our center, we could show that breastfeeding at the time of gluten introduction delays the appearance of celiac disease and makes it less likely that its presentation is predominantly gastrointestinal. Based on current evidence, it appears reasonable to recommend that gluten be introduced in small amounts in the diet between 4 and 6 months, while the infant is breastfed, and that breastfeeding is continued for at least a further 2–3 months.

Introduction

Although no official recommendation from professional societies or academic bodies is available specifically on the timing of gluten introduction, with some exceptions [1], it would appear that most commonly gluten is introduced between 4 and 6 months of age. In fact, epidemiological surveys conducted in developed countries in the last couple of decades show a progressive trend toward shifting introduction of solid foods (even 15 years ago often still introduced with other cereals before 4 months) to a later age [2], and it is generally believed that the habit of introducing gluten into the diet around that time is justified [2–4]. In the United States, typically the first solid food to be introduced into the diet is rice cereal, followed by cereal grains (oats, barley, wheat and rye).

In the healthy child who does not belong to a group at risk for development of food allergy or celiac disease, there is a paucity of data to support or contradict such practice. From a purely digestive-absorptive view point, it could be argued that gluten-containing cereals should be tolerated by the time the combined digestive abilities of pancreatic amylase, brush-border-bound glucoamylase and pancreatic and brush border-bound peptidases have reached the capacity of fully digesting 'normal' amounts of the starch and protein components of such food staples, i.e. at the remarkably early age of 4–6 weeks, in full-term babies [5]. It remains to be seen whether such an early introduction is advisable, and as mentioned no recommendations endorse such practice.

Gluten Introduction and the Risk of Food Allergy

In infants at risk for food allergy on the other hand, many studies have been conducted, and recommendations based on a large body of evidence are now available from the American Academy of Pediatrics (AAP) [6] and from a joint committee of the European Society for Pediatric Gastroenterology, Hepatology and Nutrition (ESPGHAN) and of the European Society for Pediatric Allergy and Clinical Immunology (ESPACI) [7].

Both these recommendations are largely based on evidence that early introduction of solid foods (<3–4 months) may increase the risk of developing eczema and asthma, something that a subsequent study however does not appear to confirm [8]. According to both sets of recommendations, in infants at risk of developing food allergy breastfeeding should be exclusive for 4–6 months of age, with complementary food introduced during that time window [1, 6, 7]. However, it should be stressed that to date, only one very recent study has evaluated prospectively the timing of specific dietary exposures in relation to the development of specific food allergy in a population selected for being at risk of type-1 diabetes (IDDM) and/or celiac disease (see below for

Table 1. Adjusted odd ratios for development of wheat allergy [from 9]

Characteristics	Adjusted OR (95% CI)[a]
Age exposed to cereal grains (wheat, barley, rye, oats)	
0–6 months	1.00
≥7 months	3.8 (1.18–12.28)
Age exposed to rice cereal	
0–6 months	1.00
≥7 months	1.6 (0.46–5.23)
Breastfeeding duration, 1-month increase	1.05 (1.00–1.11)
Any food allergy before 6 months of age	
No	1.00
Yes	7.6 (2.67–21.9)
Family history of allergic disorders	
No	1.00
Yes	3.9 (1.40–10.88)

[a]All variables were included simultaneously in the logistic regression model.

more details on this cohort of children enrolled in the so-called 'DAISY' study), but not at risk of allergy [9]. Most previous studies, on which current recommendations are based, have in fact focused on eczema and asthma, complex disorders not always associated with food allergy. This specific study examined the association between cereal-grain exposure (wheat, barley, rye, oats) in the infant diet and development of wheat allergy in 1,612 children from birth until the mean age of 4.7 years. One percent of these children developed wheat allergy. Surprisingly, those who were first exposed to cereals after 6 months of age had an increased risk of wheat allergy compared with children first exposed to cereals before 6 months of age (see table 1).

Interestingly, the results of this prospective study are in substantial agreement with the findings of another recent study: a large, population-based, prospective birth cohort study conducted in Germany [10], showing that delaying solid food introduction beyond the 6th month did not offer protection toward atopic dermatitis or atopic sensitization.

Thus, taken together these very recent observations support the recommendation of introducing solids between 4 and 6 months of age as endorsed by the joint European committee [7] and in agreement with the AAP Committee on Nutrition [1], whilst they do not support the widely diffused practice to recommend further delaying the introduction of cereal grains beyond that time.

Gluten Introduction and the Risk of IDDM

Another important aspect of cereal (and hence gluten) introduction into the diet has to do with its role in causing IDDM. This condition results from the destruction of the insulin-producing cells of the pancreas. Autoantibodies to the islet cells, or islet autoimmunity, which mark this destructive process, can be present for years prior to the diagnosis of IDDM. Exposure to cereal in the infant diet has been implicated, albeit inconsistently, in the etiology of IDDM. First it was cow's milk that was associated with increased risk [11, 12], although different studies have yielded conflicting results. Studies of other foods in the infant diet have also been contradictory, with some investigations finding that IDDM cases had been exposed to solid foods earlier than controls [13, 14], others found no association [15, 16]. Recently, a role for cereals has been proposed as a result of the same large epidemiological investigation cited before (the DAISY study), conducted in a cohort of children at risk for IDDM followed prospectively from birth for a mean of 4.7 years [17]. This study documented that exposure to cereals (rice, wheat, oats, barley, rye) that occurred early (≤ 3 months) as well as late (≥ 7 months) resulted in a significantly higher risk of appearance of islet cell autoimmunity compared to introduction between 4 and 6 months. Figure 1 [from 17] shows the percentages of children developing islet cell autoimmunity in function of the age at first introduction of cereals. Interestingly, this study also showed that if cereals were introduced while the child was still breastfed, the risk of islet cell autoimmunity was reduced, independently of the age at introduction of cereals. A previous large study in Germany had also shown a similar increased risk of developing islet cell autoimmunity for children born to parents with IDDM when gluten is introduced during the first 3 months of life [18]. In both these studies, no effect of the duration of breastfeeding and/or age at introduction of cow's milk was detected [17, 18].

Gluten Introduction and the Risk of Celiac Disease

Arguably the most central aspect of gluten introduction into the diet regards the issue of how this may influence the appearance and/or the presentation of celiac disease.

In the last few years, a robust new wealth of knowledge has accumulated, leading to the understanding of celiac disease as an autoimmune reaction to the ubiquitous enzyme tissue transglutaminase (tTG) in the intestinal mucosa, initiated by exposure to dietary gluten in genetically predisposed individuals. Many details of this reaction have been revealed, and a role for innate immunity in the early phases of the process has been suggested [19]. Yet basic questions about the amount of gluten needed to trigger celiac disease and the possible role of the timing of its introduction into the diet have remained unanswered.

Once the role of gluten had been clearly identified, the quest to find a relation between the timing of its introduction into the diet and the appearance of celiac disease began. At the same time, the search for a possible protective

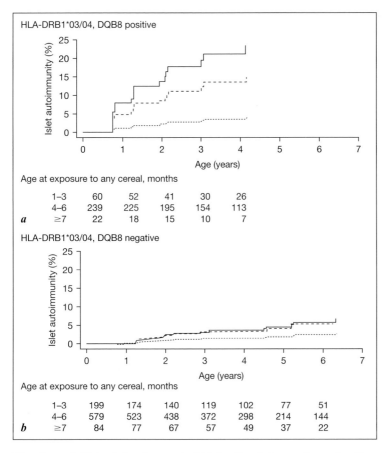

Fig. 1. a, b Risk of development of islet cell autoimmunity as function of the age at introduction of cereals [from 17]. The numbers in the tables below the graphs represent the number at risk.

role of breastfeeding was also unleashed, and the two were often conducted simultaneously.

The Protective Role of Breastfeeding

As for breastfeeding, as early as more than 50 years ago its protective role was already proposed [20]. The majority of subsequent investigations (though performed with different methodologies and thus somewhat hard to compare) did indeed find a negative correlation between its duration and the development of celiac disease [21–25], to the point that – also according to a very recent rigorous meta-analysis [26] – such a protective effect can now be considered universally accepted. For instance, the most recent study on this issue [24], a population-based case-referent study of Swedish children that examined 627

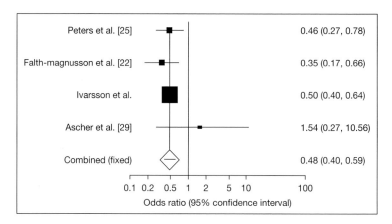

Fig. 2. Odds ratio of the effect of breastfeeding at the time of gluten introduction on the development of celiac disease [from 26].

cases with celiac disease and 1,254 referents showed that in children less than 2 years old, the median (25th, 75th centile) duration of breastfeeding was 5 months (3, 7) for cases and 7 months (4, 9) for controls (p < 0.001).

Another intriguing aspect of the protective role of breastfeeding that has recently received a great deal of attention based on the notion that breast milk may provide passive as well as active mucosal immunity [27, 28] is the possibility that breastfeeding at the time of gluten introduction may also prove to be of protective value. To test this hypothesis, several observational epidemiological studies have been conducted and reviewed in a recent meta-analysis [26]. All of them, with only one exception found in a small study [29], showed that introducing gluten during breastfeeding reduces the risk of development of celiac disease. Figure 2 [from 26] shows in a graphical manner the odds ratio of developing celiac disease if breastfed at the time of gluten introduction.

In our recent, unpublished series of 162 celiac children studied at the University of Chicago [30], we found some evidence that breastfeeding at the time of gluten introduction delays the appearance of celiac disease: in fact (see fig. 3) the age at diagnosis was slightly but significantly higher in children who had been breastfed at the time of gluten introduction as compared to those who were not. Additionally, celiac children who were breastfed at the time of gluten introduction were just as likely to develop typical (i.e. gastrointestinal) as atypical (i.e. extraintestinal) celiac disease (see fig. 4), whereas children who were not breastfed when weaned with gluten had a much higher chance of developing mostly gastrointestinal symptoms (fig. 4).

Therefore, while the evidence is there, the actual mechanism through which breast milk protects against the development of celiac disease is unclear. On an entirely speculative basis, three main theories seem plausible: (1) Continuing

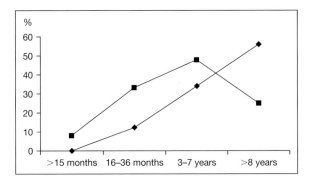

Fig. 3. Breastfeeding at the time of gluten introduction results in delayed appearance of celiac disease. ■ = Celiac children nonbreastfed at time of gluten introduction; ◆ = celiac children breastfed at time of gluten introduction (n = 162).

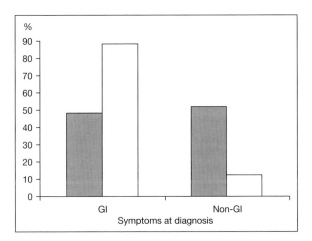

Fig. 4. Introduction of gluten while nonbreastfed is more likely to induce typical (gastrointestinal) symptoms in celiac children. □ = Celiac children nonbreastfed at time of gluten introduction; ▨ = celiac children breastfed at time of gluten introduction. Celiac children who were breastfed at the time of gluten introduction were just as likely to develop typical (i.e. gastrointestinal) as atypical (i.e. extraintestinal) celiac disease, whereas children who were not breastfed when weaned with gluten had a significantly (p < 0.01) higher chance of developing predominantly gastrointestinal symptoms (n = 162). GI = Gastrointestinal.

breastfeeding at the time of weaning results in a lower amount of gluten given to the infant, and so reduces the chances of the child developing symptoms of celiac disease. (2) Breast milk could, by preventing gastrointestinal infections, reduce the chances that they trigger pathophysiological mechanisms that may be contributing factors to the development of celiac disease. In fact, infections of the gastrointestinal tract in early life could lead to increased permeability of the intestinal mucosa, allowing the abnormal entry of gluten into the submucosal compartment. Enteric infections can also increase the expression of tTG, thus possibly increasing the production of deamidated gluten peptides. (3) Breast milk may possess unique immunomodulating effects that, by interfering with the early phases of the interaction between toxic peptides and the innate immune system of the intestinal mucosa, allow for the development of gluten tolerance.

Whatever the mechanism underlying the protective effect of breast milk, the big question that has puzzled researchers from early times remains: is such protection effective in completely aborting the onset of celiac disease in predisposed individuals, or is it simply delaying its appearance and/or causing it to appear in more subtle, less overtly symptomatic forms? To date, we have essentially no data to answer this, and larger epidemiological studies are needed.

The Specific Role of Gluten

Does the timing of gluten introduction per se, independently of breast-feeding, influence the development of celiac disease in predisposed individuals? Theoretically, this is an attractive possibility, as there might well be an age interval during which humans have a decreased ability to develop oral tolerance to a newly introduced antigen.

In reality, the results of most previous studies suggest that the age at first gluten exposure – while affecting the age at onset of symptoms – had actually no bearing on the development of celiac disease [21–23, 25]. All of the studies so far examined however had been conducted retrospectively. A recent prospective, 10-year observational study [31] conducted in the USA that enrolled 1,560 children considered at increased risk of celiac disease or IDDM came to a different conclusion, showing that initial exposure to gluten in the first 3 months or at 7 months and later significantly increased the risk of subsequent celiac disease autoimmunity (CDA), defined as a positive tTG on two or more consecutive visits or a positive tTG once with a small bowel biopsy consistent with celiac disease. The data have been generated as part of the larger study already mentioned, the so-called project DAISY (Diabetes Autoimmunity Study in the Young), aimed at prospectively describing the natural history of IDDM and CDA in genetically predisposed children. In this study, the increased risk of celiac disease or IDDM was defined as having either HLA-DR3 or DR4 alleles or a first degree relative with IDDM. The majority of children studied were identified at birth and followed for a mean of about 5 years, with serum tTG measured at 9, 15 and 24 months and yearly thereafter. Fifty-one children developed CDA. Their mean age at first positive tTG was 4.7 years. Three were exposed to wheat, barley, or rye between 1 and 3 months, 12 (23%) at 4–6 months, and 36 (71%) at 7 months or later. Among CDA-negative children, only 40 (3%),

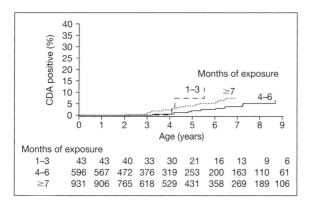

Fig. 5. Risk of CDA by months of exposure to gluten in entire cohort [from 31]. The numbers in the table below the graph represent the number at risk. Wilcoxon p = 0.04.

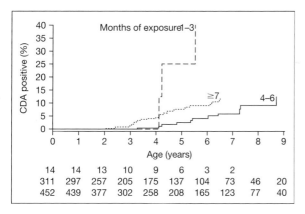

Fig. 6. Risk of CDA by months of exposure to gluten in HLA-DR3-positive children [from 31]. Wilcoxon p = 0.004.

574 (38%) and 895 (59%) were positive at the same time intervals. Adjusting for HLA-DR3 status, children exposed to gluten in the first 3 months of life had a 5-fold increased hazard of CDA compared with those exposed at 4–6 months. Figures 5 and 6 show the risk of CDA by month of exposure to gluten in the entire cohort and in those who were HLA-DR3 positive, respectively. Children not exposed to gluten until 7 months or later were at a slightly increased hazard of CDA compared with those exposed in the 4- to 6-month period (an only marginally significant difference, however).

An unexpected finding of this study was the lack of evidence for a protective effect of prolonged breastfeeding. This finding is in contradiction to the previous studies from Europe already commented upon. The discrepancy, besides being possibly due to different methodologies (most studies were done retrospectively and in populations including children not at genetic risk for celiac disease), may also be related to differences inherent in infant diets across studies, reflecting infant diet practices different from those of the United States.

But what about the amount of gluten in the diet? Does this factor also play a role? While this study completely leaves out this parameter [31], previous studies seem to suggest that indeed the amount of gluten may be a determinant in the risk of developing celiac disease. Ivarsson et al. [24] could demonstrate in their epidemiological investigation of 627 cases of celiac children and 1,254 referents that cases received a larger amount of flour, and that at 7 months of age, cases still consumed larger amounts of flour than referents. Another classical example is provided by the so-called Scandinavian paradox. In fact, it is known that a profound difference in the prevalence of celiac disease exists between the neighboring countries of Denmark, where a very low prevalence has repeatedly been found [32], and Sweden, where a much higher prevalence is reported. The explanation given for this is a striking difference in the diet of infants, who apparently receive much less gluten in Denmark [32]. Further evidence supporting the idea that the quantity of gluten is important comes again from Sweden where a so-called epidemic of celiac disease has been observed [33]. A sharp increase in symptomatic celiac disease in young children was thought to be related to a sudden increase in the consumption of gluten in infancy as a result of new dietetic guidelines (later changed for this reason). In analyzing the data from the 'epidemic' of the 1980s, and comparing them to the prevalence recorded subsequently in the same geographical areas, Carlsson et al. [34] found (see table 2) that the prevalence of celiac disease before the rules were changed (i.e. during a time of a higher amount of gluten at weaning) was overall 1.03% [35], including asymptomatic cases detected at screening and cases with gastrointestinal symptoms. This compared to a prevalence of only 0.39% in subsequent years [34], thus suggesting that indeed higher quantities of gluten in the diet of the weaning infant lead to a higher rate of appearance of celiac disease in the first 2 years of age. Although the story may be more complex than this, as new epidemiological data show that other factors have influenced the fluctuation in the prevalence of this condition in Sweden [36], we can conclude from the available evidence that the amount of gluten may be a major factor in the appearance of celiac disease.

Conclusions and Final Recommendations

It seems reasonable to conclude the following:

Table 2. Prevalence of celiac disease in 2- to 3-year-old children in Sweden [adapted from 34]

	Feeding rules of the late 1980s [35]	Feeding rules after 1996 [34]	p
Asymptomatic (diagnosed through screening)	9/960 (0.9%)	5/979 (0.7%)	NS
With gastrointestinal symptoms	22/3,004 (0.7%)	17/5,641 (0.3%)	<0.01
Total prevalence	31/3,004 (1.03%)	22/5,641 (0.39%)	<0.01

- Certainly early (0–3 months) and possibly late (>6 months) introduction of wheat into the diet is likely to increase the risk of wheat allergy.
- Early (0–3 months) and possibly late (>6 months) introduction of gluten into the diet is likely to increase the risk of IDDM in genetically predisposed children.
- Breastfeeding is likely to reduce the risk of celiac disease and/or to delay its onset.
- Introduction of gluten during breastfeeding reduces the risk of celiac disease (and/or significantly delays its onset) and influences the time and the type of presentation.
- Infants nonbreastfed at the time of gluten introduction seem to be more likely to develop typical (gastrointestinal) celiac disease.
- Introducing gluten at 4–6 months seems to be associated with the lowest risk of celiac disease.
- Introduction of 'large amounts' of gluten increases the risk of celiac disease.

From all of the above, the following final recommendations can be drawn for the prevention of celiac disease:

- Breastfeeding should be conducted for at least 6 months.
- Gluten should be introduced while the infant is breastfed between the age of 4 and 6 months.
- Gluten should be introduced in 'small amounts'.
- Breastfeeding should be conducted for at least 2–3 months after gluten introduction.

References

1 Kleinman RE: American Academy of Pediatrics recommendations for complementary feeding. Pediatrics 2000;106:1274.
2 Fewtrell MS, Lucas A, Morgan JB: Factors associated with weaning in full term and preterm infants. Arch Dis Child Fetal Neonatal Ed 2003;88:F296–F301.

3 van Odijk J, Hulthen L, Ahlstedt S, et al: Introduction of food during the infant's first year: a study with emphasis on introduction of gluten and of egg, fish and peanut in allergy-risk families. Acta Paediatr 2004;93:464–470.

4 Wilson AC, Forsyth JS, Greene SA, et al: Relation of infant diet to childhood health: seven year follow up of cohort of children in Dundee infant feeding study. BMJ 1998;316:21–25.

5 Auricchio S, Della Pietra D, Vegnente A: Studies on intestinal digestion of starch in man. II. Intestinal hydrolysis of amylopectin in infants and children. Pediatrics 1967;39:853–862.

6 American Academy of Pediatrics: Committee on Nutrition. Hypoallergenic infant formulas. Pediatrics 2000;106:346–349.

7 Host A, Koletzko B, Dreborg S, et al: Dietary products used in infants for treatment and prevention of food allergy. Joint Statement of the European Society for Paediatric Allergology and Clinical Immunology (ESPACI) Committee on Hypoallergenic Formulas and the European Society for Paediatric Gastroenterology, Hepatology and Nutrition (ESPGHAN) Committee on Nutrition. Arch Dis Child 1999;81:80–84.

8 Zutavern A, von Mutius E, Harris J, et al: The introduction of solids in relation to asthma and eczema. Arch Dis Child 2004;89:303–308.

9 Poole JA, Barriga K, Leung DY, et al: Timing of initial exposure to cereal grains and the risk of wheat allergy. Pediatrics 2006;117:2175–2182.

10 Zutavern A, Brockow I, Schaaf B, et al: Timing of solid food introduction in relation to atopic dermatitis and atopic sensitization: results from a prospective birth cohort study. Pediatrics 2006;117:401–411.

11 Savilahti E, Akerblom HK, Tainio VM, et al: Children with newly diagnosed insulin dependent diabetes mellitus have increased levels of cow's milk antibodies. Diabetes Res 1988;7: 137–140.

12 Virtanen SM, Saukkonen T, Savilahti E, et al: Diet, cow's milk protein antibodies and the risk of IDDM in Finnish children. Childhood Diabetes in Finland Study Group. Diabetologia 1994;37:381–387.

13 Kostraba JN, Cruickshanks KJ, Lawler-Heavner J, et al: Early exposure to cow's milk and solid foods in infancy, genetic predisposition, and risk of IDDM. Diabetes 1993;42:288–295.

14 Perez-Bravo F, Carrasco E, Gutierrez-Lopez MD, et al: Genetic predisposition and environmental factors leading to the development of insulin-dependent diabetes mellitus in Chilean children. J Mol Med 1996;74: 105–109.

15 Hypponen E, Kenward MG, Virtanen SM, et al: Infant feeding, early weight gain, and risk of type 1 diabetes. Childhood Diabetes in Finland (DiMe) Study Group. Diabetes Care 1999;22: 1961–1965.

16 Virtanen SM, Rasaner L, Ylonen K, et al: Early introduction of dairy products associated with increased risk of IDDM in Finnish children. The Childhood in Diabetes in Finland Study Group. Diabetes 1993;42:1786–1790.

17 Norris JM, Barriga K, Klingensmith G, et al: Timing of initial cereal exposure in infancy and risk of islet autoimmunity. JAMA 2003;290:1713–1720.

18 Ziegler AG, Schmid S, Huber D, et al: Early infant feeding and risk of developing type 1 diabetes-associated autoantibodies. JAMA 2003;290:1721–1728.

19 Hourigan CS: The molecular basis of coeliac disease. Clin Exp Med 2006;6:53–59.

20 Andersen DH, Di Sant'Agnese PA: Idiopathic celiac disease. I. Mode of onset and diagnosis. Pediatrics 1953;11:207–223.

21 Auricchio S, Follo D, de Ritis G, et al: Does breast feeding protect against the development of clinical symptoms of celiac disease in children? J Pediatr Gastroenterol Nutr 1983;2:428–433.

22 Falth-Magnusson K, Franzen L, Jansson G, et al: Infant feeding history shows distinct differences between Swedish celiac and reference children. Pediatr Allergy Immunol 1996;7:1–5.

23 Greco L, Auricchio S, Mayer M, et al: Case control study on nutritional risk factors in celiac disease. J Pediatr Gastroenterol Nutr 1988;7:395–399.

24 Ivarsson A, Hernell O, Stenlund H, et al: Breast-feeding protects against celiac disease. Am J Clin Nutr 2002;75:914–921.

25 Peters U, Schneeweiss S, Trautwein EA, et al: A case-control study of the effect of infant feeding on celiac disease. Ann Nutr Metab 2001;45:135–142.

26 Akobeng AK, Ramanan AV, Buchan I, et al: Effect of breast feeding on risk of coeliac disease: a systematic review and meta-analysis of observational studies. Arch Dis Child 2006;91: 39–43.

27 Goldman AS: Modulation of the gastrointestinal tract of infants by human milk. Interfaces and interactions. An evolutionary perspective. J Nutr 2000;130(suppl):426S–431S.
28 Hanson LA: Breastfeeding provides passive and likely long-lasting active immunity. Ann Allergy Asthma Immunol 1998;81:523–537.
29 Ascher H, Krantz I, Rydberg L, et al: Influence of infant feeding and gluten intake on coeliac disease. Arch Dis Child 1997;76:113–117.
30 Guandalini S: Influence of Diet on Presentation of Celiac Disease in Children in the USA. Chicago, University of Chicago Celiac Disease Center, 2007.
31 Norris JM, Barriga K, Hoffenberg EJ, et al: Risk of celiac disease autoimmunity and timing of gluten introduction in the diet of infants at increased risk of disease. JAMA 2005;293: 2343–2351.
32 Weile B, Cavell B, Nivenius K, et al: Striking differences in the incidence of childhood celiac disease between Denmark and Sweden: a plausible explanation. J Pediatr Gastroenterol Nutr 1995;21:64–68.
33 Ivarsson A, Persson LA, Nystrom L, et al: Epidemic of coeliac disease in Swedish children. Acta Paediatr 2000;89: 165–171.
34 Carlsson A, Agardh D, Borulf S, et al: Prevalence of celiac disease: before and after a national change in feeding recommendations. Scand J Gastroenterol 2006;41:553–558.
35 Carlsson AK, Axelsson IE, Borulf SK, et al: Serological screening for celiac disease in healthy 2.5-year-old children in Sweden. Pediatrics 2001;107:42–45.
36 Laurin P, Stenhammar L, Falth-Magnusson K: Increasing prevalence of coeliac disease in Swedish children: influence of feeding recommendations, serological screening and small intestinal biopsy activity. Scand J Gastroenterol 2004;39:946–952.

Discussion

Dr. Seidman: You talked about the risk of type 1 diabetes and its relationship to gluten but there is also the notion that untreated celiac disease is associated with an increased risk for other autoimmune diseases, particularly thyroiditis.

Dr. Guandalini: For those of you who are not too familiar with celiac disease, this is an autoimmune condition that is significantly associated with type 1 diabetes but also, as Dr. Seidman mentioned, with thyroiditis and other autoimmune conditions. In 1999 Ventura et al. [1] published a multicenter study in *Gastroenterology* showing that the later the diagnosis of celiac disease is made in time (i.e. the longer gluten was being eating while having celiac disease), the higher the cumulative prevalence of other associated autoimmune disorders. This appears as an interesting piece of evidence in favor of some link between celiac disease and the development of other autoimmune conditions. There are, however, no data that I am aware of regarding the timing of gluten and the onset of other autoimmune conditions aside from celiac disease and type 1 diabetes. As for thyroiditis, the prevalence of celiac disease in this condition is certainly higher than in the normal population, and is estimated to be around 3–4% [2, 3]. In this specific case, there are still doubts that celiac disease is really acting as a trigger [4].

Dr. Krebs: I am curious about the findings in relation to the introduction of complementary food in that the most common cereal introduced first in the US is rice. How carefully has it been documented that there are other sources of gluten and what are those sources? Norris et al. [5] have good dietary data.

Dr. Guandalini: Indeed rice is the cereal most commonly introduced first, followed then by grain cereals like wheat mostly; rye, barley and oats are uncommonly used early in life. In the paper by Norris et al. [5] the data refer to any cereal introduction, and they do comment, however, that even considering those who only have wheat as the first cereal, the same results hold true. It doesn't have to be gluten per se, for instance there is a very recent paper by Mojibian et al. [6] showing that individuals who have type 1 diabetes have higher levels of antibodies against a wheat storage protein called glb1 than patients who do not have type 1 diabetes, suggesting there may be other wheat storage proteins.

Dr. Ziegler: Can you enlighten us on the relationship between wheat allergy and celiac disease?

Dr. Guandalini: Very simply stated, there is no relationship. Wheat allergy is one of the many food allergic conditions, mostly of transient nature, that frequently affect babies, while celiac disease is a permanent, autoimmune-induced sensitivity to gluten.

Dr. Seidman: I was intrigued by your comments on rotavirus infection and the onset of celiac disease. Are you saying that individuals who are already on gluten when they have a rotavirus infection are more likely to develop celiac disease afterwards?

Dr. Guandalini: I included rotavirus among the possible environmental factors because of a recent epidemiological investigation by the Denver group [7], retrospectively showing a significantly higher prevalence of rotavirus infection in the second semester of age in patients who then develop celiac disease versus matched controls. The authors' speculation is that the enteritis, which is well know to cause a profound disruption in small intestinal permeability, might have favored the onset of celiac autoimmunity in predisposed individuals by allowing a much higher entry of toxic gluten epitopes.

Dr. Seidman: One of the focuses of this workshop is childhood exposure to foods and the onset of disease later in life. It is fair to say that most celiac patients are diagnosed as adults, not as children or infants, yet most human beings have rotavirus infection during childhood and infancy. We know that these patients have predisposing genes, HLA DQ2 or DQ8, and that they ingest gluten and yet they present with celiac disease in adulthood, long after a rotavirus infection.

Dr. Guandalini: Your point is well taken. However, we should note that it takes time for celiac autoimmunity to develop. In fact, even in the study by the same Denver group that prospectively followed genetically predisposed babies from birth, it was apparent that nobody actually had any detectable antibody levels before the age of 3 and half or so. Of course I understand your point, it is difficult to accept the concept that you have a rotavirus infection when you are 6 months old and then you develop celiac disease at 25 years. However, not much is known about the timing of the development of autoimmunity in any such condition.

Dr. Seidman: Is there any evidence that the feeding practices you discussed, breastfeeding and introduction to gluten, in fact have an impact on adult onset of celiac disease?

Dr. Guandalini: Very good question that I am afraid cannot be answered yet. I had the opportunity to discuss this issue with Dr. Peter Green at Columbia University in New York. His group is now looking into the relationship between early feeding habits and the development of celiac disease in adulthood. A major undertaking, as you can imagine, given the uncertainty about lucid history after many years.

Dr. Domellöf: Ivarsson [8] is currently performing a screening study of schoolchildren born before and after the Swedish celiac epidemic, and the preliminary results show that children born before the change in dietary recommendations have a high prevalence of celiac disease. The interesting part is the screening of the children born after the change in recommendations, and we are still awaiting those results.

Dr. Shahkhalili: What is the prevalence of celiac disease and type 1 diabetes in developing and developed countries? Should we have different recommendations for the introduction of gluten-containing cereal for different ethnic groups?

Dr. Guandalini: Basically all of my presentation was related to the situation in developed countries, all of these data have been generated there. I am not aware of data on type 1 diabetes, but to answer your question in terms of celiac disease, the disease is so strongly associated with HLA DQ2 and DQ8 that the current thinking is that, in practical terms, there is no celiac disease outside these haplotypes. Now these haplotypes are found in about 30–35% of the white population regardless of where in the world they were born. However, if you then go to the black population the prevalence of these haplotypes is close to zero, so the current thinking is that you cannot develop celiac disease in those areas.

Dr. Haschke: What you are saying is in contradiction to the WHO recommendations, so we need a debate on this. Do you think that, at the present time, the data are strong enough to be transferred to scientific committees for evaluation, and then to enter into discussion whether in the respective developed countries with Caucasian populations the feeding recommendations should be modified? The WHO recommendations are for the sake of the children in the whole world, therefore they are being introduced in Europe and in the United States. If there are good reasons in this cost-benefit ratio calculation, how many children more will suffer from celiac disease if gluten is introduced later versus earlier, say 4–6 months; this has to be taken into consideration. Are we far enough advanced in our understanding to start such a debate?

Dr. Guandalini: Of course it is not for me to propose changes to the WHO guidelines. I will simply give you my opinion. Firstly, one needs to consider that actually, whether we want it or not, whether our official academic bodies want it or not, in developed countries children are weaned before 6 months in spite of current WHO recommendations. I believe this is not going to change significantly. Secondly, I think we have sufficient evidence that if children in developed countries are weaned after 6 months according to the WHO recommendations, this would expose us to the obvious risk of introducing gluten at a time when breastfeeding is no longer given. In all the most recent studies the prevalence of celiac disease autoimmunity has been estimated to be close to 1% [9], so we are probably talking about the most common genetic condition of the white population. Thus, it does not appear trivial. Additionally, studies have shown that if gluten is introduced after 6–7 months of age the amount of gluten is larger [10]. So not only do we end up introducing gluten after breastfeeding has stopped, but it is also given in a larger amount. In my humble opinion I think that the time has arrived for academic panels to discuss this and possibly carve out a slightly different set of recommendations for Caucasian children. Rather than going 'against' the WHO recommendations, here the matter is to suggest a rethinking of recommendations for a specific, albeit very large part of the world population. This is something that, for example, has already been successfully done with the composition of oral rehydration solutions (ORS). I was on the panel that in 1992 recommended a new low osmolality ORS for developed countries then promulgated by ESPGHAN [11]. It took the WHO 12 years, and in 2004 they essentially accepted the same composition for ORS that we recommended, even for children with cholera [12]. It seems to me that large bodies such as the WHO, that have a global vision, are by definition slower in adopting new recommendations. I think nevertheless that whenever the scientific evidence is there, and especially if it were endorsed, as has been the case for ORS, by scientific societies like ESPGHAN, even the WHO should feel the need to examine all the evidence and come up, if necessary, with a revised set of recommendations that again might be applicable to only part of the world, in our case the Caucasian population that is at a significant risk for celiac disease. I repeat, after all, current practices already do follow such a pattern for the most part.

Dr. Gailing: Last year during the nutrition CODEX committee meeting we adopted the CODEX standard on cereal-based food with the recommendation to start at 6 months and to have these accordingly labeled on the products so it will be now translated into all the regulations throughout the world. How do you recommend managing this issue? We will be discussing this again next week in the CODEX committee meeting in Thailand. We will also discuss the gluten-free food standard and again we will probably have the same results with the introduction after 6 months.

Dr. Guandalini: I hear your urgency but I am not a political man, I am not a representative who can make decisions. So unfortunately it is not me you should ask.

Dr. Solomons: Returning to the point of preventing gluten exposure at an inappropriate time for susceptible individuals, and referring back to the screening issue. Since it is all HLA subtype-related, presumably people without that subtype can have gluten anytime or never without any effect. Therefore what is the cost of a plan in which a susceptible population, i.e. Europeans, would be screened prior to 4 months, let's say, and depending upon their positive/negative HLA appropriate type how should they be advised specifically by their pediatricians? So that means that anyone else who is immune, who doesn't have the HLA, can just do whatever nature and their mothers want.

Dr. Guandalini: There are a lot of implications to your question, and two come to mind, one is the issue of cost. At least in the United States, checking for HLA DQ2 DQ8 is very expensive, in the order of several hundred dollars for one test. So if you want to extend these to every newborn, the cost would be prohibitive. On the other hand, restricting HLA testing to the offspring of celiac patients might be a more reasonable approach because then you would identify those who are at a direct risk for celiac disease and only they will have to follow the recommendations. As an alternative, dietetic advice for each newborn could be given to every parent with celiac disease.

Dr. Solomons: Is there a possibility to lower the cost?

Dr. Guandalini: From a technical standpoint, perhaps.

Dr. Solomons: You said the prevalence is 1 in 150.

Dr. Guandalini: The prevalence of celiac disease is currently estimated to be around 1% [9].

Dr. Solomons: You could calculate the annual cost based on the birth rate in a country multiplied by the current cost, and you could calculate the cost burden for that kind of screening. Obviously again technological solutions are needed to get a cheaper screening because the implications of everyone following the recommendations for only 1 in 100 is relevant. It is another ethical issue.

Dr. Guandalini: I totally understand. I think the issue is well raised and the answer might come from looking more in depth at cost-benefit ratios before making new recommendations. That said, however, I frankly fail to see a great risk in following the dietetic recommendations of the sort I indicated.

Dr. Solomons: The risk is following recommendations that violate the dictums of the WHO in a 'politically correct' sense of the word, and that is to the extent that you are suggesting that the black or the brown or the yellow or the red pigmented ethnic groups are exempted from the same recommendations. This could set up a situation of suspicion among those groups excluded from your preventive considerations.

Dr. Vieira: It is interesting that you did not mention oats. Here in Brazil and probably in some other countries, mothers add oats to fruits or other complementary foods. Although oats have been shown not to be damaging for celiac patients in vitro and in vivo, do you think we should stick to the idea of not recommending oats in the diet of these infants?

Dr. Guandalini: From data, not only in vitro but also in vivo, and from a number of papers over the last 12 years or so, I have a strong conviction that oats are perfectly safe for the vast majority of celiac children. All my patients eat oats, and to the best of my knowledge, none of them has unexpectedly developed high levels of autoantibodies or anti-gliadin antibodies or has experienced any side effect. One needs to be aware, however, that there is the remote possibility, well documented in a paper by Arentz-Hansen et al. [13], that a tiny subset of, probably extremely rare, celiac patients may react to a chronic ingestion of large amounts of oats. More commonly, the issue with oats is that one must be sure that there is no cross-contamination in the manufacturing line between wheat-containing flours and oats because this might be the case.

Dr. Uy: I am wondering about autoimmunity in the development of type 1 diabetes. Were those children screened for DQβ? I understand that they were screened for DR3 but were they screened for DQβ Asp57, and was it is positive or negative?

Dr. Guandalini: In Caucasians, the susceptibility to type 1 diabetes strongly correlates with the absence of aspartic acid at position 57 on the DQβ chain. The formation of a putative DQ susceptibility molecule (such as DQβ Asp57−) accounts best for the disease association. That said, I am not aware if the children described in the studies by the Denver group were also screened for DQβ Asp57−. They certainly were assessed for their HLA DR3 status.

Dr. Uy: If they are positive, they are more protected from having the autoimmunity.

Dr. Guandalini: As mentioned, my recollection of the paper is that they were HLA DR3 positive, I am not sure if the DQβ status was checked.

References

1 Ventura A, Magazzu G, Greco L: Duration of exposure to gluten and risk for autoimmune disorders in patients with celiac disease. SIGEP Study Group for Autoimmune Disorders in Celiac Disease. Gastroenterology 1999;117:297–303.
2 Berti I, Trevisiol C, Tommasini A, et al: Usefulness of screening program for celiac disease in autoimmune thyroiditis. Dig Dis Sci 2000;45:403–406.
3 Volta U, Ravaglia G, Granito A, et al: Coeliac disease in patients with autoimmune thyroiditis. Digestion 2001;64:61–65.
4 Sumnik Z, Cinek O, Bratanic N, et al: Thyroid autoimmunity in children with coexisting type 1 diabetes mellitus and celiac disease: a multicenter study. J Pediatr Endocrinol Metab 2006;19:517–522.
5 Norris JM, Barriga K, Hoffenberg EJ, et al: Risk of celiac disease autoimmunity and timing of gluten introduction in the diet of infants at increased risk of disease. JAMA 2005;293: 2343–2351.
6 Mojibian M, Chakir H, MacFarlane AJ, et al: Immune reactivity to a glb1 homologue in a highly wheat-sensitive patient with type 1 diabetes and celiac disease. Diabetes Care 2006;29: 1108–1110.
7 Stene LC, Honeyman MC, Hoffenberg EJ, et al: Rotavirus infection frequency and risk of celiac disease autoimmunity in early childhood: a longitudinal study. Am J Gastroenterol 2006;101:2333–2340.
8 Ivarsson A: The Swedish epidemic of coeliac disease explored using an epidemiological approach – some lessons to be learnt. Best Pract Res Clin Gastroenterol 2005;19:425–440.
9 AGA Institute: AGA Institute Medical Position Statement on the Diagnosis and Management of Celiac Disease. Gastroenterology 2006;131:1977–1980.
10 Ivarsson A, Hernell O, Stenlund H, Persson LA: Breast-feeding protects against celiac disease. Am J Clin Nutr 2002;75:914–921.
11 Recommendations for composition of oral rehydration solutions for the children of Europe. Report of an ESPGAN Working Group. J Pediatr Gastroenterol Nutr 1992;14:113–115.
12 Joint Statement World Health Organization and UNICEF: Clinical management of acute diarrhoea. WHO Bulletin. Geneva, WHO, 2004.
13 Arentz-Hansen H, Fleckenstein B, Molberg O, et al: The molecular basis for oat intolerance in patients with celiac disease. PLoS Med 2004;1:e1.

Agostoni C, Brunser O (eds): Issues in Complementary Feeding.
Nestlé Nutr Workshop Ser Pediatr Program, vol 60, pp 157–169,
Nestec Ltd., Vevey/S. Karger AG, Basel, © 2007.

Allergic Infants: Growth and Implications while on Exclusion Diets

Kirsi Laitinen[a,b,d], *Erika Isolauri*[c,d]

[a]Department of Biochemistry and Food Chemistry, [b]Functional Foods Forum and
[c]Department of Pediatrics, University of Turku and [d]Department of Pediatrics, Turku
University Central Hospital, Turku, Finland

Abstract

The complex nature of allergic disease exposes infants to an increased risk of nutritional inadequacies. Allergic inflammation requiring extensive dietary regimens may underlie the poor growth frequently reported. Nutritional management is directed towards the prevention of explicitly diet-related deficiencies, the mainstay of treatment of food allergy being strict avoidance of offending antigens in the diet. The advantage of elimination diets lies in silencing the specific allergic inflammation induced by the food responsible, the effect thus being antigen-specific. Concomitantly, food may also contain immunomodulatory factors, and indeed research into the management of allergic disease is evolving from passive allergen avoidance to the invention of novel dietary compounds with specific effects in alleviating the immunoinflammatory reaction and stabilizing the gut mucosal barrier. Active schemes include supplementation of nutrients, particularly fatty acids and antioxidant vitamins, and probiotics with properties influencing immunoregulatory pathways. However, the conceivable joint effects of a range of nutrients and other potentially active components in the subject's habitual diet cannot be ruled out. Prior to implementation of these concepts in management regimes or products for infants, further exploration of their effects and mechanisms, including both short- and long-term safety evaluation, is called for.

Introduction

Food allergy frequently constitutes the first manifestation of allergic disorders. Moreover, food allergy regularly accompanies atopic diseases at an early age, particularly atopic eczema. Concomitantly, however, food may contain a variety of immunomodulatory factors providing protection against allergic disease.

Food is linked to current theories explaining the increasing prevalence of atopic diseases, atopic eczema, allergic rhinoconjunctivitis and asthma over recent decades throughout the industrialized world. First, the hygiene hypothesis stating that the increase is related to reduced exposure to microbes at an early age also holds true for human nutrition. The shift in food preservation from drying and natural fermentation to industrial pasteurization and sterilization has reduced the microbial exposure associated with food intake [1]. More recently, the increase in the incidence of allergic diseases has been explained by western dietary habits. There are data suggesting that dietary lipids, especially long-chain polyunsaturated fatty acids, regulate immune function and may contribute to the development and severity of the symptoms of allergic diseases [2]. An inflammatory process results in endogenously generated oxidative stress and tissue injury, and exogenous oxidants may further exacerbate existing allergic manifestations, which underlines the importance of diet-derived antioxidant defense [3].

The basic foundation here lies in a healthy, balanced diet which follows dietary recommendations and guides healthy development and normal growth [2]. Nutritional management aims to prevent direct diet-related deficiencies, acknowledging the fact that the disease state, food allergy, may make specific requirements for energy and nutrients necessary, a deficiency in which may contribute to the deterioration of nutritional status and growth failure in children. The mainstay in the treatment of food allergy is indeed strict avoidance of offending antigens in the diet [4]. The advantage of elimination diets appears to lie in silencing the specific allergic inflammation induced by the food responsible, the effect thus being antigen-specific. Elimination diets have, however, been applied in attempts both to prevent and treat the allergic condition in early childhood. Despite the persuasive rationale of thereby reducing exposure to the most important source of antigens early in life, results have been disappointing [5]. The fact that allergies to foods of vital importance, including cow's milk, predominate in early childhood, together with the recent demonstration of nutritional repercussions of such dietary regimens, calls for an improved understanding of the nutritional needs of the allergic child. Consequently, the management of allergic disease evolves from passive allergen avoidance to the introduction of novel dietary compounds with specific effects in alleviating the immunoinflammatory reaction and stabilizing the gut mucosal barrier (fig. 1).

Is Allergy Manifested by Poor Growth?

A number of studies in children have indeed shown that food allergy and atopic eczema are related to poor growth [6–10]. In addition to direct effects on height and weight, body composition, mainly muscle mass [11] and bone growth [6, 8], may be adversely affected, which is also reflected in serum

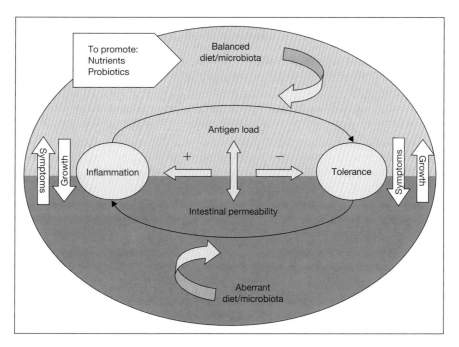

Fig. 1. The complex nature of the dietary management of food allergy. Dietary antigens induce local hypersensitivity reaction impairing the barrier function of the intestine and leading to perpetuation of the inflammation and hampering tolerance induction. Nutritional management includes elimination and a balanced diet with immunomodulatory agents.

nutritional markers [7, 9]. Even though poor growth is evinced in allergy, growth failure would not appear to be a feature of allergy (atopic eczema) per se and would not be irreversible considering the adult height attained [12]. Factors related to the severity of the disease, to inflammation and to the type of dietary management may be more relevant, which possibly explains the relatively high prevalence of short stature, ranging from 2 to 15%, in allergic patients [6, 8, 11, 12].

Link to Poor Growth: Impaired Gut Barrier Function in Allergic Disease

Food allergy can affect several organ systems. Symptoms commonly arise from the gut, skin and respiratory tract. Clinical manifestations include acute-onset skin reactions such as urticaria, pruritus and exanthema, bowel disorders such as vomiting and diarrhea, and in the respiratory tract wheezing and

159

sneezing. Delayed-onset eczematous or gastrointestinal reactions such as loose stools, chronic diarrhea, malabsorption and failure to thrive are also frequently seen [13].

Patients with early onset of symptoms, manifesting during the first few months of life, compared to later onset, 6–10 months of age [9], appear to be more seriously affected and the delay in growth may be more pronounced. Further, skin more widely or severely affected by atopic dermatitis [6, 8, 10], associated asthma [6] or multiple food allergies in comparison to single food allergies [14] appear to affect the growth of patients. This may reflect allergy-related inflammation, which if sustained may result in reduced bioavailability or loss of nutrients, while metabolic requirements may be increased.

Indeed, notwithstanding the wide variation in symptoms and immune responder types, food allergy consistently affects the gut barrier, which means that dietary antigens penetrate the mucosal barrier of the intestine, and that the antigens absorbed induce an immunoinflammatory response [4]. Dietary antigens induce a local hypersensitivity reaction which impairs the barrier function of the intestine. Mucosal dysfunction may lead to aberrant absorption of intraluminal antigens. Targets in the treatment of cow's milk allergy include elimination of the antigen responsible, alleviation of the immunoinflammatory reaction and stabilization of the gut mucosal barrier.

Elimination

Apart from alleviation of symptoms, antigen elimination preserves the barrier function of the intestine and prevents aberrant antigen absorption [as reviewed in 4]. Antigen elimination reverses the disturbance of the humoral and cell-mediated immune response, seen in a fall in serum total and specific IgE concentrations and a reduction in the proliferative response of peripheral blood mononuclear cells to the antigen. Antigen elimination improves the capacity of T lymphocyte regulation and immune elimination of dietary antigens in the gut. Uncoordinated elimination, again, may carry a risk of general nutritional inadequacy or deficiency in essential single nutrients, which for its part may even amplify the risk of sensitization. Hence the advantage of elimination diets appears to lie in silencing the specific allergic inflammation induced by the food responsible, the response being antigen-specific. The completeness of antigen elimination remains, however, questionable, as immunoreactive components of dietary protein can be detected in all substitute formulas currently available and even in breast milk. In any case therapeutic elimination diets may be potentially hazardous; recent case reports document fatal allergy as a possible consequence of a long-term elimination diet [15] and acute allergic reactions in children with atopic eczema/dermatitis syndrome after prolonged cow's milk elimination diets [16].

Alleviation of the Inflammatory Response

The growth of allergic breastfed infants has been shown to differ from that expected for age [17]. Restoration of nutritional parameters and normal growth is achieved concomitantly with alleviation of the symptoms of allergic disease, which would imply that sustained food allergy may cause poor growth. Indeed, the target organs of allergic inflammation, the skin and the gut, are tissues with a rapid turnover even in the normal state. Persistent unnoticed inflammation in the skin or in the gut may cause ongoing nutrient loss. In an experimental animal model, active inflammation, via release of proinflammatory cytokines, has recently been shown to directly impair linear bone growth, independent of nutritional intake [4, 18].

Promotion of the Barrier

It has been shown that a positive oral food challenge reaction results in albumin secretion in the gut, increased fecal α_1-antitrypsin and tumor necrosis factor-α concentrations, as well as increased intestinal permeability [4]. Data on atopic patients with multiple food allergies indicate that altered macromolecular absorption in the gut may proceed even when the patient is on an elimination diet [19]. It is conceivable, however, that persistent unnoticed intestinal inflammation in these patients could have deranged the intestinal barrier. In a like manner, differences in the neonatal gut microbiota, in particular the balance between *Bifidobacterium* and *Clostridium* microbiota, may precede the manifestation of the atopic responder type with heightened production of antigen-specific IgE antibodies, suggesting a crucial role for the balance of the indigenous intestinal bacteria in the maturation of human immunity to a nonatopic mode. The establishment of an indigenous microbiota has a particularly strong impact on the immunophysiological regulation in the gut. The importance of the immunoregulatory potential of the gut microbiota is emphasized in a recent demonstration of cross-talk between the innate and the adaptive immune systems; the nature of the initial immune response governs the homeostasis of the adaptive immune response. The gut microbiota provides maturational signals for the gut-associated lymphoid tissue, particularly for the IgA plasma cells, conferring the first line of host immunological defense. Realization of this has led to the introduction of novel modes of therapeutic intervention based on the consumption of mono- and mixed cultures of beneficial live microorganisms as probiotics.

A number of probiotics have a long history of safe use and a demonstrated safety record in human consumption, and no health concerns have been observed [20]. The numerous immunological properties of probiotics have, however, raised concern over possible effects on the growth of infants. In our 4-year follow-up study the height of children was unaffected, but there was a tendency for their weight to be lower in the group perinatally receiving probiotics [11].

Diet-Related Causes for Poor Growth

The management of food allergy by elimination diet may not be without risks, particularly in cases where the avoidance of nutritionally significant foods such as milk or cereals is necessary. Undesirably, alongside the management of documented food allergies, elimination diets are also used in attempts to control the symptoms of a wider range of allergic conditions, most often in a self-determined manner [21]. The consequences of such dieting may be severe and even manifest themselves in a failure to thrive, as demonstrated in children whose parents chose to implement elimination diets [22]. In point of fact, inadequate or unbalanced intakes of energy and particular nutrients in food allergy [7, 14, 23] and to a lesser extent in atopic eczema [11] have been demonstrated in studies analyzing dietary intake from food records. On the other hand, dietary treatment, i.e. intakes of nutrients [7], number of foods eliminated from the diet and substituted by other foods of the same group [8, 9], or type of feeding, whether breastfed or formula-fed [10], has not explained poor growth or has only marginally influenced growth impairment. Feeding practices in infancy, including breast- or formula feeding, and the age at introduction of complementary foods have been related to the risk of allergy, but their relation to growth is more intricate, which most likely reflects the lack of randomized studies owing to ethical considerations and the difficult task of relating dietary intake to growth. Generally the intake over only a few days may be analyzed, whereas disturbances in growth may manifest with delay. Clearly long-term insufficiency of intake contributes to a deterioration in nutritional status and growth failure in children. Reduced energy availability originates from three main sources: reduced food intake due to poor appetite or symptoms of the disease such as gastrointestinal complaints or poor utilization of nutrients, increased losses, e.g. due to steatorrhea, or increased requirements, e.g. due to infections [2]. On the other hand, reduced physical activity due to ill health may compensate for the increased energy requirements. Appropriate guidance and monitoring of elimination diets and nutritional status are essential to the successful management of the disease, since the regulation of food intake may result in both quantitative and qualitative changes in dietary composition with effects which extend beyond growth. The current challenge lies in evaluation of the possible effects of dietary composition not only on growth but, in a wider perspective, on immune function.

Balanced Diet for the Allergic Infant

Diet may play a more significant role in the management of allergy than traditionally assumed. The natural interest in dietary factors in relation to allergic diseases has centered on proteins, the antigens, since their exclusion from the diet forms the basis for management of documented food allergies.

With scientific knowledge accruing the significance of the diet for the maturing immune system in early infancy to ensure normal growth and development has received increasing attention. Specific nutrients and supplemental dietary compounds with immunomodulatory properties, including lipids, antioxidants and probiotics, have been exploited in therapeutic interventions. Food may not only be a source of dietary antigens causing sensitization, but may also contain protective factors. This may be particularly important in the case of food allergies in balancing the restricted diet ensuing upon the management of the disease, i.e. elimination.

Realization of a link between dietary lipids and health dates from studies with Eskimos showing an association between the consumption of fatty fish and a low prevalence of cardiovascular diseases and asthma. Since then, the mechanisms whereby long-chain polyunsaturated fatty acids may modulate health have been extensively studied and evidence has accrued for their immunomodulatory properties [24], amenable to application in both the regulation of symptoms and reduction of the risk of allergic disease. Equally, antioxidants, including ascorbic acid, β-carotene, α-tocopherol, selenium and zinc, may counteract endogenously generated oxidative stress resulting from inflammatory processes in allergic disease [3]. In sequence, probiotics, added dietary compounds or compounds resulting from traditional food preparation methods, i.e. fermentation, exhibit a range of properties influencing health, among them their ability to avert deviant microbiota development, strengthen the immature or impaired gut barrier function and alleviate abnormal immune responsiveness [1]. Current practice focuses on active prevention schemes, including supplementation of nutrients and probiotics with properties influencing immunoregulatory pathways and thus with potential health effects. However, the diversity of nutrients and other potentially active components in the subject's habitual diet and their conceivable joint effects may not be ruled out. A combination of dietary compounds would indeed appear to exert effects on the child's health outcome [11]. The route for the first allergic responses arises from the gastrointestinal tract, and early modification of the diet towards a balanced intake of nutrients, with account taken of interactions amongst nutrients and microbes, may thus offer a tool for either prevention or management in addressing the increasing problem of allergic disease.

Fatty Acids, Vitamins and Probiotics to Balance the Diet

The most frequently reported abnormality in cell fatty acid composition in allergy, an imbalance between series n-6 and n-3 fatty acids, has been addressed in an attempt to modify the dietary lipid composition, mainly by an increase in intake of n-3 fatty acids; the expected effect was reduced production of the n-6 fatty acid-derived mediator, prostaglandin E_2 (PGE_2),

163

which has been linked to elevated IgE synthesis due to the induction of B cell differentiation in the presence of IL-4 [25]. A recent systematic review failed, however, to show consistent associations between consumption of n-3 polyunsaturated fatty acids, their sources being fish or fish oil supplements, and asthma [26]. Likewise, according to a meta-analysis, the severity of atopic eczema was not improved by fish oil supplementation [27]. In more controlled settings, infusion of n-3 fatty acid-based lipid emulsion for adult patients with atopic dermatitis has resulted in an improvement in symptoms [28]. The conflicting results may be explained by the different roles of fatty acids depending on the end-organ manifestations, skin or respiratory, or the types of allergy, namely atopic and nonatopic eczema [29]. Further, despite their apparent proinflammatory role, n-6 fatty acids may also contribute to an anti-inflammatory intestinal environment, as antigen stimulation up-regulates PGE_2 production from the n-6 fatty acid arachidonic acid, with ensuing suppression of antigen-specific T cell proliferation in gut-associated lymphoid tissue [30]. Polyunsaturated fatty acids may also exert their effects at the site of antigen introduction, since they are known to influence the integrity of the intestinal epithelium by regulating tight junction permeability [31].

Evidence for the joint action of dietary compounds comes from studies showing that polyunsaturated fatty acids affect the growth and adhesion of probiotics to the mucus and epithelial cells, thus modifying the fatty acid milieu within the intestine, the inflammatory mediators derived from them being thus readjusted by the intestinal microbiota [32]. With respect to mucosal function other nutrients, particularly glutamine, important for replication and functioning of the gastrointestinal cells, and vitamin A, may also have protective effects. In allergic disease, vitamin A has been found to inhibit IgE production in mouse peripheral blood mononuclear cells [33]. Additionally, supplementation with vitamin A in mice has resulted in depression of interferon-γ and IL-4, the potential cytokines in allergic disease, and in an increase in mucosal IgA, with the capacity to protect mucosal surfaces [34]. Further, vitamin A may play a role in strengthening the host microbe interaction known to control intestinal epithelial homeostasis. The link between vitamins and fatty acid metabolism arises from the capacity of vitamin A to alter the activation of the arachidonic acid cascade and hence suppress PGE_2 production in vitro [35].

Probiotics are live microbial food supplements or components of bacteria which have been demonstrated to have beneficial effects on human health [1]. Modification of the gut microbiota by probiotics and the immunomodulatory effects of specific probiotic strains may be taken as an alternative to attain a prophylactic or therapeutic effect in allergic disease in early childhood. The effects of probiotics in allergic disease have been attributed to restoration to normal of increased intestinal permeability and unbalanced gut microecology, improvement in the intestine's immunological barrier functions, alleviation of the intestinal inflammatory response, and reduced generation of proinflammatory cytokines characteristic of local and systemic allergic inflammation [1]. Moreover, the potential of specific strains of the gut microbiota to contribute to the generation of T helper 1- and T helper 3-type immune responses counterregulating the T helper 2-type immune responses in atopic disease may create optimal conditions to redirect the polarized immunological memory of the newborn to a healthy balance and thereby reduce the risk of atopic disease. The objective of probiotic intervention in allergy is to control the allergic inflammatory response, before the T helper 2-type immune responsiveness to environmental antigens is consolidated and before altered structure and function develop in the target organ.

Conclusions

Infants with allergic disease are at risk of nutritional inadequacies resulting from the complex nature of the disease. Careful dietary planning and monitoring allow the growth of infants to reach their genetic potential and population reference range. Failure to thrive may result from inadequate monitoring, as the reasons for growth failure are various, mainly related to elimination diets and disease-related inflammation. The challenge for the future lies in discovering an appropriate combination of active compounds and exploring their mechanisms of action for use as dietary supplements within a balanced diet or in modifying the infant's diet to reinforce the development of innate immunity in the infant and management of allergic disease. A novel approach in the management is offered by joining the forces of nutrients and probiotics as dietary components, i.e. active prevention management as opposed to passive elimination diets. Particularly patients with extensive disease whose growth is most seriously affected may benefit from such an approach. Prior to applying these concepts in management regimes or products for infants, further exploration of their effects and their mechanisms, including both short- and long-term safety evaluation, is of the essence.

References

1 Isolauri E: Probiotics in human disease. Am J Clin Nutr 2001;73:1142S–1146S.
2 Laiho K, Isolauri E: Biotherapeutic and nutraceutical agents; in Guandalini S (ed): Textbook of Pediatric Gastroenterology and Nutrition. London, Taylor & Francis, 2004, pp 525–537.
3 Greene LS: Asthma, oxidant stress, and diet. Nutrition 1999;15:899–907.
4 Isolauri E: The treatment of cow's milk allergy. Eur J Clin Nutr 1995;49:49–55.
5 Zeiger RS, Heller S: The development and prediction of atopy in high-risk children: follow-up at age seven years in a prospective randomized study of combined maternal and infant food allergen avoidance. J Allergy Clin Immunol 1995;95:1179–1190.

6 Kristmundsdottir F, David TJ: Growth impairment in children with atopic eczema. J R Soc Med 1987;80:9–12.

7 Paganus A, Juntunen-Backman K, Savilahti E: Follow-up of nutritional status and dietary survey in children with cow's milk allergy. Acta Paediatr 1992;81:518–521.

8 Massarano AA, Hollis S, Devlin J, et al: Growth in atopic eczema. Arch Dis Child 1993;68:677–679.

9 Isolauri E, Sütas Y, Salo MK, et al: Elimination diet in cow's milk allergy: risk for impaired growth in young children. J Pediatr 1998;132:1004–1009.

10 Agostoni C, Grandi F, Scaglioni S, et al: Growth pattern of breastfed and nonbreastfed infants with atopic dermatitis in the first year of life. Pediatrics 2000;106:e73.

11 Laitinen K, Kalliomäki M, Poussa T, et al: Evaluation of diet and growth in children with and without atopic eczema: follow-up study from birth to four years. Br J Nutr 2005;94:565–574.

12 Patel L, Clayton PE, Jenney MEM, et al: Adult height in patients with childhood onset atopic dermatitis. Arch Dis Child 1997;76:505–508.

13 Hill DJ, Firer MA, Shelton MJ, et al: Manifestations of milk allergy in infancy: clinical and immunological findings. J Pediatr 1986;109:270–276.

14 Christie L, Hine RJ, Parker JG, et al: Food allergies in children affect nutrient intake and growth. J Am Diet Assoc 2002;102:1648–1651.

15 Barbi E, Gerarduzzi T, Longo G, et al: Fatal allergy as a possible consequence of long-term elimination diet. Allergy 2004;59:668–669.

16 Flinterman AE, Knulst AC, Meijer Y, et al: Acute allergic reactions in children with AEDS after prolonged cow's milk elimination diets. Allergy 2006;61:370–374.

17 Isolauri E, Tahvanainen A, Peltola T, et al: Breast-feeding of allergic infants. J Pediatr 1999;134:27–32.

18 Konaris SG, Fisher SE, Rubin CT, et al: Experimental colitis impairs linear bone growth independent of nutritional factors. J Pediatr Gastroenterol Nutr 1997;25:137–141.

19 Majamaa H, Isolauri E: Evaluation of the gut mucosal barrier: evidence for increased antigen transfer in children with atopic eczema. J Allergy Clin Immunol 1996;97:985–990.

20 Borriello SP, Hammes WP, Holzapfel W, et al: Safety of probiotics that contain lactobacilli or bifidobacteria. Clin Infect Dis 2003;36:775–780.

21 Eggesbo M, Botten G, Stigum H: Restricted diets in children with reactions to milk and egg perceived by their parents. J Pediatr 2001;139:583–587.

22 Roesler TA, Barry PC, Bock SA: Factitious food allergy and failure to thrive. Arch Pediatr Adolesc Med 1994;148:1150–1155.

23 Henriksen C, Eggesbo M, Halvorsen R, et al: Nutrient intake among two-year-old children on cow's milk-restricted diets. Acta Paediatr 2000;89:272–278.

24 Cabral GA: Lipids as bioeffectors in the immune system. Life Sci 2005;77:1699–1710.

25 Roper RL, Brown DM, Phipps P: Prostaglandin E_2 promotes B lymphocyte Ig isotype switching to IgE. J Immunol 1995;154:162–170.

26 Thien FCK, Woods RK, De Luca S, et al: Dietary marine fatty acids (fish oil) for asthma in adults and children. Cochrane Database Syst Rev 2002;3:CD001283.

27 van Gool CJAW, Zeegers MPA, Thijs C: Oral essential fatty acid supplementation in atopic dermatitis – a meta-analysis of placebo-controlled trials. Br J Dermatol 2004;150:728–740.

28 Mayser P, Mayer K, Mahloudjian M, et al: A double-blind, randomized, placebo-controlled trial of n-3 versus n-6 fatty acid-based lipid infusion in atopic dermatitis. J Parenter Enteral Nutr 2002;26:151–158.

29 Laitinen K, Sallinen J, Linderborg K, et al: Serum, cheek cell and breast milk fatty acid compositions in atopic and nonatopic eczema. Clin Exp Allergy 2006;36:166–173.

30 Newberry RD, Stenson WF, Lorenz RG: Cyclooxygenase-2-dependent arachidonic acid metabolites are essential modulators of the intestinal immune response to dietary antigen. Nat Med 1999;5:900–906.

31 Usami M, Muraki K, Iwamoto M, et al: Effect of eicosapentaenoic acid (EPA) on tight junction permeability in intestinal monolayer cells. Clin Nutr 2001;20:351–359.

32 Kankaanpää PE, Salminen S, Isolauri E, et al: The influence of polyunsaturated fatty acids on probiotic growth and adhesion. FEMS Microbiol Lett 2001;194:149–153.

33 Worm M, Herz U, Krah JM, et al: Effects of retinoids on in vitro and in vivo IgE production. Int Arch Allergy Immunol 2001;124:233–236.

34 Albers R, Bol M, Bleumink R, et al: Effects of supplementation with vitamins A, C, and E, selenium, and zinc on immune function in a murine sensitization model. Nutrition 2003;19:
   940–946.
35 Halevy O, Sklan D: Inhibition of arachidonic acid oxidation by ß-carotene, retinol, and alpha-
   tocopherol. Biochim Biophys Acta 1987;918:304–307.

Discussion

Dr. Haschke: When talking about probiotics, I think we need to know more about
the strains you were using in your studies. You have very good and interesting results
with certain strains. This is very important, as for probiotics, there is wide variety in
breast milk, and we have little idea of what they are really doing. We are just starting
to understand this. As we learned yesterday for probiotics; one strain might have a
specific function in terms of prevention of allergy, another prevents diarrhea, the third
helps to treat diarrhea. Can you elaborate a little on the strains you are working with?

Dr. Laitinen: Thank you for raising this important point. The studies done in
Turku by Dr. Isolauri's team mainly used *Lactobacillus* GG, and indeed the intervention study for prevention of allergy and investigation of the joint effects of nutrients
and probiotics used *Lactobacillus* GG [1].

Dr. Haschke: This is the first time that you refer to a 'system'; it is not only the probiotic strain to be added which helps, you also mention other factors in the diet. How
did you determine this? Is it shown by statistical methods that these components
might also have an effect? Why do you mention this now as this is relatively new, this
'system'.

Dr. Laitinen: Generally in research we tend to look at single nutrients, food items
or probiotics and their health effects instead of the diet as a whole. Often it is thought
that supplementing with something makes everything alright, but this is not the case.
Certainly the diet as a whole, compared to, e.g., single nutrients, appears to have joint
or even additive properties influencing health outcome, whether it is a question of the
prevention or management of allergy. By performing multivariate analyses we have
been able to generate new hypotheses and now it may be the time for intervention
studies to explore the matter in more detail. Certainly some studies have been done
in vitro, e.g. looking at how polyunsaturated fatty acids can influence probiotics [2],
and this is a good start for studies of this kind.

Dr. Fisberg: There is a recent editorial in the *Pediatric Allergy and Immunology*
by Wjst [3] in which he made a statement about the relationship of vitamin D and
allergy, especially with regard to the relationship between decreased levels of rickets
and the levels of vitamin D supplementation, and the increased levels of allergy, especially asthma, in many countries. Do you have any data on this?

Dr. Laitinen: In our research team we have no data on this, but there is at least
one Finnish epidemiological study were the association was shown between vitamin D
supplementation and an increased risk of allergies in later life [4].

Dr. Morelli: Congratulations on your presentation because it has introduced some
new aspects on the work of Dr. Isolauri about atopic dermatitis and *Lactobacillus* GG.
Your data now suggest that the protective action observed against atopic dermatitis in
the very large work that was published in the *Lancet* and other papers, is to be attributed not only to the feeding of *Lactobacillus* GG but also to other supplementations.
So we have to presume that what was observed is not only the result of the
Lactobacillus GG action, it is also related to the presence of other supplements.

Dr. Laitinen: The study did not actually involve supplements; except probiotics,
we were looking at the diets that infants were habitually consuming and we didn't

have an intervention concerning nutrients. But yes, it appears that there may be synergistic effects of different nutrients and probiotics. If you look at these vitamins on their own, e.g. vitamin A is important for the gut and zinc for growth and so on, thus there appears to be a rationale behind the effects and the interactions as well.

Dr. Seidman: Your group has pioneered studies using probiotics to prevent atopic disease in high risk infants. One study in Switzerland [5, 6] suggested that it may be interesting to intervene even in children who are not at risk for atopy. This is based on the understanding that the 30% of all infants that are at risk would be in equal number to the 70% who don't have a parental history. What is your opinion about the general use of probiotics in all infants, whether or not at risk, for preventing atopic disease?

Dr. Laitinen: Here it is best to approach the issue by considering whether there might be any concerns related to the use of probiotics. According to our data, there doesn't appear to be any problem in terms of growth. If the child can eat normal food, there doesn't appear to be any concern that would prevent eating probiotics. In the literature there are only a few cases where the use of probiotics may not be advisable, these are individuals compromised by immune defense. So from the point of view that there might be benefits, why not.

Dr. Brunser: You said that intestinal microorganisms and probiotics may work together. When you say intestinal microbes, do you mean the resident microbiota or those bacteria in transit along the gastrointestinal tract? I think these are two different situations, and probably from the functional point of view they operate on the gut in completely different ways.

Dr. Laitinen: I was mainly thinking of inflammatory responses that might occur due to microbiota and how the host–microbe interaction works, what might be the inflammatory responses there, and how could probiotics influence that process.

Dr. Brunser: Tomorrow I am going to show some experimental work by Menard et al. [7] showing that, if probiotics are given, the resident microbiota exert a depressing effect on the responses of blood mononuclear cells to lipopolysaccharide stimulation, and that it is possible to establish a clear distinction between the effects of the resident microbiota and that of the probiotics. The resident microbiota is a system that operates 'in the background'. But individuals who live in an environment contaminated by bacteria produce another type of response, what we call chronic environmental enteropathy, that apparently protects the individuals against allergic reactions because it is probably the result of stimulation of the Th1 mechanisms by the passing organisms. In Chile, which has gone through a very rapid improvement in environmental sanitation, we no longer see intense histological manifestations of chronic environmental enteropathy, but instead we are experiencing a tremendous increase in asthma and eczema, and this in a span of less than 30 years.

Dr. Laitinen: Perhaps that goes back to the original hygiene hypothesis. We certainly don't want back the diseases we used to have, so now probiotics may be the answer for modifying intestinal microbiota and thus health promotion. Coming back to the safety issue, as far as I understand probiotics do not colonize the intestine permanently, so if you stop consuming probiotics, you stop the effects.

Dr. Domellöf: I was very intrigued by your data from the multivariate analysis. If you were to design a supplementation trial with a combined probiotic and multinutrient supplement, which components would you include?

Dr. Laitinen: I don't think I have an answer but I would probably take the diet as a whole and not any particular nutrient. Perhaps meeting the general dietary recommendations could be a good starting point, if we were even able to change the fat composition of the diet and meet the optimal intake of the nutrients. Perhaps for an intervention I would have a cocktail of nutrients, particularly those influencing gut integrity, glutamine and vitamin A. But there is more work to be done before there is an answer to your question.

References

1 Laitinen K, Kalliomäki M, Poussa T, et al: Evaluation of diet and growth in children with and without atopic eczema: follow-up study from birth to 4 years. Br J Nutr 2005;94:565–574.
2 Kankaanpää P, Yang B, Kallio H, et al: Effects of polyunsaturated fatty acids in growth medium on lipid composition and on physicochemical surface properties of lactobacilli. Appl Environ Microbiol 2004;70:129–136.
3 Wjst M: The vitamin D slant on allergy. Pediatr Allergy Immunol 2006;17:477–483.
4 Hyppönen E, Sovio U, Wjst M, et al: Infant vitamin D supplementation and allergic conditions in adulthood: northern Finland birth cohort 1966. Ann NY Acad Sci 2004;1037:84–95.
5 Exl BM, Deland U, Secretin MC, et al: Improved general health status in an unselected infant population following an allergen-reduced dietary intervention programme: the ZUFF-STUDY-PROGRAMME. Part II: Infant growth and health status to age 6 months. ZUg-FrauenFeld. Eur J Nutr 2000;39:145–156.
6 Exl BM, Deland U, Secretin MC, et al: Improved general health status in an unselected infant population following an allergen reduced dietary intervention programme. The ZUFF-study-programme. Part I: Study design and 6-month nutritional behaviour. Eur J Nutr 2000;39:89–102.
7 Menard S, Candalh C, Bambou JC, et al: Lactic acid bacteria secrete metabolites retaining anti-inflammatory properties after intestinal transport. Gut 2004;53:821–828.

Agostoni C, Brunser O (eds): Issues in Complementary Feeding.
Nestlé Nutr Workshop Ser Pediatr Program, vol 60, pp 171–184,
Nestec Ltd., Vevey/S. Karger AG, Basel, © 2007.

Weaning Infants with Malnutrition, Including HIV

Noel W. Solomons

Center for Studies of Sensory Impairment, Aging and Metabolism (CeSSIAM),
Guatemala City, Guatemala

Abstract

A normal pregnancy and adequate lactation performance should produce at 6 months of life a healthy baby, who has a weight and height within the limits of international growth norms. When that does not happen and the child is either too small (or too big), i.e. 'malnourished', strong determinants will have been maternal health, combined with environmental stress to the baby. In discussing differential strategies for weaning and complementary feeding, the distinction must first be made between true *clinical* malnutrition and simply *deviant growth*. The former needs rehabilitation therapy, which is beyond the scope of this discussion. For deviant poor growth, one must devise a regimen that removes an infant from any low-weight danger zone for increased early mortality risk. Thereafter, one can address the emerging scientific evidence that rapid accelerated catch-up growth has implications for increased metabolic derangement and chronic disease risk in childhood and beyond. Human immunodeficiency virus (HIV), infecting either mother or mother and offspring, is one of the emerging situations that will produce malnutrition before a child is due to be weaned. It will also often induce early weaning. Attention to specific micronutrient supplementation is recommended in HIV-seropositive and malarial infants.

Copyright © 2007 Nestec Ltd., Vevey/S. Karger AG, Basel

Introduction

Adequate early nutrition is the most essential element in assuring adequate growth and appropriate cognitive and functional development of the infant. Given the evolutionary nature of maternal milk, its ability to support normative growth is axiomatic. Moreover, it is the consensus of public health opinion that exclusive breastfeeding through at least the first 4 [1], if not a full 6 months of life [2], followed by timely and appropriate introduction of foods to complement maternal milk intake, is the ideal dietary pattern during the first year of life.

171

The nutritional status of a fetus and nursing infant is almost totally dependent upon the mother and maternal factors. If maternal health and nutrition are satisfactory during gestation, and adequate lactation and exclusive breastfeeding are established, a 6-month-old infant should be well-nourished at the moment of initiating the weaning process. Given the degree to which appropriate early feeding *should* be protective both of normal growth and good health [3], the association of the term 'malnutrition' with the initiation of weaning may seem somewhat tautological on its face.

Hence, to get oriented on logical bearings of this topic, we must take a step backwards and consider the implicit query: *Under what circumstances would a child emerging from the early months of life, and presumably exclusively breastfed, be classified as* 'malnourished' *at the point of the life course at which complementary feeding is first indicated?* To address this, requires an examination of the multiple definitions of 'malnutrition' in order to understand the connotations and implications of each, and their application in evaluation. Moreover, if growth or body composition have been truly retarded or distorted despite exclusive breastfeeding, we must identify any noxious process(es) that compromised the usually protective and privileged situation of exclusive breastfeeding.

What Constitutes 'Malnutrition' at the Initiation of Weaning?

The primary indicator of adequate nutrition during infancy is adequate growth, that is having anthropometric indices (length and weight) that fall within the boundaries of a standard reference growth curve, and having a trajectory of growth that tracks an appropriate velocity month by month. The National Center for Health Statistics growth curve [4], the traditional international standard for decades, was criticized for the influence of energy-dense formula feeding and lack of ethnic diversity in its constituent population. In April 2006, United Nations agencies adopted a new standard for growth [5]. The reference populations for the first 2 years of life were a combination of select cohorts from 6 geographic locations, maintaining ideal practices of infant and toddler feeding practices, including 4 months of exclusive breastfeeding and at least 1 year of maternal milk offering [6]. According to the framers of the new World Health Organization (WHO) growth curve, it is meant to be 'prescriptive', that is to be the universal standard for all children independent of social class, ethnicity or geographical origin [6].

Micronutrient malnutrition adds another dimension to nutritional adequacy at the time of weaning. The breast milk content of certain nutrients, such as iron and zinc, is low and becomes progressively more marginal with the passage of lactation. To the extent that the complementary feeding regimen chosen will correct any deficits in micronutrients, however, any utility of diagnosing iron or zinc deficits would be impractical and academic.

Table 1. Three distinct scenarios of nonnormative growth attainment below the standards of operative infant growth standards

(1) Clinical protein-energy malnutrition (kwashiorkor, marasmus)
(2) Anthropometric deficits, without latent disease
(3) Anthropometric deficits, with a latent infectious or hereditary disease

Poor Growth in Early Infancy

Beyond the appropriate macronutrient forms and micronutrient content of human milk, infants benefit from the passive immunity transferred in utero from the mother's circulation via the placenta and from the hygienic nature of maternal milk, combined with its immunoprotective properties. Hence, substantial infections should be a rarity during the first months of life. It is important to distinguish three scenarios of 'malnutrition' (table 1).

Severe Protein-Energy Malnutrition in Infancy
The aforementioned biological factors generally protect a breastfed infant through the first semester of life, but unique situations of early infectious stress or true maternal lactation failure can produce the clinical protein-energy malnutrition syndromes of kwashiorkor (edematous) and marasmus (inanition). In such situations, one common principle is to continue breastfeeding through the child's recuperation. So, to some extent, the therapeutic recovery feeding regimen is a variety of complementary feeding.

However, with this severity of malnutrition and clinical illness the regimens are unique and specialized. A consultancy of the WHO and the Nestlé Foundation renewed a focus on the nuances of rehabilitation of severe protein-energy malnutrition [7]. This regimen has improved child survival [8]. A consideration of the clinical management of severe malnutrition is beyond the scope of the present discussion. Suffice it to say, however, that the principles discussed in the rest of this chapter and in other contributions to this volume come into practice when the severely malnourished child emerges from intensive therapy, and is returned to an age-appropriate diet.

Pathological Factors Contributing to Poor Growth
before 6 Months of Age
When severe growth faltering is observed in supposedly exclusively breastfed 6-month-old children of privileged circumstances, the leading possibilities to be considered are: (1) not indeed having received exclusive lactation, (2) presence of congenital or hereditary anomalies, or (3) infant abuse. When it occurs in underprivileged conditions, the leading possibilities to be considered are: (1) having suffered substantial fetal malnutrition (small birth size), (2) not indeed having received exclusive lactation, and (3) presence of an infection.

What infections are relevant in the first 6 months of life? It should be remembered that breastfed infants are relatively resistant to some of the more notorious tropical diseases. For instance, intestinal helminths are not usually contracted until a child begins to crawl, and it takes months for the eggs to mature into adult worms. Recurrent diarrheal disease emerges when the weaning period begins, but is not likely to have occurred during exclusive breastfeeding. Infancy is a period of unique susceptibility to two epidemic diseases, however; we shall use them as examples in this analysis. Malaria can begin early in life, insofar as the children have not yet acquired immunity; it adversely affects growth early in life [9]. Human immunodeficiency virus (HIV) can be transmitted in utero, during birth or from the breast milk of an infected mother, but convenient early diagnosis is confounded by the presence of maternal antibodies.

Ecological and Environmental Factors Contributing to
Poor Growth before 6 Months of Age

It was shown in elegant studies with Peruvian infants from Lima's squatter slums that, despite exclusive breastfeeding, growth may not follow the same trajectory as in their peers in the United States [10]. Based on poor growth in poultry and livestock raised in unsanitary conditions, we postulated that chronic immunostimulation might explain some of the variance of poorer growth, even of appropriately fed infants [11]. This scenario was based on a presumed mechanism of 'damage', i.e. metabolic disruption by the burden of ambient microbes.

A complementary (and not mutually exclusive) alternative scenario for slow early growth is based on a proposition of programmed '*adaptation*' [12]. This theory postulates that the fetus senses (predicts) – and fetal growth responds to – the conditions of the external environment in which it will have to survive. The prospect of deprivation predisposes to adapting with a more compact body habitus and a more efficient metabolism.

Unhygienic and deprived ecological circumstances of rural agrarian or urban slum communities invoke modulators of – or signaling of messages for – limited early-life growth. In the face of enduring squalid deprivation, it would seem preferable, moreover, to influence growth by removing the adverse conditions, rather than by pushing trophic stimulation strategies to force attainment of the standard growth pattern.

Guidelines for Complementary Feeding in 'Infant Malnutrition'

The foregoing discussion raises some doubts on the assurance with which, short of overt clinical signs and symptoms, we can label a certain pattern of growth as constituting 'malnutrition'; meanwhile, we recognize that a certain 'hidden hunger' for sufficient intake of micronutrients may coexist with – or without – states of slower growth. Ongoing research provides us with emerging consideration on the causes and consequences of deviant growth patterns in infancy, but the practical aspects of improving complementary feeding are still grounded in what household economics, cultural acceptability and established science and experience will allow for.

Theoretical Considerations for Anthropometric 'Deviation'

When is being small in size a consequence of injury or damage, and when is it an attempt at adaptation to adverse ambient circumstances? The need to ponder such a question has arisen with the emergence of the school of biological thinking known as developmental origins of health and disease. The theory of predictive adaptive responses is predicated on a life-long, phenotypic programming of metabolic response in relation to accessing and storing nutrients [12]. If the prediction is for nutrient scarcity, the phenotype for nutrient management will be one of compulsive retention. If the environmental signal projects abundance, then a looser control of nutrient disposal will dominate the metabolic phenotype.

It now seems, however, that it is not only smallness of size, but also undergoing a period of intense and rapid compensatory growth, that forms and solidifies the life-long metabolic disposition toward excessive nutrient retention and chronic disease [13]. Multiple epidemiological observations, recently summarized [14], confirm an association between early small size, rapid 'catch-up' growth or both and risks of obesity, metabolic disorders and malignancies from childhood onward. This predisposition to disease is now attributed to the fetal and infant adaptations for scarcity becoming *dys*adaptive at a point in later life when, unanticipated, the dietary offering of sodium, sugar, fat, and energy becomes abundant.

These considerations raise the philosophical quandary as to whether the feeding regimen for a child who was born small or faltered in growth trajectory during the first semester of life should aim: (1) to *stimulate* growth despite the ecological conditions (trophic intent), or (2) to *release* the infant from environmental barriers to growth providing an adequate offering of nutrients (enabling intent). The former is prescriptive *for* the host; the latter is adaptive *by* the host. A series of correlates for the latter assumption of adaptation are provided in table 2.

Future food technology research could seek to develop simple techniques to provide a filler substance to an infant's diet that would dilute its caloric density without jeopardizing micronutrient status nor severely impairing growth and development. Additional cost, cultural acceptability, infant's discomfort from hunger, and disruption of family dining patterns are among the considerations to be addressed in such dietary modulation of infant growth.

Balanced against the concern for long-term chronic disease risk are a series of *clear and present dangers* from low body size and slow growth for

Table 2. Admonitions for the protection of the infant born under adverse circumstances in a low-income developing society

---

- Do not be so small as to be at higher risk of death from infectious diseases
- Achieve and maintain a 'protective' relative weight compatible with survival
- Beyond that, however, do not be in a hurry – nor in an obligation – to achieve the median weight for your age (or higher), especially if your length has not extended in a normative fashion
- Rather maintain a normative partition between lean and fat tissues in relation to your attained length
- Seek a dietary pattern consistent with your in utero adaptation, restricted if you were of low birth weight or there was a rapid early growth spurt, and more liberal if you were of normal birth weight and early growth

---

infants in developing countries. The clinical consequences of low birth weight and growth faltering for mortality risk have been well documented for decades. Pelletier et al. [15] documented that underweight (low weight for age) is a contributing factor in over half the deaths in children under 5 years of age. Whether the low weight is a marker of a child at risk or a true mediator of his demise, this association has inculcated a clinical and public health imperative to grow a small child out of the weight zone of high mortality risk. We confront the paradox that (1) being below a certain weight in infancy conveys a certain excess risk of infectious mortality [15], whereas (2) rapid accelerated growth in infancy conveys a predisposition to metabolic derangement in childhood [14] and chronic morbidity in adult life [13]. To the extent that small body size truly exposes infants to risk of adverse outcomes for infections in the unsanitary and derived environments of developing countries, it would be at some peril to infant health if we would too lightly discard conventional wisdom and practice of rapidly recovering normative weights.

*Practical and Prescriptive Considerations for
Anthropometric Deviation*

Whatever the theoretical considerations for a child that is small, there cannot – and should not – be substantial deviation from the WHO's practical principles of adapting a child to the household dietary scheme [16]. The constraints on nutrient density and bioavailability in the common grains and tubers, milled and mashed to produce traditional weaning foods in developing countries, have been meticulously documented in a classic analysis by Brown and coworkers [17, 18] for United Nations agencies' publications, and are discussed elsewhere in this workshop.

As to the limits of absorbing the zinc and iron in contemporary complementary diets, premasticated meat was presumably the basis for the evolutionary complementary food of hunting clans. Solving the low nutrient density and poor bioavailability issues for diverse micronutrients should cause us to heed recent calls for early introduction of animal protein [19], and even consider cooked meat and visceral organs for initiating weaning [20].

Good caring practices in the household are indispensable for successfully feeding an infant of whatever growth attainment. Social scientists at the Cornell University developed a 'best-practice complementary feeding behaviors' framework which identified the following elements: 'what is fed, how food is prepared and given, who feeds the child, when food is fed (frequency and scheduling), and the feeding environment (where)' [21]. Clearly many household members, including slightly older siblings, participate in infant feeding. Factors such as the microbiological purity of the water used to prepare porridges and gruels need to be assured.

Theoretical Considerations for Infection-Related Growth Retardation

We have isolated two contemporary infectious scourges – malaria and HIV – that can impair infant growth virtually from the time of conception through early infancy. In fact, even if an infant is not infected with the HIV virus, exposure to maternal antiretroviral medications in utero and in breast milk can adversely affect growth. These infections represent situations where the nuances of feeding and care at the initiation of weaning have more profound, and weighty considerations for the health of the infant and the well-being of the family is in the balance.

In these two diseases of intracellular pathogen origin, theoretical concerns for adverse effects of iron and zinc exposure have arisen. A recent supplement field trial in a malarial area of Africa confirmed excess mortality with oral iron supplementation [22], with no adversity from oral zinc. Trials elsewhere on the continent in HIV-infected infants and toddlers uncovered no untoward effects with either zinc [23] or iron [24], but theoretical concerns remain.

Practical and Prescriptive Considerations for Infection-Related Growth Retardation

The emotional and financial burdens of malaria and HIV call for pragmatism and practicality in the management of complementary feeding. Moreover, as shown in a recent study in Côte d'Ivoire, when weaning was initiated much earlier by HIV-seropositive mothers, there were negative consequences for growth [25]. Nevertheless, the basic principles of complementary feeding are as operative in these infections as with all infants [16–18].

When financial and logistical conditions permit, however, some additional strategies in complementary feeding may improve outcomes. For instance, since avoiding ambient infections, especially in the immune deficiency states of infants living with HIV is a priority, even more attention to water purity and food hygiene is desirable. Probiotics and hyperimmune bovine colostrum, moreover, may have a role in prophylaxis and treatment of diarrhea [26]. For instance, the protozoa, *Cryptosporidium parvum*, produces a profuse,

Table 3. Elements of a research agenda to address outstanding issues for complementary feeding in relation to 'preweaning malnutrition'

- Safe and ethical manner to restrict the rate of growth – but not the ultimate growth attainment – by manipulating energy density in complementary feeding regimens
- Extend studies and surveillance to refine knowledge regarding safety and dosage forms of zinc and iron in infant HIV and iron in infant malaria
- Examine potential interactions between foods and dietary supplements with antiretroviral medications in infancy, to maximize synergistic effects and minimize any antagonistic effects
- Prospectively examine the safety, efficacy, effectiveness and efficiency (cost-effectiveness) of meat and organ meats as the first complementary food item
- Follow-up cohorts of infants with below normative body size at 6 months (anthropometric deviants) into childhood, adolescence and adulthood to assess any associations between rates of early growth and biomarkers of chronic disease risk and eventual chronic disease occurrence

---

intractable diarrheal state resistant to antimicrobials, but susceptible to the antibodies in bovine colostrum concentrates.

Periodic vitamin A supplementation has proven protective of growth and health in both HIV- and malaria-infected infants and toddlers and is recommended [27, 28]. Zinc supplementation may also be protective [23]. In infected infants, there is untapped promise in a series of supplement formats, such as sprinkles (a powder), spreads (analogous to nut butters), and foodLETS (crushable flavored tablets), recently devised to provide selected micronutrients directly to complementary dishes or diets prepared at home [29].

Elements for a Research Agenda

The fundamental public health goal surrounding considerations for infants with poor growth is assuring their short-term survival and health through their second semester of infancy and into the toddler period. Thereafter, appropriate growth and full psychomotor and physiological development are to be encouraged. Balancing practical issues of early mortality risk with predicted adverse long-term health outcomes in the management of low weight, we lack complete knowledge and wisdom for assessing our patients and setting optimal goals for dietary intake and growth. We also lack tools and recipes for formulating diets to achieve less rapid weight recovery without endangering health, nutrition or ultimate height attainment. Based on the sum of present considerations, elements of a research agenda to address the pressing issues have been outlined in table 3.

Conclusion

It is not expected that an exclusively breastfed infant would be lagging in growth attainment or velocity after the 6th month of life when complementary feeding should begin. Not all growth failure and nonnormative body composition, moreover, represent 'malnutrition' in a universal connotation. It may be due variously to phenotypic adaptation *or* nutrient imbalance, each of which has differential relevance to short-term survival and long-term health. Our first imperative is to understand the theoretical principles that would influence assessment of nutritional implications of observed growth. We then need to dominate the practicalities of current best practices for routine feeding and application of micronutrient supplements. A review of the topic reveals a number of uncertainties and unresolved issues that lend themselves to continuing investigation. The end would be refining assessment of 'small' infants to assign the most appropriate goals for their growth velocity and micronutrient nutrition while developing affordable and acceptable complementary feeding guidelines and practices to achieve the safest and most harmonious outcomes.

References

1 American Academy of Pediatrics Committee on Nutrition: Complementary feeding; in Kleinman RE (ed): Pediatric Nutrition Handbook. Elk Grove Village, American Academy of Pediatrics, 2004, pp 103–115.
2 World Health Organization/UNICEF: Global Strategy for Infant and Young Child Feeding. Geneva, WHO, 2003.
3 Dewey KG, Cohen RJ, Brown KH: Exclusive breast-feeding for 6 months, with iron supplementation, maintains adequate micronutrient status among term, low-birthweight, breast fed infants in Honduras. J Nutr 2004;134:1091–1098.
4 Hamill PV, Drizd TA, Johnson CL, et al: Physical growth: National Center for Health Statistics percentiles. Am J Clin Nutr 1979;32:607–629.
5 World Health Organization: Child Growth Standard Charts, April 27, 2006. www.who.int/childgrowth.
6 Garza C: New growth standards for the 21st century: a prescriptive approach. Nutr Rev 2006;64:S55–S59.
7 World Health Organization: Management of Severe Malnutrition: a Manual for Physicians and other Senior Health Workers. Geneva, WHO, 1999.
8 Ashworth A, Chopra M, McCoy D, et al: WHO guidelines for management of severe malnutrition in rural South African hospitals: effect on case fatality and the influence of operational factors. Lancet 2004;363:1111–1115.
9 Mamiro PS, Kolsteren P, Roberfroid D, et al: Feeding practices and factors contributing to wasting, stunting, and iron-deficiency anaemia among 3–23-month old children in Kilosa district, rural Tanzania. J Health Popul Nutr 2005;23:222–230.
10 Dewey KG, Peerson JM, Heinig MJ, et al: Growth patterns of breast-fed infants in affluent (United States) and poor (Peru) communities: implications for timing of complementary feeding. Am J Clin Nutr 1992;56:1012–1018.
11 Solomons NW, Mazariegos M, Brown KH, Klasing K: The underprivileged, developing country child: environmental contamination and growth failure revisited. Nutr Rev 1993;51:327–332.
12 Gluckman PD, Hanson MA, Spencer HG: Predictive adaptive responses and human evolution. Trends Ecol Evol 2005;20:527–533.

13 Uauy R, Solomons NW: Role of the international community: forging a common agenda in tackling the double burden of malnutrition. SCN News 2006;32:24–37.

14 Singhal A, Cole TJ, Fewtrell M, et al: Is slower early growth beneficial for long-term cardiovascular health? Circulation 2004;109:1108–1113.

15 Pelletier DL, Frongillo EA Jr, Schroeder DG, Habicht JP: The effects of malnutrition on child mortality in developing countries. Bull World Health Organ 1995;73:443–448.

16 World Health Organization: Complementary Feeding. Family Foods for Breastfed Children. Geneva, WHO, 2000.

17 Brown KH, Allen LH, Dewey KG: Complementary Feeding of Young Children in Developing Countries: A Review of Current Scientific Knowledge. Geneva, WHO, 1998.

18 Dewey KG, Brown KH: Update on technical issues concerning complementary feeding of young children in developing countries and implications program. Food Nutr Bull 2003;24:5–28.

19 Bwibo NO, Neumann CG: The need for animal source foods by Kenyan children. J Nutr 2003;133(suppl 2):3936S–3940S.

20 Krebs NF, Westcott JE, Butler N, et al: Meat as a first complementary food for breastfed infants: feasibility and effect on zinc intake and status. J Pediatr Gastroenterol Nutr 2006;42: 207–214.

21 Pelto GH, Levitt E, Thairu L: Improving feeding practices: current patterns, common constraints, and the design of interventions. Food Nutr Bull 2003;24:45–82.

22 Sazawal S, Black RE, Ramsan M, et al: Effects of routine prophylactic supplementation with iron and folic acid on admission to hospital and mortality in preschool children in a high malaria transmission setting: community-based, randomised, placebo-controlled trial. Lancet 2006;367:133–143.

23 Bobat R, Coovadia H, Stephen C, et al: Safety and efficacy of zinc supplementation for children with HIV-1 infection in South Africa: a randomised double-blind placebo-controlled trial. Lancet 2006;367:814–815.

24 Olsen A, Mwaniki D, Krarup H, Friis H: Low-dose iron supplementation does not increase HIV-1 load. J Acquir Immune Defic Syndr 2004;36:637–638.

25 Becquet R, Leroy V, Ekouevi DK, et al; ANRS 1201/1202 Ditrame Plus Study Group: Complementary feeding adequacy in relation to nutritional status among early weaned breastfed children who are born to HIV-infected mothers: ANRS 1201/1202 Ditrame Plus, Abidjan, Cote d'Ivoire. Pediatrics 2006;117:e701–e710.

26 Solomons NW, Orozco M: Modulación del sistema inmune y respuesta a patógenos por concentrados de calostro bovino; in Marcos A, Montero A, Wärnberg J (eds): Malnutrición en el Mundo. Madrid, Editec@red, 2003, pp 141–156.

27 Villamor E, Mbise R, Spiegelman D, et al: Vitamin A supplements ameliorate the adverse effect of HIV-1, malaria and diarrheal infections on child growth. Pediatrics 2002;109:E6.

28 Shankar AH, Genton B, Semba RD, et al: Effect of vitamin A supplementation on morbidity due to *Plasmodium falciparum* in young children in Papua New Guinea. Lancet 1999;354: 203–209.

29 Nestel P, Briend A, de Benoist B, et al: Complementary food supplements to achieve micronutrient adequacy for infants and young children. J Pediatr Gastroenterol Nutr 2003;36: 316–328.

Discussion

Dr. Michaelsen: You mentioned that you have some problems with prescriptive growth, but I didn't really understand. Are you suggesting an alternative?

Dr. Solomons: I have a problem with the notion of prescriptive in many ways. I never mentioned them but I am glad you asked the question. What they basically say is that you should be within a certain channel on a reference growth chart. Let us go back to how the children were selected and treated to become part of the data-set. There was a master prescription. The prescription is to be well fed, to be perfectly fed by contemporary standards, including a period of being exclusively breastfed. It is unfair to assume to be on a trajectory created by exposure to an optimum environment and feeding regime, if he or she has a different start in life. We need to focus on the conditions that permit the growth pattern on the WHO standards, not on the channels within the standards themselves. That is my problem with prescriptive growth. In my opinion, prescriptive has to start with the conditions and not the trajectory.

Dr. Cabus: I have read some papers about people with AIDS who interrupt breast-feeding, and when breastfeeding is combined with food, it is easier to get the virus. Could you comment on this?

Dr. Solomons: There is science and very systematic observations. Up to 4 months for any suckling, there is a certain risk of the mother passing on the virus to the child. If the mother is not willing to undertake that risk she should never let the milk flow from her breast into the child. The evidence suggests, however, that up to 4 months of age, if she doesn't get things like mastitis or cracking of the nipples that will enhance the infection, the child will have a minimum risk of contracting the virus as long as she doesn't use any other food besides breast milk. We mean truly exclusive breastfeeding. Now at 4 months other foods are going to be started anyway, so at that point rather than continuing to give breast milk, which is the recommendation for any other situation, breastfeeding should abruptly stop because the combination of milk and solid foods produces more risk of viral transmission. This could be related to changes in permeability of the intestinal wall. Now the other thing to discuss is how safe artificial formula feeding from day zero is, and to me this is a question of the purity of the water. The products are fine, but can water sanitation be managed? It is possible, then that is a viable alternative. The question if there is more risk of death when artificial formulas are used is valid if the water is infected, but if the water is pure there is no risk, as in a developed country. It is not an easy scenario but if it can be managed then that is another successful way to prevent the transmission. Of course the child could already be infected and that is something that is easily discovered with all the sophistication of virus counts done by antigen detection. The child has the maternal antibody, or children who have positive mothers will have the antibody until that clears in the child's own antibody. So resources and the direction of resources is the major issue of consideration in an AIDS-infected environment. This is my understanding of why abrupt weaning at 4 months or never breastfeeding are the only two recommended alternatives, and mixed feeding is definitely not recommended.

Dr. Haschke: The WHO has a clear policy on this. We should not assume that the majority of mothers, in particular in southern Africa, are living under conditions where they don't have access to clean water. In South Africa, for example, it is the program of the government that more than 90% of the population should have access to clean water, including all the people living in settlements and even in big cities where the HIV rate is very high. So here the government has clearly decided to offer food programs for these children. The same is true for Botswana and other countries where HIV rates are high. For informal settlements, I think that there definitely should be an alternative to food programs, for example exclusive breastfeeding, which is the other way to enhance child survival.

Dr. Pazvakavambwa: I just wanted to clarify the issue of formula feeding in HIV. There was a CDC study in Botswana in which the government provided formula and antiretrovirus drugs to HIV-infected children. But then there was a study in which the mortality in formula-fed babies, where the water was said to be freely available and of good quality, was compared with the mortality in breastfed babies, and it was found that the mortality in breastfed babies was much lower than in exclusively formula-fed babies [1]. So I think that even in the so-called richer developing countries one has to be very careful before prescribing exclusive formula feeding in the presence of HIV.

Dr. Solomons: As a confounder there is of course a self-selective nature. On the one hand, there are mothers who choose to breastfeed and those who choose to formula feed; so you can never truly eliminate the maternal confidence factor from an observation.

Dr. Bulusu: Going back to this WHO prescriptive growth that you were mentioning. In the child development program in India, these growth charts are being used, and today each and every village community level worker is aware of grades 1, 2, 3, and 4 malnutrition because the charts are more like a guideline for them. Growth monitoring is done at the village level, so even an illiterate worker or mother can see just on the basis of the charts that her child has fallen, so improvement is needed. In the positive deviance program of UNICEF, which is being tried in India, just by showing the care and feeding practices of one mother sets an example for the other mothers in the village. When one mother with the same socioeconomic status is able to improve her child's condition why can't the other mothers do so? Perhaps I am wrong, but I look at this growth chart not as a directive that your child has to be there but probably as a guideline to see where your child stands and how best can we improve the status of the child.

Dr. Solomons: It would be different, if 'standards' were taken as a guideline, or 'reference' means knowing where the child is in relationship to where he might be going. We have to be very careful when using those two concepts. Prescriptive to me means standard [2]; 'reference' is compared to anything that can be considered to be a comparative reference. The choice of words is important. What I assert is that it is dangerous and a motive for action when a child is losing channels. But maintaining one's channels or gaining channels are different. So either of those two is all right. What I am concerned about is gaining channels too rapidly; that is to start below the red line and be about the green line in 4 months. Now the next question is at age 7, 8, 15 years and so forth, as to what has that rapid growth brought. Especially in India where, as I mentioned yesterday in my response to your talk, there is the Indian paradox which means that body composition is quite different. As a regional phenomenon mothers have a median BMI of 18.5, that is what we consider the lower limit of normal. So half your population is by definition chronically energy malnourished. I don't believe they are, I don't believe that term fits. Similarly you have the so-called thin-fat babies [3]. Babies are small but they are fatty, and the fat is both visceral and subcutaneous. Both of which seem to be primed for metabolic insulin-resistant. So what happens when a thin-fat baby is born to a mother who is eating high glycemic index food? Then the situation is worse for that baby than for the one in Paris whose evolution and adaptation has been conditioned for over the last 500 years. The French baby is better off in opulence than the rural migrant in India. Now it may only require one generation for Indian babies to receive an external message of affluence, so they will no longer be programmed for retention but programmed for easy excretion.

Dr. Shahkhalili: What would happen if small babies did not have catch-up growth during the suckling and weaning period? Could it happen later? Would these babies with delay/lack of early catch-up growth have a risk for later metabolic disease?

Dr. Solomons: I can't give you a general answer, and I don't want to because I don't think the science guides us well. But clinically, if you take two children with exactly the same situation, one of them may do well with growth and the other may not. So I don't know the predictors of the diagnostic subtleties to determine which type is which. But I hope we can learn that and then it would be a management issue, not on a public health level but on an individualized level by a practitioner or care taker. What I am basically saying – which the public health people don't want to hear from me – is that to respond to low size at birth, we need to depend upon more of the art of clinical judgment rather than the standard of prescriptive management to determine how the child should grow. The battle is not to be so small as to be at risk of death and dying early, because it is better to be alive and diabetic later rather than to be dead early. But using that as a principle on how to manage growth, I think the study by Demmelmair et al. [4] is very important because it should give us a handle on both the ethical considerations and the dietary management that can make people grow more slowly. There are certain ways that if you give children complementary feeding they will cross channels and grow right back up to the green line, at least in weight, in a very short period of time. I think at least the science suggests that this pattern has more adverse consequences. Slower growth, however, is harder to produce. We don't have a lot of experience with controlled slow growth. I think randomized trials, such as the one happening in Europe [4], should perhaps happen in developing countries like India, which produces two patterns of growth that should be looked at in terms of the metabolic consequences in later life. As I emphasized it is better to survive to be able to think about going on to later life. So the global imperative is for the child to survive, and then worry about how they are going to be metabolically better off, because we now have the science and the concepts to think of a better quality of life after surviving.

Dr. Ibe: Why does the WHO describe this growth chart as prescriptive?

Dr. Solomons: I don't know; go to the website or look at Dr. Garcia's talk [2]. The WHO calls it prescriptive, I don't.

Dr. Ibe: We use the growth chart as a medical tool and it is called the route to a healthy child for the mothers because it is visual. They look at it and see how their babies are doing; they show esthetic growth.

Dr. Solomons: Living in our country (Guatemala), the goal would be to show steady growth: don't lose growth, don't go down. That would be my first mandate, and my second would be don't grow upwardly on the curve too fast if there is the option to grow more slowly. But going down, weighing less than before, that is a bad sign. It is a sign of immediateness and then all the therapeutic efforts to save the children from death have to be quickened. But if they are growing on a good slope on the chart, I don't care whether they are between the red lines or below the red lines of the center of the reference distribution. I do care if they are above the red lines (i.e. overweight). That was in my paper but I didn't talk about macrosomia and large babies, another problem, not so much a problem in Nigeria, India and Guatemala, but maybe in Paris where an occasional baby can weigh more than 5 kg at birth.

Dr. Michaelsen: You mentioned the CHOP study [4] and several others have also mentioned it. It is a randomization study, randomization to formulas with different protein contents starting from early after delivery, so it will not really give us an answer on an effect during the weaning period which is a period where we don't know very much about programming.

Dr. Solomons: At 6 months, they get off the low protein or the higher protein diet. But it is still about growth and not about feeding. So the notion then would be to learn. I hoped that that was embodied in my research agenda. There is also follow-up formula but they still have to eat solid foods with it. How do you then maintain the moderate and not accelerated growth once you start feeding other than infant formula? That is the question.

Dr. Agostoni: May I give you some details on this since we are part of the protein trial with infant formulas that has just been mentioned (the CHOP project). The low protein group and the high protein group go on up to 12 months because they switch to two follow-on formulas with low and high protein content, respectively, so they stop the low and the high protein schedule at 12 months. As far as their dietary intakes from solids and other sources, they are going to be integrated too.

Dr. Brunser: As I want to close the session, I want to say two things to Dr. Solomons. First of all, your lecture was, as always, very thought-provoking. The second thing is that you will have to change the picture of your mosquito: you wanted me to say that the mosquito in your slide was the malaria mosquito, Anopheles, but as it turns out, it is the yellow fever mosquito, *Stegomya fasciata*.

References

1 Kuhn L, Peterson I: Options for prevention of HIV transmission from mother to child, with a focus on developing countries. Paediatr Drugs 2002;4:191–203.
2 Garza C: New growth standards for the 21st century: a prescriptive approach. Nutr Rev 2006;64:S55–S59; discussion S72–S91.
3 Yajnik CS, Fall CH, Coyaji KJ, et al: Neonatal anthropometry: the thin-fat Indian baby. The Pune Maternal Nutrition Study. Int J Obes Relat Metab Disord 2003;27:173–180.
4 Demmelmair H, von Rosen J, Koletzko B: Long-term consequences of early nutrition. Early Hum Dev 2006;82:567–574.

Agostoni C, Brunser O (eds): Issues in Complementary Feeding.
Nestlé Nutr Workshop Ser Pediatr Program, vol 60, pp 185–199,
Nestec Ltd., Vevey/S. Karger AG, Basel, © 2007.

Adverse Effects of Cow's Milk in Infants

Ekhard E. Ziegler

Fomon Infant Nutrition Unit, Department of Pediatrics, University of Iowa,
Iowa City, IA, USA

Abstract

The feeding of cow's milk has adverse effects on iron nutrition in infants and young children. Several different mechanisms have been identified that may act synergistically. Probably most important is the low iron content of cow's milk. It makes it difficult for the infant to obtain the amounts of iron needed for growth. A second mechanism is the occult intestinal blood loss, which occurs in about 40% of normal infants during feeding of cow's milk. Loss of iron in the form of blood diminishes with age and ceases after 1 year of age. A third factor is calcium and casein provided by cow's milk in high amounts. Calcium and casein both inhibit the absorption of dietary nonheme iron. Infants fed cow's milk receive much more protein and minerals than they need. The excess has to be excreted in the urine. The high renal solute load leads to higher urine concentration during the feeding of cow's milk than during the feeding of breast milk or formula. When fluid intakes are low and/or when extrarenal water losses are high, the renal concentrating ability of infants may be insufficient for maintaining water balance in the face of high water use for excretion of the high renal solute. The resulting negative water balance, if prolonged, can lead to serious dehydration. There is strong epidemiological evidence that the feeding of cow's milk or formulas with similarly high potential renal solute load places infants at an increased risk of serious dehydration. The feeding of cow's milk to infants is undesirable because of cow's milk's propensity to lead to iron deficiency and because it unduly increases the risk of severe dehydration.

Introduction

The feeding of cow's milk to infants has undesirable consequences in two unrelated areas. One is iron nutrition, where several characteristics of cow's milk combine to produce a strong propensity to cause iron deficiency. The other area is body water economy, where the unduly high potential renal solute load of cow's milk increases the risk of severe dehydration.

Cow's Milk and Iron Deficiency

There is an extensive body of evidence beginning in the 1970s showing that the feeding of cow's milk to infants (and to young children) is strongly associated with diminished iron stores and an increased probability of iron deficiency. Many of the studies were conducted in the USA [1–6] and Great Britain [7–11], but studies have also been reported from Denmark [12], Australia [13], Ireland [14], Sweden [15], Iceland [16] and a cross section of European countries [17].

The study of Male et al. [17] involved 488 normal infants in 11 different countries. When iron status was assessed at 12 months of age, 7.2% of the subjects had iron deficiency and 2.3% had iron deficiency anemia. Feeding of cow's milk was a strong determinant of iron status, with each month of cow's milk feeding increasing the risk of iron deficiency by 39%. In a study in Iceland [16] involving 180 normal infants, iron status at 12 months of age was found to be strongly negatively associated with cow's milk consumption between 9 and 12 months of age. Infants in the highest quintile of milk consumption were in significantly worse iron status than infants consuming lesser amounts of cow's milk.

In most studies, the iron status of infants fed cow's milk is compared with that of infants fed formula, which is usually fortified with iron. However, in two studies [1, 2] formulas were used that were not fortified with iron. These formulas still led to better iron nutritional status than cow's milk. These studies thus provide evidence that cow's milk affects iron status adversely not just through its low iron content and suggest that additional mechanisms are involved in producing poor iron status. Two such mechanisms are known. One is occult intestinal blood loss. The other is inhibition of absorption of dietary nonheme iron by components of cow's milk. The relative importance of the known mechanisms cannot be determined from existing data. Although it appears that the low iron content of cow's milk is most important, it is likely that all three mechanisms act in concert to produce iron deficiency.

Low Iron Content of Cow's Milk

One reason why cow's milk causes iron deficiency is its low iron content (about 0.5 mg/l). Taking into account the iron endowment at birth, the infant needs to absorb on average about 0.7 mg (0.55–0.75 mg) of iron each day in the first year of life in order to avoid iron deficiency [18]. If 10% of ingested iron is absorbed, the infant needs to ingest about 7 mg of iron each day, and if 30% is absorbed (which is unlikely but possible), the intake still needs to be about 2.3 mg/day. In either case it is obvious that cow's milk can at best make an insignificant contribution to the needed iron intake. (In contrast, formulas with iron concentrations between 6 and 12 mg/l easily meet infants' iron needs.) The infant fed cow's milk thus depends almost entirely on complementary foods to provide the needed iron. If the infant consumes iron-fortified complementary foods (e.g., cereals) or meat, the iron intake can be high enough to meet needs. But nonfortified complementary foods seldom provide enough iron. Thus, the infant fed cow's milk is at risk of iron deficiency, even if the efficiency of iron absorption is high, as it is apt to be when iron stores are becoming depleted.

Occult Intestinal Blood Loss

Normal infants lose small quantities of blood in their feces at all times. In the past, investigators were able to measure fecal blood loss quantitatively using the radiochromium (^{51}Cr) technique. With this technique, erythrocytes are withdrawn from the subject, labeled in vitro with ^{51}Cr and reinjected. Measurement of radioactivity simultaneously in blood and feces then permits quantitative determination of the amount of blood lost in feces. Using this technique, Elian et al. [19] found that blood loss averaged 0.59 ml/day in infants hospitalized for various nonintestinal infectious illnesses. Each infant had measurable blood loss. In infants with gastroenteritis blood loss averaged 1.85 ml/day. Wilson et al. [20] were the first to recognize that the feeding of cow's milk can lead to an increase in intestinal blood loss. Studying iron-deficient infants and toddlers with the ^{51}Cr method, they found that in a sizable number of infants there was a clear and reproducible increase in fecal blood loss caused by the feeding of cow's milk. In other iron-deficient subjects blood loss occurred sometimes during cow's milk feeding but not at other times. In infants with consistent cow's milk-induced blood loss, the amount of blood lost averaged 1.7 ml/day. When the same subjects were fed formula (milk-based or soy-based), blood loss decreased to 0.3 ml/day. Blood loss of 1.7 ml/day is equivalent to iron loss of 0.53 mg/day, which, if it is not causing an outright negative iron balance, makes it at least very difficult for the infant to achieve a net iron gain of 0.7 mg/day as is necessary to prevent iron depletion.

As the studies of Wilson et al. [20] concerned infants and toddlers with iron deficiency, it remained unclear how common cow's milk-induced blood loss was in infants with normal iron stores. To answer this question, Fomon et al. [21] performed a study in which normal 4-month-old infants were randomly assigned to pasteurized cow's milk, or heat-treated cow's milk (heat-treated to the same extent as ready-to-feed infant formula), or iron-fortified ready-to-feed infant formula. Between 112 and 196 days of age, stool specimens were collected weekly and tested for the presence of blood by the guaiac test. During the first 4 weeks of the trial, 39% of infants fed cow's milk had one or more guaiac-positive stools and 17% of all stools were guaiac positive. In contrast, among infants fed formula or heat-treated cow's milk, only 9% of infants had one or more guaiac-positive stools (p < 0.01) and only 2.4% of all stools were guaiac positive (p < 0.001). During month 2 and 3 of the trial, differences between feeding groups were smaller and not statistically significant. There were no differences in iron nutritional status, possibly because iron intake was generous in all groups.

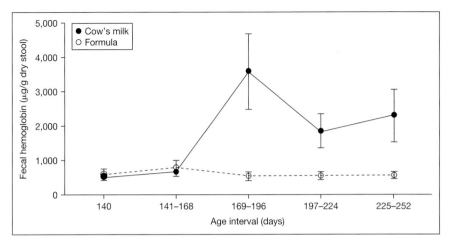

Fig. 1. Fecal hemoglobin concentration in infants fed formula and infants fed cow's milk beginning at 168 days of age (mean ± SE). Drawn from data of Ziegler et al. [22].

While the study by Fomon et al. [21] showed that a sizable minority of normal infants had intestinal blood loss when fed cow's milk, it provided no information about the quantity of blood lost during feeding of cow's milk, and it concerned relatively young infants. A subsequent study [22] of similar design employed a quantitative method for determination of fecal hemoglobin. Also, it initiated the feeding of cow's milk at a later age (5½ months). There were two feeding groups, one fed cow's milk and one fed iron-fortified milk-based formula. Infants had initially been breastfed or had been fed milk-based or soy-based formulas, but for at least 1 month before entering the trial all infants were fed a milk-based formula. As in the earlier study, the percentage of guaiac-positive stools rose from a baseline value of 3% to 30% during the first month of the trial (p < 0.01), whereas among infants fed formula the proportion of guaiac-positive stools remained low (5%). The concentration of hemoglobin in stool increased in infants fed cow's milk from 622 µg/g dry stool before cow's milk to a mean of 3,598 µg/g (SD 10,479) dry stool during the first month of feeding cow's milk (as illustrated in fig. 1). In infants fed formula stool hemoglobin concentration did not change from baseline and remained significantly (p < 0.01) lower than in infants fed cow's milk. Again, a large minority (38%) of infants fed cow's milk reacted to cow's milk ('responders') and accounted for all the observed increase in mean stool hemoglobin concentration. As before, the majority of infants ('nonresponders') were indistinguishable from formula-fed control infants. Among the responders, fecal hemoglobin concentration varied widely, as indicated by the large SD value.

One responder infant in the study of Ziegler et al. [22] had massive hemoglobin loss during the first month of the study (average iron loss of 2.04 mg/day). This infant developed iron deficiency anemia after just 1 month on cow's milk and was taken out of the study and given iron treatment, to which she responded promptly and completely. The remaining 9 responders lost on average 0.24 mg of iron/day, an amount that is not trivial in infants whose ability to gain 0.7 mg of iron/day is already compromised by low iron intake due to being fed cow's milk. It is of note that intestinal blood loss was clinically silent and that feeding-related behaviors did not differ between responders and nonresponders. Also of note is that infants who were fed milk-based formula from birth were less likely (p = 0.059) to respond to cow's milk with intestinal blood loss than infants who were breastfed from birth.

Subsequent studies [23, 24] answered the question whether cow's milk-induced intestinal blood loss occurs also in older infants. Infants were fed cow's milk for 2 months starting at 7½, 9 and 12 months of age. About half the study participants were initially breastfed for various lengths of time, while the other half of infants were fed formula only (including soy-based formula). During the feeding of cow's milk beginning at 7½ months (224 days) of age, fecal hemoglobin concentration rose significantly (p < 0.05), but the increase was on average less pronounced than at 5½ months of age. Among the 26% of infants who were classified as responders, average fecal hemoglobin was 3,010 µg/g dry stool (fig. 2). Among the responders were 2 infants with persistent high fecal hemoglobin concentration that averaged 7,430 and 8,156 µg/g dry stool, respectively.

When cow's milk was introduced at 9 months (280 days) of age, 29% of infants showed a response and had average stool hemoglobin concentration of 2,711 µg/g (SD 1,732) dry stool, which was significantly (p < 0.01) higher than at baseline when concentration averaged 1,395 µg/g (SD 856) dry stool. In contrast, introduction of cow's milk at 12 months of age produced no increase in fecal hemoglobin above baseline (fig. 2). Two infants (7%) showed a response, but it was quite mild and short-lived. Of note is that baseline fecal hemoglobin concentrations showed a marked increase with age. They averaged 657 µg/g dry stool at 5½ months of age and rose steadily until they reached 1,395 µg/g dry stool at 9 months of age and 1,194 µg/g dry stool at 12 months of age (fig. 2). The increase probably reflects the increasing presence of unabsorbed food heme (e.g. from meat) rather than increased baseline blood loss, but the latter possibility cannot be excluded.

Inhibition of Absorption of Iron by Components of Cow's Milk

In contradistinction to heme iron, the absorption of nonheme iron, which constitutes the bulk of dietary iron, is subject to inhibition by a number of substances that commonly occur in the diet. Cow's milk contains much higher amounts of calcium and casein than, for example, breast milk. It is well established that calcium is a potent inhibitor of iron absorption [25]. In adult

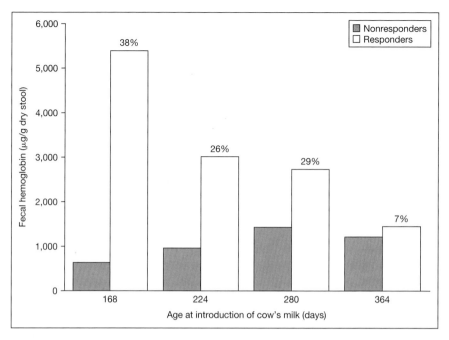

Fig. 2. Summary of results from 3 studies [22–24] with introduction of cow's milk at different ages. Infants fed cow's milk who did not respond and those responding to cow's milk with increased fecal hemoglobin are shown. Numbers on top of bars indicate percent responders.

subjects, iron absorption from human milk was 37.3% and from cow's milk 15.5% [26]. When the calcium concentration of human milk was raised to the same level as in cow's milk, iron absorption from human milk was only 19.2%. Thus, calcium explained about 70% of the difference in iron bioavailability between human and cow's milk [26]. No similar studies have been reported for infants. Hurrell et al. [27] showed that casein and other milk proteins strongly inhibit the absorption of iron. Thus it is evident that cow's milk with its high calcium and casein content is likely to have an adverse impact on the availability of iron which the infant and young child obtains from complementary foods.

Cow's Milk and Renal Solute Load

Waste substances of endogenous and dietary origin that require excretion by the kidneys are collectively referred to as renal solute load (RSL). Most of the RSL is of dietary origin and is related to the protein and electrolyte

Table 1. PRSL of various milks and formulas [modified from 29]

Feeding	Components of PRSL					PRSL	
	Na mmol/l	Cl mmol/l	K mmol/l	P mmol/l	urea mmol	mosm/l	mosm/ 100 kcal
Human milk	7	11	13	5	57	93	14
Milk-based formula	8	12	18	11	86	135	20
Soy-based formula	13	16	19	9	103	160	24
Two thirds cow's milk	14	20	26	20	124	204	30
Whole cow's milk	21	30	39	30	188	308	46

content of the diet. Potential renal solute load (PRSL) refers to solutes of dietary origin that need to be excreted in the urine except for a small proportion that is used for synthesis of new tissues and that is lost through nonrenal routes. Solutes are expressed in milliosmols and the concentration of the urine (osmolality) is expressed in milliosmols per kilogram of water.

Excretion of the RSL requires water and the minimum amount of water needed to excrete a given amount of RSL depends on the concentrating ability of the kidneys. When an infant is well and feeding ad libitum, his ability to excrete unneeded solutes and maintain water balance is more than adequate, even if the feeding has a high PRSL, for example cow's milk. However, there are circumstances in which the PRSL of the feeding is an important factor in maintaining water balance. In acute illnesses, food intake and hence fluid intake is generally decreased while evaporative loss of water is increased if there is fever. Water loss is further increased if there is diarrhea. In these circumstances the size of the PRSL determines whether or not water balance can be maintained.

Calculation of PRSL of the Diet

Nitrogenous compounds (mostly urea), the three electrolytes and phosphate make up the bulk of the RSL of infants. Therefore, an approximation of PRSL may be obtained as follows:

PRSL = N/28 + Na + Cl + K + P,

where the units are in millimoles (or milliosmols), except for N, which is total nitrogen in milligrams, and the term, N/28, represents nitrogenous solutes. The PRSL provided by various milks and formulas is presented in table 1. The value for mature human milk is 93 mosm/l (14 mosm/100 kcal). The value of 135 mosm/l (20 mosm/100 kcal) for the PRSL provided by milk-based formulas is representative and is somewhat lower than the PRSL of soy-based formulas (160 mosm/l; 24 mosm/100 kcal). The PRSL of whole cow's milk is 308 mosm/l (46 mosm/100 kcal) [28, 29].

Water Balance

As reviewed by Ziegler and Fomon [28] and Fomon and Ziegler [29], the physiological and clinical significance of the RSL rests on the impact it can have on body water economy. Water is ingested with milk, formula and other foods. At the caloric concentration of 67 kcal/100 ml, breast milk, cow's milk and formula provide about 90 ml of preformed water plus about 5 ml of water derived from the oxidation of fat and carbohydrate, for a total of 95 ml of water for each 100 ml of feeding. Water is inevitably lost from the body by evaporation and in feces. Evaporative water loss is increased considerably by fever and by elevated environmental temperature. Fecal water loss, which normally amounts to about 10 ml/kg/day, is greatly increased in diarrhea. Water not lost via feces or evaporation is available to the kidneys for urine formation. The amount of water available is diminished when evaporative and/or fecal water losses are increased. The capacity of infants to concentrate urine is not fully developed and is generally limited to 900–1,000 mosm/kg of water, with some normal infants being unable to achieve even 900 mosm/kg water [30–33].

Relation of PRSL to Urine Osmolality and Water Balance

An understanding of the PRSL of the infant's diet is of practical importance, as is evident from theoretically based calculations and from epidemiological data. Urine osmolality of infants may be predicted from the PRSL. The actual RSL is the PRSL minus the portions used for growth and lost through nonrenal routes. The latter losses, except during episodes of diarrhea, are small and may be ignored. The RSL may be estimated by subtracting from the PRSL solutes used for growth, i.e. 0.9 mmol (or mosm)/g of weight gain. An estimate of the RSL may therefore be calculated as RSL = PRSL − (0.9 × gain). Urine volume may be estimated from intake of milk or formula minus evaporative water loss. Urine osmolality can then be calculated. The data in table 2 show that predicted urine concentrations of hypothetical infants agree reasonably well with observed urine concentrations. Therefore, predictions of urine osmolality can be used to model urine osmolality and water balance in situations where the water balance is under stress.

In normal infants consuming commonly fed diets, water balance is easily maintained because, even with the infant's limited renal concentrating ability, the quantity of water is sufficient to excrete all the RSL. Figure 3 depicts urine osmolality (predicted) of a hypothetical infant. The strong effect of PRSL of the infant's diet on urine osmolality is evident. The effect of complementary foods (data not shown) is to increase urine osmolality except in the case of cow's milk, where the effect is to decrease predicted urine osmolality. If the child experiences a febrile illness, the amount of water available for

Table 2. Urine osmolality (predicted and observed) of infants in relation to PRSL of the diet

Feeding	PRSL mosm/l	Urine osmolality	
		predicted mosm/kg	observed mosm/kg
Human milk	93	120	157
Milk-based formula	135	204	–
Soy-based formula	160	272	–
Two thirds cow's milk	204	342	396
Whole cow's milk	308	550	–

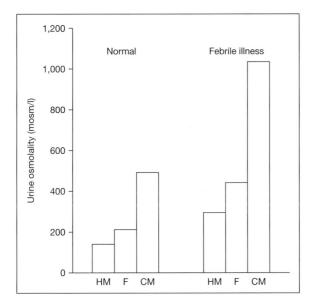

Fig. 3. Effect of feeding on calculated urine osmolality of a hypothetical infant (12 months old; 10.5 kg) under normal conditions or during a febrile illness (see text for details). HM = Human milk; F = formula; CM = cow's milk.

urine formation is diminished and urine osmolality increases dramatically, as the right panel of figure 3 illustrates. In the latter scenario it is assumed that the volume of intake from all sources is decreased by 25% and that evaporative water loss is increased by 33%. Even with these rather modest deviations from normal, there is a marked effect on urine osmolality. And now the PRSL of the infant's feeding makes a crucial difference. With human milk or formula, the osmolality is still well within the infant's concentrating ability. But with cow's milk, the urine osmolality will be close to the infant's urinary concentrating ability. If the osmolality that would be necessary to excrete all renal solutes exceeds the infant's concentrating ability, maximally concentrated urine will be excreted and the infant will go into negative water balance. If the decrease in intake and/or the increase in evaporative water loss are higher than assumed in the example, the infant fed cow's milk will be in more strongly negative water balance. Persistent negative water balance leads to dehydration. Infants fed cow's milk are therefore at greater risk of significant dehydration than infants fed human milk or formula.

Epidemiological Evidence

Epidemiological data indicate that infants fed formulas providing PRSL of 39 mosm/100 kcal or more are at much greater risk of hypertonic dehydration during illness than are breastfed infants (average PRSL of human milk is about 14 mosm/l) or those fed currently marketed formulas (PRSL about 20–24 mosm/ 100 kcal). In the United Kingdom, whole cow's milk and formulas with only slightly lower PRSL were widely fed to infants until 1974, when health authorities recommended feedings with lower PRSL. This recommendation was widely followed and the use of feedings with high PRSL declined sharply. A number of reports documented a decrease in the incidence of hypernatremic dehydration occurring in the years following the change [34–37]. The close temporal relation between changes in feeding practices and the decline in the incidence of hypernatremic dehydration strongly suggests that hypernatremic dehydration occurs more frequently when feedings provide an unduly high PRSL. In the United States, the change in feeding practices that led to the use of formulas with relatively modest PRSL occurred more gradually, and epidemiological data comparable to those for the United Kingdom are not available. Nevertheless, there is little doubt that the incidence of hypernatremic dehydration has decreased as formulas with more modest PRSLs replaced evaporated milk formulas in the 1970s. In hospitals in the Bronx, diarrhea with dehydration was reported to account for about 12% of infant admissions from the 1960s through the 1980s. The dehydration was hypernatremic in 19.5% of these infants in 1963–1972, 9.3% in 1973–1980, and 4.5% in the 1980s [38].

Recommended Upper Limit for PRSL of the Infant's Diet

Thus, as discussed in more detail by Ziegler and Fomon [28], both theoretically based calculations and epidemiological evidence suggest that a PRSL of about 39 mosm/100 kcal or greater places the infant at risk of hypernatremic dehydration, whereas feedings providing 20–24 mosm/100 kcal appear to offer a satisfactory margin of safety with respect to water balance. It seems reasonable to limit the PRSL of feedings for infants to 30–35 mosm/100 kcal. RSL considerations entered prominently into the recommendation in 1992 of the Committee on Nutrition of the American Academy of Pediatrics [39] that infants should be breastfed or fed formulas rather than whole cow's milk (PRSL 46 mosm/100 kcal) during the first year of life.

Conclusion

Because of its adverse effects on iron status and because it increases the risk of severe dehydration, unmodified cow's milk should not be fed to infants. One of the main objections to the feeding of cow's milk, its negative effect on iron status, could be overcome by the use of iron-fortified cow's milk or by providing iron supplements. The dehydration risk can be reduced by lowering the PRSL to less than 35 mosm/100 kcal. That can be accomplished by simply diluting cow's milk and by adding a source of energy (e.g., carbohydrate), i.e. making it into a formula. But the feeding of unmodified pasteurized cow's milk places infants and toddlers at high risk of iron deficiency and increases the risk of severe dehydration.

References

1 Smith NJ, Hunter RE: Iron requirements during growth; in Hallberg L, Harwerth H-G, Vannotti A (eds): Iron Deficiency. New York, Academic Press, 1970, pp 199–211.
2 Woodruff CW, Wright SW, Wright RP: The role of fresh cow's milk in iron deficiency. Am J Dis Child 1972;124:26–30.
3 Tunnessen WW, Oski FA: Consequences of starting whole cow milk at 6 months of age. J Pediatr 1987;111:813–816.
4 Penrod JC, Anderson K, Acosta PB: Impact on iron status of introducing cow's milk in the second six months of life. J Pediatr Gastroenterol Nutr 1990;10:462–467.
5 Fuchs GJ, Farris RP, DeWier M, et al: Iron status and intake of older infants fed formula vs cow milk with cereal. Am J Clin Nutr 1993;58:343–348.
6 Kwiatkowski JL, West TB, Heidary N, et al: Severe iron deficiency anemia in young children. J Pediatr 1999;135:514–516.
7 Morton RE, Nysenbaum A, Price K: Iron status in the first year of life. J Pediatr Gastroenterol Nutr 1988;7:707–712.
8 Wharf SG, Fox TE, Fairweather-Tait SJ, Cook JD: Factors affecting iron stores in infants 4–18 months of age. Eur J Clin Nutr 1997;51:504–509.
9 Lawson MS, Thomas M, Hardiman A: Iron status of Asian children aged 2 years living in England. Arch Dis Child 1998;78:420–426.
10 Williams J, Wolff A, Daly A, et al: Iron supplemented formula milk related to reduction in psychomotor decline in infants from inner city areas: randomised study. Br Med J 1999;318: 693–697.
11 Thane CW, Walmsley CM, Bales CJ, et al: Risk factors for poor iron status in British toddlers. Public Health Nutr 2000;3:433–440.
12 Michaelsen KF, Milman N, Samuelson G: A longitudinal study of iron status in healthy Danish infants: effects of early iron status, growth velocity and dietary factors. Acta Paediatr 1995;84: 1035–1044.
13 Mira M, Alperstein G, Karr M, et al: Haem iron intake in 12–36 month old children depleted in iron: case-control study. Br Med J 1996;312:881–883.
14 Gill DG, Vincent S, Segal DS: Follow-on formula in the prevention of iron deficiency: a multi-centre study. Acta Paediatr 1997;86:863–869.
15 Bramhagen A-C, Axelsson I: Iron status of children in southern Sweden: effect of cow's milk and follow-on formula. Acta Paediatr 1999;88:1333–1337.

16 Thorsdottir I, Gunnarsson BS, Atladottir H, et al: Iron status at 12 months of age – effects of body size, growth and diet in a population with high birth weight. Eur J Clin Nutr 2003;57: 505–513.

17 Male C, Persson LA, Freeman V, et al; Euro-Growth Iron Study: Prevalence of iron deficiency in 12-mo-old infants from 11 European areas and influence of dietary factors on iron status (Euro-Growth study). Acta Paediatr 2001;90:492–498.

18 Fomon SJ: Nutrition of Normal Infants. St Louis, Mosby-Year Book, 1993, p 252.

19 Elian E, Bar-Shani S, Liberman A, Matoh Y: Intestinal blood loss: a factor in calculations of body iron in late infancy. J Pediatr 1966;69:215–219.

20 Wilson JF, Lahey ME, Heiner DC: Studies on iron metabolism. V. Further observations on cow's milk-induced gastrointestinal bleeding in infants with iron-deficiency anemia. J Pediatr 1974;84:335–344.

21 Fomon SJ, Ziegler EE, Nelson SE, Edwards BB: Cow milk feeding in infancy: gastrointestinal blood loss and iron nutritional status. J Pediatr 1981;98:540–545.

22 Ziegler EE, Fomon SJ, Nelson SE, et al: Cow milk feeding in infancy: further observations on blood loss from the gastrointestinal tract. J Pediatr 1990;116:11–18.

23 Ziegler EE, Jiang T, Romero E, et al: Cow's milk and intestinal blood loss in late infancy. J Pediatr 1999;135:720–726.

24 Jiang T, Jeter JM, Nelson SE, Ziegler EE: Intestinal blood loss during cow milk feeding in older infants. Quantitative measurements. Arch Pediatr Adolesc Med 2000;154:673–678.

25 Hallberg L: Does calcium interfere with iron absorption? Am J Clin Nutr 1998;68:3–4.

26 Hallberg L, Rossander-Hultén L, Brune M, Gleerup A: Bioavailability in man of iron in human milk and cow's milk in relation to their calcium contents. Pediatr Res 1992;31:524–527.

27 Hurrell RF, Lynch SR, Trinidad TP, et al: Iron absorption in humans as influenced by bovine milk proteins. Am J Clin Nutr 1989;49:546–552.

28 Ziegler EE, Fomon SJ: Potential renal solute load of infant formulas. J Nutr 1989;119: 1785–1789.

29 Fomon SJ, Ziegler EE: Renal solute load and potential renal solute load in infancy. J Pediatr 1999;134:11–14.

30 Winberg J: Determination of renal concentrating capacity in infants and children without renal disease. Acta Paediatr Scand 1959;48:318–328.

31 Edelmann CM Jr, Barnett HL, Troupkou V: Renal concentrating mechanisms in newborn infants. J Clin Invest 1960;39:1062–1069.

32 Drescher AN, Barnett HL, Troupkou V: Water balance in infants during water deprivation. Am J Dis Child 1962;104:366–379.

33 Polacek E, Vocel J, Neugebauerova L, et al: The osmotic concentrating ability in healthy infants and children. Arch Dis Child 1965;40:291–295.

34 Arneil GC, Chin KC: Lower-solute milks and reduction of hypernatraemia in young Glasgow infants. Lancet 1979;ii:840.

35 Davies DP, Ansari BM, Mandal BK: The declining incidence of infantile hypernatraemic dehydration in Great Britain. Am J Dis Child 1979;133:148–150.

36 Sunderland R, Emery JL: Apparent disappearance of hypernatraemic dehydration from infant deaths in Sheffield. Br Med J 1979;2:575–576.

37 Manuel PD, Walker-Smith JA: Decline of hypernatraemia as a problem in gastroenteritis. Arch Dis Child 1980;55:124–127.

38 Finberg L: Comment on Ziegler & Fomon. J Nutr 1992;119:1788.

39 American Academy of Pediatrics, Committee on Nutrition: The use of whole cow's milk in infancy. Pediatrics 1992;89:1105–1109.

Discussion

Dr. Fisberg: I think there is no doubt that cow's milk is not suited for children especially at very young ages. One of the main concerns, especially in developing countries where the prices are not subsidized, is the high cost of the formulas. So what would be an alternative to this situation in those countries?

Dr. Ziegler: On the iron side cow's milk could be fortified with iron. Chile is doing it and I think Argentina is also doing it. It is not expensive. On the renal solute load side, a formula can be made out of cow's milk by diluting it with water and adding a source of energy, preferably also a source of iron. That would improve the ratio of renal solute load to water. I suspect that is done in Brazil widely, cow's milk is not fed as straight cow's milk, it is fed as a formula. Of course the ultimate answer is to breast-feed because, besides all other advantages, the economics of breastfeeding are highly favorable.

Dr. Gailing: What are your considerations on renal solute load and the eventual dehydration and iron losses with the consumption of diary products? After 6 months a lot of babies are switched from a part of the milk or the infant formula to normal fresh dairy products based on cow's milk. Do you have the same conclusion when the babies are eating this type of product in a large amount?

Dr. Ziegler: If you are asking me about cheese, would cheese cause blood loss? I suspect not, but I don't know, I have not studied any dairy products other than whole pasteurized cow's milk. The concern about the lack of iron is the same with all dairy foods. But I must emphasize that a low iron content is only a concern when a food is the predominant source of energy, as would be the case in a 6-month-old infant fed cow's milk.

Dr. Domellöf: What do you think is the mechanism behind the cow's milk-induced blood loss; is it related to cow's milk allergy?

Dr. Ziegler: I told you that babies who were exposed to modified cow's milk anti-gens from birth had a low incidence of blood loss. This suggests perhaps that there is tolerance that develops in those babies who are exposed to cow's milk antigens from early on.

Dr. Shahkhalili: Could the different effects of sterilized cow's milk (heat treated at 115°C) and pasteurized milk be due to a lack of live bacteria in sterile milk?

Dr. Ziegler: Although pasteurized milk is not completely sterile whereas milk treated to 115°C is, neither form of milk is a source of bacteria for the infant.

Dr. Agostoni: I am always very curious about these unknown compounds. Do you have any information whether it is from whey or casein, or do you know whether by supplying yogurt or fermented milk you have the same effect?

Dr. Ziegler: A colleague of ours in Russia has studied fermented milk. The name of it is kefir, and he found that there is blood loss when it is given to young infants.

Dr. Simell: If I am not totally mistaken, if children who are receiving cow's milk are properly supplemented with iron, the bleeding to the gut is stopped. There are some adult studies looking at the same phenomenon and clearly it looks as though this is happening. Do you know anything more?

Dr. Ziegler: I know which study you are referring to, it was done in the 1960s, but there is an alternative interpretation. The study concluded that if you are anemic you lose blood. I think the alternative interpretation, that you lose blood and therefore you are anemic, is just as viable and fits the data. So I don't believe that anemia makes you lose blood, I think it is the other way round.

Dr. Pazvakavambwa: I want to know if the high UHT milk, the long-life milk, is different from ordinary cow's milk?

Dr. Ziegler: I don't know the answer, I have not studied UHT milk. How high is the temperature in UHT? 115°C, that would suggest that it does not induce bleeding.

Dr. Solomons: I was interested in your initial run through of requirements for absorption. I am always interested in something that doesn't have the standard devia-tion. So you were giving some single numbers, is this an average number, is this a max-imum number that is the highest number in the range of what children need? First of all I don't believe it is a single number, I believe that infants have a range to be absorbed and that range also is dependent on other things, for instance on their difference in growth rates and tissue requirements for iron. This has been illustrated by some recent studies on mice at Davis California [1]. To interpret it, we must acknowledge all of the caveats in extrapolating from a rodent to a human in terms of maturation equivalency. Nevertheless, the observation suggested that iron adsorption is more sensitive to interference from zinc in early life. I think what we are learning from both experiments in animal and human research is that there are a number of intricate factors beyond calcium and the gut that might texture, produce more nuances in requirements from infant to infant for iron. I am skeptical about a single number that you multiply by another number and get another number and call that number universal for all humanity.

Dr. Ziegler: I agree with your point that there has to be a range and that which I showed is at best an average. But I used it mainly to illustrate the fact that there is a substantial requirement for iron that cannot be met by cow's milk. Now that 170-mg increase from birth obviously has a large range because we know that some babies are born with low iron stores and some are born with high iron stores. So if you want you can calculate from the lowest possible iron content at birth to the highest possible iron content at 1 year and you come up with a large number. Then you could do the converse and assume a baby with large iron stores will end up with a low iron content at 1 year. They will obviously have very different increments.

Dr. Morelli: I don't know if I remember well, but whey protein could be negatively affected by the UHT process, especially if it is real UHT and not UHST. There are two methods for this kind of heat treatment. The old one was UHT and now we have UHST, which takes a very short time; in a couple of seconds steam is injected into the milk, and this treatment is very soft for casein, but not for globulin. So this could be a tool to isolate and identify unknown components.

Dr. Ziegler: Since we don't know what the offending agent is, the only way to find out whether UHT-treated milk causes blood loss is to do a test.

Dr. Giovannini: Do you have any data on the consumption of whole cow's milk and its incidence in obesity? We talked about obesity and breastfeeding, but in Western countries whole milk is still used today, not only for economic reasons. Are there any data which could explain to our colleagues who are sometimes the first not to believe too much in breastfeeding and don't believe too much in formulas?

Dr. Ziegler: I don't think that anyone has done long-term follow-up studies to see what the incidence of obesity is in childhood or adulthood. I know Dr. Michaelsen has data on the relationship of milk consumption to obesity or adiposity at 4 years. There is adult literature that says if weight-loss diets include a large amount of dairy foods, there is a more pronounced loss of percent body fat, but that is only in the situation of weight loss. For children nothing of that sort is known. But that is current intake of cow's milk, and you are asking if consuming cow's milk during infancy has anything to do with obesity later on, and I don't think anyone knows.

Dr. Cardoso: Could you comment on parasitic infections and blood loss in the developing countries?

Dr. Ziegler: If you have parasitic infections then obviously there are some that can cause substantial blood loss, but I can't comment.

Dr. Solomons: Intestinal parasites are unlikely to establish adult worms within the first 6 months in the life of an infant; it takes longer for the parasitic egg to develop into a worm than it takes the child to develop into an older infant. Hookworm comes to the skin and if a baby is left lying around, it might get infected. Hookworm causes bleeding and is contacted by the fecal oral route. The child has to be crawling, so this a disease that is well above the infant period.

Dr. Barclay: I would just like to come back to the relationship between calcium and iron absorption. The studies done by Hallberg and Rossander [2] were acute absorption studies. Acute single meal studies show a dramatic effect of calcium intake on iron absorption. However, more recent data from longer term studies, over several weeks or months, show that the effect of calcium intake on iron absorption actually disappears. Is there now a consensus on this relationship between calcium intake and iron absorption?

Dr. Ziegler: Cow's milk causes iron deficiency. If we dismiss blood loss and dismiss inhibition of iron absorption, we are left with the low iron content of cow's milk as the mechanism. But something is causing infants fed cow's milk to be iron deficient, there is no question.

Dr. Michaelsen: We made an intervention study with calcium in pubertal girls in order to look at bone metabolism and iron status [3]. We asked them to take calcium with the evening meal to increase compliance, and there was absolutely no effect on iron status after 1 year.

References

1 Kelleher SL, Lonnerdal B: Zinc supplementation reduces iron absorption through age-dependent changes in small intestine iron transporter expression in suckling rat pups. J Nutr 2006;136:1185–1191.
2 Hallberg L, Rossander L: Absorption of iron from Western-type lunch and dinner meals. Am J Clin Nutr 1982;35:502–509.
3 Molgaard C, Kaestel P, Michaelsen KF: Long-term calcium supplementation does not affect the iron status of 12-14-y-old girls. Am J Clin Nutr 2005;82:98–102.

Agostoni C, Brunser O (eds): Issues in Complementary Feeding.
Nestlé Nutr Workshop Ser Pediatr Program, vol 60, pp 201–219,
Nestec Ltd., Vevey/S. Karger AG, Basel, © 2007.

Whole Cow's Milk: Why, What and When?

Kim Fleischer Michaelsen, Camilla Hoppe,
Lotte Lauritzen, Christian Mølgaard

Department of Human Nutrition and LMC Centre for Advanced Food Studies,
Faculty of Life Sciences, University of Copenhagen, Copenhagen, Denmark

Abstract

There are differences between at what age industrialized countries recommend that cow's milk can be introduced to infants. Most countries recommend waiting until 12 months of age, but according to recommendations from some countries (e.g. Canada, Sweden and Denmark) cow's milk can be introduced from 9 or 10 months. The main reason for delaying introduction is to prevent iron deficiency as cow's milk is a poor iron source. In one study mainly milk intake above 500 ml/day caused iron deficiency. Cow's milk has a very low content of linoleic acid (LA), but a more favorable LA/α-linolenic ratio, which is likely to be the reason why red blood cell docosahexaenoic acid (DHA) levels seem to be more favorable in infants drinking cow's milk compared to infants drinking infant formula that is not supplemented with DHA. It has been suggested that cow's milk intake can affect the later risk of obesity, blood pressure and linear growth, but the evidence is not convincing. There are also considerable differences in recommendations on at what age cow's milk with reduced fat intake can be introduced. The main consideration is that low-fat milk might limit energy intake and thereby growth, but the potential effects on development of early obesity should also be considered. Recommendations about the age for introduction of cow's milk should take into consideration traditions and feeding patterns in the population, especially the intake of iron and long-chain polyunsaturated fatty acids and should also give recommendations on the volume of milk.

Introduction

It has for decades been discussed at what age cow's milk can be introduced to the diet of the infant or young child, at what age milk with reduced fat content can be introduced, and how much the recommended daily intake should be. The discussion is ongoing.

The role of cow's milk in the complementary feeding diet was also discussed at a joint meeting between ESPGHAN and the International Paediatric Society (IPA) in Casablanca in 1999 [1]. In the proceedings from the meeting some of the main issues on cow's milk were highlighted and the following research questions were mentioned [2]:

1 What is the appropriate age for the introduction of cow's milk?
2 What is a reasonable daily amount during 'late' lactation, and when the diet has been diversified?
3 Is there a need for special modified formulas for young children (toddlers' formulas)?
4 Is there an effect of the fatty acid composition of cow's milk on the risk of developing cardiovascular disease later in life?
5 Do fermented milk products have significant positive effects on morbidity and growth in countries with poor hygiene or in industrialized countries?
6 Does cow's milk protein have a role in the development of diabetes?

Some of these issues will be discussed in this article in the light of new evidence. The aim is to give an update on the scientific evidence for some of the potential negative and positive effects of giving cow's milk to infants and young children. The potential effect of a high renal solute load in cow's milk and the data suggesting that cow's milk can provoke microscopic intestinal bleeding will only be briefly mentioned as these two topics are discussed in detail in the article in this volume by Ziegler (pp. 185–195). The effects of fermented milk products are discussed in the article by Brunser et al. (pp. 235–247).

This article discusses both short-term and potential long-term effects of using whole cow's milk in complementary feeding. However, very few randomized studies are available and although there is an increasing literature on the potential programming effect of early diet it is still not known to what degree late infancy and young childhood are also periods sensitive to programming.

Recommendations on Age of Introduction

The main reason for delaying the introduction of cow's milk is to prevent the development of iron deficiency. Recommendations on age of introduction will thus have to take into account the risk of iron deficiency in the population, the iron content of the remaining diet, recommendations on iron supplements, alternatives to cow's milk, and the amount of milk given.

In most countries it is now recommended that cow's milk is not introduced before the age of 12 months, whereas some countries recommend that it can be introduced from the age of 9 months [3, 4] or 10 months [5].

The American Academy of Pediatrics Committee on Nutrition published recommendations on the use of whole cow's milk in 1992 in which the main statement was that whole cow's milk (and low iron formulas) should not be used during the first year of life [6]. The main argument was the low iron content and the risk of iron deficiency. In the recommendations it was also noted that infants fed whole cow's milk have low intakes of linoleic acid (LA) and vitamin E, and excessive intakes of sodium, potassium, and protein.

In Canada the official recommendations for healthy term infant feeding were updated in 2005 [3]. The guidelines are issued by a joint working group including the Canadian Paediatric Society, Dieticians of Canada and Health Canada. The recommendations are that pasteurized whole cow's milk may be introduced at 9 months. The text reads: 'Infants weaned from breastfeeding before 9 months of age should receive iron-fortified formula. Non-fortified formula and cow's milk are unsuitable alternatives as they contain very little natural iron which is poorly absorbed. When milk is combined with other dietary sources of iron, such as iron-fortified infant cereals, puréed liver, meat, fish, legumes and egg yolk, it may be possible to avoid iron deficiency and anemia. However, there are limited data to support or refute this estimation. After 9 months of age, when a wider variety of foods is being ingested, the introduction of cow's milk is not associated with any risk of iron deficiency.'

According to the recommendations from the health authorities in Denmark cow's milk can be gradually introduced as drinking milk from the age of 9 months, but there is no advice against continuing with infant formula until the age of 12 months. The potential negative effect on iron status of an early introduction is solved by a general recommendation in Denmark that any infant that does not receive at least 400 ml of iron-fortified infant formula per day from the age of 6–12 months should have medicinal iron as drops. This recommendation covers also breastfed infants. Thus, there is a choice between using either cow's milk and iron drops or using infant formula, which in Denmark, as in all European countries, is fortified with iron.

In Sweden it is recommended that cow's milk can be introduced from the age of 10–12 months. In the paper giving the background for these ages it is argued that it is important to wait until 10–12 months to introduce cow's milk, because earlier introduction would have a negative effect on iron status [5].

Recommendations on when to use cow's milk with reduced fat content are discussed in the section on fat quantity.

Current Intake

Many studies have presented data on the prevalence of feeding cow's milk at different ages during infancy. Here a few examples are given.

In the Euro-Growth study 2,245 infants participated from 22 centers in 11 countries during the period of 1990–1996 [7]. At the age of 4, 5, 6, 9 and 12 months 4, 6, 9, 18 and 31%, respectively, were fed cow's milk as the only milk source. At 6, 9 and 12 months the percentage of children receiving any cow's milk was 18, 33 and 50%, respectively. Of those receiving cow's milk the

Table 1. Content of energy and selected nutrients in cow's milk, infant formula and breast milk (per 100 ml)

	Breast milk	Formula	Full-fat milk
Energy, kJ	270–290	280–290	270
Energy, kcal	65–70	67	65
Protein, g	0.9	1.2–1.8	3.4
Carbohydrates, g	6.7	70–80	4.4
Oligosaccharides, g	1.3	0	0
Fat, g	3.5	3.8	3.5
Calcium, mg	20–25	42	116
Phosphorus, mg	12–14	21	93
Sodium, mg	12–25	16	45
Potassium, mg	40–55	55	144
Iron, mg	0.03–0.09	0.4–0.7	0
Zinc, mg	0.1–0.3	0.4	0.42
Vitamin A, μg	30–60	50	29
Vitamin C, μg	10	7–9	1.2
Vitamin D, μg	0.03	1.0	0.1
Vitamin K, μg	0.2–0.5	2.8	1.6
Folic acid, μg	80–140	6.5	11

percentage receiving low fat cow's milk at 6, 9, 12, 24 and 36 months were 24, 20, 25, 31 and 33%, respectively.

In a recent study from Canada it was found that 13% of mothers said that they were feeding their infant cow's milk as the primary source of milk before the age of 9 months [8]. This was mainly the case in families with younger mothers, with lower annual incomes, and families that were less likely to have attended prenatal classes. These families were also more likely to have introduced solid foods or skimmed milk before the recommended ages.

In a study from Iceland 7% of the infants received cow's milk at the age of 5 months but at the age of 6 months as many as 40% of the infants received cow's milk [9]. At the time of the study the recommendation was that cow's milk could be introduced from the age of 6 months. The intake of cow's milk during the age period from 9 to 12 months was divided into quintiles with a median intake of 289 ml, and the median intake in the two upper quintiles being 412 and 583 ml. At the age of 2 years 16% of the children had an intake above 500 ml.

Iron

The main reason for delaying the introduction of cow's milk is a concern about the iron status of the infant and young child. Cow's milk has a low iron content (table 1) combined with a low availability. Furthermore, several studies have shown that feeding cow's milk to infants can cause microscopic bleeding from the gastrointestinal tract, in some cases up to about 9 months of age.

Many studies have shown the association between intake of cow's milk and low iron status. In the large Euro-Growth study including 488 infants from 11 European centers 7.2% had iron deficiency and 2.3% iron deficiency anemia at the age of 12 months. Early introduction of cow's milk was a strong negative determinant of iron status and the use of infant formula a positive determinant [10]. This has also been shown by other studies [11].

In a study from Iceland the association between the daily intake of whole cow's milk and iron status was examined. At the age of 12 months 1 in 5 infants had low serum ferritin and 2.7% were also anemic [9]. Cow's milk intake from 9 to 12 months was negatively associated with iron status, but only significantly, if the intake was above 460 ml/day. At the age of 2 years iron deficiency had declined to 9% with 1.4% having iron deficiency anemia [12]. Of the 11 infants being iron deficient only 1 had a daily milk intake below 500 ml, and among those with an intake above 500 ml, half were iron deficient.

Protein

Cow's milk has a protein content that is more than 3 times as high as that in breast milk, 3.5 compared to 1% or lower in mature breast milk. The content in infant formula is much closer to the level in breast milk. Calculated as protein energy percent the values are about 5–6, 9–10 and 20–21 for human milk, infant formula and cow's milk, respectively.

When the fat content of milk is reduced, the relative contribution of protein to the energy content (protein energy percentage) is increased. If the intake of low-fat milk is the same as the intake of whole milk, the protein intake from milk will be the same, but if the lower energy intake from low-fat milk is compensated by a higher milk volume, then the protein intake will increase. If an infant drinks 350 ml of whole milk (3.5%) and changes to skimmed milk (0.3%) with the same energy intake, the infant will have to drink 600 ml of skimmed milk and the protein intake will increase from 12 to 20 g.

The potential effects of protein intake on later health are discussed in the sections on overweight and obesity, blood pressure and linear growth.

Fat Quality

A marked difference between cow's milk, infant formula and breast milk is the fatty acid composition [13–15]. One of the important differences is a high content of saturated fatty acids in cow's milk, about 65–70% of the weight of total fatty acids. For comparison the content of saturated fatty acids is about

40–50% in human milk. It is especially the content of 14:0, 16:0 and 18:0 that are higher in cow's milk.

A high intake of saturated fatty acids from milk increases the cardiovascular risk in adults and it has been discussed whether the early intake of saturated fat also influences cardiovascular risk factors. In a large study from Finland [16] the intervention group was recommended to use skimmed milk from the age of 7 months and to compensate the low fat intake by adding vegetable oil to the diet. However, the intervention group was also advised to continue a diet with a reduced saturated fat intake later in childhood. At the age of 9 years there was still a significant difference in fat intake with a lower intake of total fat and saturated fat in the intervention group compared to the control group [17]. Thus, it is not possible to determine whether the low saturated fat intake during late infancy has also been a determinant of the more advantageous results in the intervention group of insulin sensitivity (HOMA index) at 9 years and endothelial function at 11 years [17, 18]. However, the evidence that there are any adverse long-term effects of a high intake of milk fat in early life is, however, weak [19].

Another main difference in fat quality is that the content of LA (18:2n-6) is considerably lower in cow's milk (about 2%) compared to the content in human milk (8–13%) or infant formula (10–19%). The content of LA (18:2n-3) is also somewhat lower (0.2–1.2%) in cow's milk, but very variable. In human milk it is about 0.7–1.1% and in infant formula 1.2–2.0%. The ratio 18:2n-6/18:3n-3 can therefore vary a lot in cow's milk from values at the same level as infant formula, 8–10, down to around 4, when the level of LA is high. Thus, despite a low level of n-3 fatty acids the n-6/n-3 ratio in cow's milk is quite favorable.

Cow's milk does not contribute to the intake of long-chain polyunsaturated fatty acids (LCPUFA), whereas both docosahexaenoic acid (DHA) and arachidonic acid (AA) are present in human milk. However, the content varies considerably with the diet of the mother. Population mean values of DHA in human milk vary from 0.15 to 1.0% and of AA from 0.4 to 0.8% [13]. Traditionally there was no LCPUFA in infant formula, but now more and more formulas are supplemented with DHA and in some cases also with AA.

The effect of cow's milk intake on LCPUFA status in infants and young children is not well documented. Many infants fed on cow's milk will have a very low intake of DHA as a high fish intake is not common in many populations during the complementary feeding period. On the other hand, it has also been suggested that a high intake of short-chain polyunsaturated fatty acids (PUFA), especially LA (18:2n-6), which is much lower in cow's milk than in human milk and infant formula, can have a negative effect on the LCPUFA status. In one study piglets were randomized to formula with different ratios of LA to α-LA (ALA, 8:3n-3) from 0.5:1 to 10:1 and with LA kept constant at 13% of fat content [20]. The highest incorporation of DHA in brain and other tissues was seen at ratios of 4:1 and 2:1. In rats fed oils with a different content of ALA it was the oil with the lowest ALA content that resulted in the highest DHA levels in the heart tissue and plasma. The explanation suggested for this was that the low ALA intake resulted in a decreased competition for delta-6-desaturase [21]. In one study comparing breastfeeding, formula feeding and a group fed evaporated cow's milk, the red blood cell DHA level at 3 and 6 months was highest in the breastfed group, but higher in the cow's millk group than the formula group [22]. Thus, regarding DHA status in the infant it is likely that cow's milk with its favorable n-6/n-3 ratio and low PUFA content can result in DHA tissue values at the same level as formula that is not supplemented with DHA.

Cow's Milk with Reduced Fat Content

When is it appropriate to introduce cow's milk with a reduced fat content? In several countries the recommendation is that fat-reduced milk should not be introduced during the first 2–3 years of life, while others recommend that semi-skimmed milk can be introduced earlier. The main concern is that reducing the fat content might also reduce total energy intake because the infant might not be able to compensate the lower energy intake by eating more. In an analysis of fat intake and growth in 19 countries from Central and South America it was concluded that it was only when the dietary fat content was below 22% that there was a problem with growth [23]. Other concerns have been that low-fat milk might result in an increased protein intake as explained in the section on protein. Furthermore, it has been suggested that the high intake of saturated fatty acid from whole milk might increase the cardiovascular risk in later life as discussed in the section on fat quality.

The ESPGHAN nutrition committee has made recommendations on fat intake during the first years of life. It was concluded that fat intake should not be reduced before the age of 3 years [19].

In the WHO guiding principles for feeding nonbreastfed children 6–24 months of age [24] it is stated that whole milk is a good source of fat during the first 2 years of life, that semi-skimmed milk may be acceptable after 12 months of life, but skimmed milk is not recommended as a major food source during the first 2 years of life.

In the United Kingdom it is recommended that semi-skimmed milk (1.5–1.8% fat) should not be introduced before 2 years and skimmed milk (<0.3%) not before the age of 5 years [25]. On the official website (www.eatwell.gov.uk/ageandstages/baby/weaning) it is argued that full-fat milk should not be used before 12 months as it does not have the right balance of nutrients and that semi-skimmed milk can be introduced from 2 years, if the child is a good eater and has a varied diet.

According to the Canadian recommendations [3] partly skimmed milk (1 and 2%) is not routinely recommended in the first 2 years, and skim milk is found inappropriate in the first 2 years. The arguments are that skim milk provides no essential fatty acids and has a very low energy density. With high intakes, protein and solute intake would be significantly higher than the infant needs. It is stated that approximately 15% of Canadian infants are on 2% milk around 1 year of age and although there is no clear indication of negative consequences, there is no medical or nutritional indication to recommend the routine use of partially skimmed milk. Although whole cow's milk is recommended for the second year of life, it is also stated that 2% milk may be an acceptable alternative provided that the child is eating a variety of foods and growing at an acceptable rate.

In Denmark it is recommended that if cow's milk is used it should be full-fat milk up to the age of 12 months, but after that age it is recommended that milk should preferably be semi-skimmed, which in Denmark has a fat content of 1.5% [4]. The background for recommending a reduced fat content, already from the age of 12 months was (1) that this reduction in fat intake in an amount of milk that was not supposed to be more than 500 ml was not likely to bring the fat content of the total diet down to a level that would affect energy intake, (2) that in this age group there was no documented positive effects of a high saturated fat intake and (3) that is was important to get young children used to drinking low-fat milk.

Milk Volume

Not many recommendations on milk intake during infancy include recommendations on the preferred volume or give an upper limit.

In the WHO guiding principles for feeding nonbreastfed children 6–24 months of age [24] there are recommendations on the volume of intake. Using linear programming analysis it was calculated that if the diet was not fortified or supplemented 200–400 ml were needed per day if there were other animal source foods in the diet and 300–500 ml if there were no other animal source foods.

One of the problems with a large milk intake is that it can take up a considerable part of the energy intake, leaving only limited space for other foods and thereby a diversified diet. In table 2 the energy content of 350 and 500 ml of cow's milk with different fat contents has been calculated as a percentage of the recommended energy intake of a 12-, 24- or 36-month-old child. If a 12-month-old child drinks 500 ml of whole cow's milk daily, it takes up about 36% of the recommended energy intake, and thus leaves 64% of the energy intake for other foods. An intake of 1,000 ml a day will thus take up as much as 72% of the energy intake, leaving only 28% for other foods. No one will recommend such a high intake, but there are children who drink very large amounts of milk, so called milkaholics. It is not known how common this is, but these young children are know at pediatric departments where they are occasionally admitted with severe iron anemia.

Table 2. Percentage of energy requirements covered by an intake of 500 or 350 ml of cow's milk with different fat content

	Whole cow's milk (3.5% fat)		Semi-skimmed milk (1.5% fat)		Skimmed milk (0.3% fat)	
	500 ml	350 ml	500 ml	350 ml	500 ml	350 ml
12 months	36	25	28	20	21	15
2 years	29	21	23	16	17	12
3 years	26	18	20	14	15	11

The energy requirement was calculated as the energy requirement per kilogram body weight (Nordic Nutrient Recommendations) multiplied by the median weight of Danish children. The values are averages for boys and girls.

In a 2-year-old child 500 ml of whole cow's milk provides 29% of the recommended energy intake, but if the volume is reduced to 350 ml and the fat content to 1.5% (semi-skimmed milk), milk will only cover 16% of the recommended energy intake. This can be less than optimal if the remaining diet is of poor quality and with little food of animal origin. But if the diet is diverse with a fat content above 25 energy percent, there should be no problem.

It is difficult to recommend what is a reasonable energy intake from milk and when the intake is so high that it will interfere with a varied intake of other healthy foods. It depends on the composition of the remaining diet. A daily intake of about 500 ml of cow's milk seems to be a reasonable upper limit, although the evidence for such a limit is not strong. The data from Iceland on milk intake and iron status [9, 12] support that it is only if the volume is above 400–500 ml that there is a problem with iron deficiency, in a society with no recommendations on routine iron supplementation. As 500 ml whole cow's milk is covering about one third of the energy requirements during the second year of life, there is a reasonable amount of space left for a diversified diet.

Overweight and Obesity

It has been suggested that a high protein intake early in life could result in an increased risk of developing overweight or obesity later in life. The proposed mechanism is that a high protein intake stimulates secretion of insulin-like growth factor-1 (IGF-1) and thereby triggers precocious cell multiplication and accelerates maturation. The increased IGF-1 levels may then accelerate growth and increase muscle mass and adipose tissue, and thus induce an early adiposity rebound, the time point at which the BMI increases after its nadir in childhood.

An early adiposity rebound is then associated with a higher risk of obesity later in childhood and possibly also in adulthood [26]. In a longitudinal study from France it was found that the protein energy percentage at the age of 2 years was positively correlated with BMI and subscapular skinfold thickness at 8 years after adjustment for energy intake at 2 years and parental BMI [24]. The protein-adiposity hypothesis was supported by an Italian study, in which Scaglioni et al. [27] examined the influence of the intake of macronutrients in early life on the development of overweight at 5 years. Those with a BMI above the 90th percentile at age 5 years had a significantly higher protein intake at 1 year of age than children with a lower BMI. In this population, the protein intake was very high, 22 protein energy percent (PE%) in the overweight group against 20 PE% in the nonoverweight group. Also, the proportion of overweight was very high. However, a study from the United Kingdom of factors affecting timing of adiposity rebound, in which almost 900 children were followed from birth to 5 years of age, there was no evidence of associations between protein intake and timing of adiposity rebound [28]. The average PE% at 18 months was about 14.5. Also, in our study of 105 Danish children, analyzing whether diet at 9 months of age was associated with adiposity at 10 years of age, there were no significant associations between protein intake at 9 months and body fat percentage (DEXA scan) or BMI at 10 years [29]. The average PE% at 9 months of age was 14 in this study. Thus, the data on the relationship between protein intake and adiposity is inconclusive. In a recent review Agostoni et al. [30] suggested that it was only when the protein intake was above 15 energy percent that there was an significant association between protein intake and development of adiposity.

The protein hypothesis is at present being tested in a large multicenter randomized controlled trial where nonbreastfed infants are randomized to infant formula with different protein contents (www.danoneinstitute.org/EUchildhoodobesity). This study tests whether moderate differences in protein content of infant formula will have an effect in formula-fed infants and if this is the case whether it is possible that the differences in protein content between human milk and infant formula could be an explanation for the lower prevalence of childhood overweight and obesity in breastfed infants seen in some studies. As the intervention will have its main effect during the first part of infancy, the results from this study will not be able to determine directly whether differences in protein intake during late infancy and young childhood have an effect on later development of overweight.

In relation to the potential effect of protein and milk intake on the risk of developing obesity later in life the recent paper by Moore et al. [31] is of interest. They found that low dairy intake in early childhood predicts excess body fat gain. Dietary intakes recorded during the 3- to 5-year age period with BMI and skinfolds measured from 10 to 13 years were compared. They found that those in the lowest tertile of dairy intake had a BMI that was approximately two units higher and had an extra 25 mm of subcutaneous fat in the sum of 4 skinfolds. The effects were stronger after controlling for intake of energy and saturated fat, suggesting that there was a protective effect in the nonfat part of the dairy products. An effect of calcium has been suggested by several authors [32, 33], mainly based on findings from studies in adults, but in the study by Moore et al. adding calcium to the multivariate analysis strengthened the results, suggesting that the effect did not come from calcium.

Several other studies have suggested that milk intake is inversely associated with body weight and obesity. However, it is unknown which components in milk possess the bioactivity associated with weight loss. As mentioned, the milk minerals, such as calcium, might play a role in the regulation of body weight [32, 34], through decreased absorption of fat from the intestine or through regulating the fat metabolism by influencing lipolysis, fat oxidation and lipogenesis. Other components in milk, such as milk peptides, might also be of importance in the regulation of body weight. Protein diets are popular for reducing obesity, because they seem to increase satiety [35]. Protein digestion leads to stimulation of many physiological and metabolic responses known to be involved in the regulation of food intake, and effects are found to be dependent on the protein source. Mechanisms by which peptides from protein digestion exert their effect on food intake via the gut include slowing stomach emptying, perhaps via opioid receptors and direct or indirect stimulation of gut hormone receptors. Milk protein hydrolysis products of relevance to regulation of food intake include casomorphins and caseinomacropeptide. Casomorphins are peptides released upon the digestion of casein and are known to interact with gastric opioid receptors thus slowing gastrointestinal motility [36]. Casomorphins may play a role in regulating food intake because the opioid antagonist was found to prevent reduction in food intake after a casein preload was given to rats [37].

The data supporting the protein-obesity hypothesis are still not convincing and it is above all not clear to what degree this hypothesis is relevant for the intake of cow's milk at the age from 9 to 18 months. Likewise, the data suggesting that low-fat dairy products have a beneficial effect on the development of obesity should still be considered as a hypothesis and if it is confirmed, there are at present no data to elucidate whether such an effect is relevant for the 9- to 18-month age period.

Blood Pressure

The type of milk intake at 3 months has been associated with blood pressure as young adults. The Barry Caerphilly Growth study cohort, involving infants born between 1972 and 1974, was followed up at the age of 23–27 years [38]. In the 1970s infants that were not breastfed were given formulas based on dried whole cow's milk, which consequently had a high protein and sodium content. In this study there was a significant positive association between the amount of whole cow's milk given at the age of 3 months and systolic blood pressure as young adults. As it is an observational study it is not known if this effect is caused by a programming effect of a high protein intake, a high sodium intake or other factors in milk or if it is caused by a bioactive effect of human milk, as also pointed out by the authors. Giving unmodified cow's milk at 3 months of age is very 'unphysiological' and infants at this early age are likely to be much more sensitive to a programming effect than during late infancy.

We have examined the effect of dietary intake in young children at age 2½ years on blood pressure measured at the same age. We found that protein intake measured as protein energy percentage was significantly negatively associated with both systolic and diastolic blood pressure. The average protein intake in this group was about 42 g/day or 12 energy percent and milk intake about 400 ml/day [39]. Thus, approximately one third of the protein intake came from cow's milk. This effect of protein intake on blood pressure has also been shown in older children and in adults [39].

These data suggest that a very early high protein intake might have a programming effect on blood pressure and at the same time that a high protein intake in young children could be associated with a reduction in current blood pressure. As with many other issues about programming the sensitive age window is not known and it is in particular not known whether the age period from 9 to 18 months is a sensitive period for this kind of programming.

Linear Growth

In a recent review summarizing epidemiological and intervention studies it was concluded that cow's milk seems to have a positive effect on linear growth [40]. The strongest evidence that cow's milk stimulates linear growth comes from observational studies in both infants and preschool children, and from intervention studies in developing countries that show considerable effects. Additionally, observational studies from well-nourished populations also show an association between milk intake and growth [41]. These results suggest that milk has a growth-stimulating effect even in situations where the nutrient intake is adequate. This effect is supported by intervention studies that show that milk intake stimulates circulating levels of the growth factors insulin [42] and IGF-1 [43], which suggests that the growth-stimulating effects of cow's milk are at least partly due to the stimulation of the IGFs. We speculate that this stimulating effect is the reason why at least three studies have shown that formula-fed infants have higher levels of IGF-1 than breastfed infants [44–46]. This is in accordance with studies showing that formula-fed infants have a linear growth velocity which is slightly, but significantly, higher than breast-fed infants [47, 48]. We are not aware of studies comparing the IGF-1 levels of infants fed formula and cow's milk. Although we do not know which compounds in milk stimulate IGF-1 levels, we speculate that the effect of cow's milk is stronger than that of formula because of its high content of protein and minerals.

There are emerging data suggesting that the IGF axis can be programmed by early diet, and it is possible that the type of milk intake during early life also has a role in this programming [48, 50]. Despite the lower IGF-1 levels in breastfed compared to formula-fed infants, studies have suggested that breastfed infants have both higher IGF-1 levels during childhood [51] and are taller as adults [52, 53].

We speculate that cow's milk intake compared to infant formula intake, also during late infancy and early childhood, will increase IGF-1 levels and thereby perhaps also increase linear growth velocity. However, it is not known whether this has positive or negative effects in the long-term and whether this age period is also sensitive to programming of the IGF-1 axis. In adults high levels of IGF-1 are associated with an increased risk of several cancers [54, 55], whereas low levels of IGF-1 are associated with an increased risk of cardiovascular disease [56].

Conclusions

There is no doubt that the most important implication of giving cow's milk in late infancy and early childhood, compared to infant formula, is the potential negative effect on iron status. If cow's milk is given instead of infant formula, a sufficient iron intake should be secured either through a diet with sufficient meat or iron-fortified foods or through iron supplements. The age at which cow's milk can be introduced depends on to what degree the iron needs of the infant or young child can be met by other iron sources.

One of the problems mentioned in giving cow's milk is the low level of LA [6]. However, cow's milk has a favorable n-6/n-3 ratio and it is likely that feeding cow's milk will results in DHA tissue concentrations at the same level as feeding infant formula which is not fortified with DHA. Late infancy and young childhood represent a period during which the brain still develops and a sufficient DHA intake is, therefore, important. However, there are insufficient data on how diet affects LCPUFA status and functional outcomes during this age period. There is a need to know more about the relative impact of cow's milk versus infant formula, the effect of infant formula fortified with DHA and the effect of fish intake.

Important nutrients during the complementary feeding period are iron and fatty acids. To what degree the intake of these nutrients should rely on a diversified diet or should be covered by formula will be different in different populations, depending on economic status, infant feeding habits and tradition.

When cow's milk is given to infants and young children, it is important to make sure that cow's milk intake does not compete with breast milk intake, as is also the case with infant formula.

The complementary feeding period is a period when the infant should be accustomed to a diversified diet. If the intake of cow's milk is very high, there is less space for a diversified diet. A maximum intake of about 500 ml seems a prudent recommendation. A reasonable intake will also reduce the risk of too high a protein intake.

Cow's milk with reduced fat intake should not be introduced too early as it will have a negative impact on the energy density of the diet, which might affect growth. On the other hand, in view of the current obesity epidemic, young children should be accustomed to a low fat diet at an early age.

There are some data suggesting that cow's milk intake during the complementary feeding period, perhaps through the high protein intake, has long-term effects on risk factors for noncommunicable diseases. However, the available data point in many directions and at present it is not possible to draw any firm conclusions. Data on the long-term implications of diet during the complementary feeding period are scarce and should be studied more in the future. There has been a shift in focus of research in programming from the intrauterine to the postnatal period. Much data is available on the long-term implications of feeding and growth during early infancy, but very little about the effects of diet and growth during the complementary feeding period.

References

1 Aggett PJ: Research priorities in complementary feeding: International Paediatric Association (IPA) and European Society of Paediatric Gastroenterology, Hepatology, and Nutrition (ESPGHAN) workshop. Pediatrics 2000;106:1271.
2 Michaelsen KF: Cow's milk in complementary feeding. Pediatrics 2000;106:1302–1303.
3 Canadian Paediatric Society: Dietitians of Canada and Health Canada: Nutrition for Healthy Term Infants. Ottawa, Minister of Public Works and Government Services, 2005.
4 The National Board of Health (Denmark): Recommendations for the Nutrition of Infants; Recommendations for Health Personnel (in Danish). Copenhagen, The National Board of Health (Denmark), 2005.
5 Axelsson I, Gebre-Medhin M, Hernell O, et al: Recommendations for preventing infantile iron deficiency; delay cow's milk intake until 10–12 months of age (in Swedish). Läkartidningen 1999;96:2206–2208.
6 American Academy of Pediatrics Committee on Nutrition: The use of whole cow's milk in infancy. Pediatrics 1992;89:1105–1109.
7 Freeman V, van't Hof M, Haschke F: Patterns of milk and food intake in infants from birth to age 36 months: the Euro-growth study. J Pediatr Gastroenterol Nutr 2000;31:S76–S85.
8 Coleman BL: Early introduction of non-formula cow's milk to southern Ontario infants. Can J Public Health 2006;97:187–190.
9 Thorsdottir I, Gunnarsson BS, Atladottir H, Michaelsen KF: Iron status at 12 months of age – effects of body size and diet in a population of high birth weight. Eur J Clin Nutr 2003;57:505–513.
10 Male C, Persson LA, Freeman V, et al; Euro-Growth Iron Study Group: Prevalence of iron deficiency in 12-mo-old infants from 11 European areas and influence of dietary factors on iron status (Euro-Growth study). Acta Paediatr 2001;90:492–498.
11 Michaelsen KF, Milman N, Samuelson G: A longitudinal study of iron status in healthy Danish infants: effects of early iron status, growth velocity and dietary factors. Acta Paediatr 1995;84:1035–1044.

12 Gunnarsson BS, Thorsdottir I, Palsson G: Iron status in 2-year-old Icelandic children and associations with dietary intake and growth. Eur J Clin Nutr 2004;58:901–906.

13 Straarup EM, Lauritzen L, Færk J, et al: The stereospecific triacylglycerol structures and fatty acid profiles of human milk and infant formulas. J Pediatr Gastroenterol Nutr 2006;42: 293–299.

14 Lauritzen L, Jørgensen MH, Michaelsen KF, Hansen H: The essentiality of long chain n-3 fatty acids in relation to development and function of the brain and retina. Prog Lipid Res 2001; 40:1–94.

15 Jensen RG: Handbook of Milk Composition. Academic Press, San Diego, 1995.

16 Niinikoski H, Viikari J, Ronnemaa T, et al: Prospective randomized trial of low-saturated-fat, low-cholesterol diet during the first 3 years of life. The STRIP Baby Project. Circulation 1996;94: 1386–1393.

17 Kaitosaari T, Ronnemaa T, Viikari J, et al: Low-saturated fat dietary counseling starting in infancy improves insulin sensitivity in 9-year-old healthy children: The Special Turku Coronary Risk Factor Intervention Project for Children (STRIP) study. Diabetes Care 2006;29: 781–785.

18 Raitakari OT, Ronnemaa T, Jarvisalo MJ, et al: Endothelial function in healthy 11-year-old children after dietary intervention with onset in infancy: The Special Turku Coronary Risk Factor Intervention Project for children (STRIP). Circulation 2005;13:3786–3794.

19 Aggett PJ, Haschke F, Heine W: Committee report: childhood diet and prevention of coronary heart disease. ESPGAN Committee on Nutrition, European Society of Paediatric Gastroenterology and Nutrition. J Pediatr Gastroenterol Nutr 1994;19:261–269.

20 Blank C, Neumann MA, Makrides M, Gibson RA: Optimizing DHA levels in piglets by lowering the linoleic acid to alpha-linolenic acid ratio. J Lipid Res 2002;43:1537–1543.

21 Cleland LG, Gibson RA, Pedler J, James MJ: Paradoxical effect of n-3-containing vegetable oils on long-chain n-3 fatty acids in rat heart. Lipids 2005;40:995–998.

22 Courage ML, McCloy UR, Herzberg GR, et al: Visual acuity development and fatty acid composition of erythrocytes in full-term infants fed breast milk, commercial milk, or evaporated milk. J Dev Behav Pediatr 1998;19:9–17.

23 Uauy R, Mize CE, Castillo-Duran C: Fat intake during childhood: metabolic responses and effects on growth. Am J Clin Nutr 2000;72S:1354S–1360S.

24 World Health Organization: Guiding Principles for Feeding Non-Breastfed Children 6–24 Months of Age. Geneva, WHO, 2005.

25 Department of Health: Report on Health and Social Subjects: Weaning and the Weaning Diet. London, HMSO, 1994, No 45.

26 Rolland-Cachera MF, Deheeger M, Akrout M, Bellisle F: Influence of macronutrients on adiposity development: a follow-up study of nutrition and growth from 10 months to 8 years of age. Int J Obes 1995;19:573–578.

27 Scaglioni S, Agostoni C, Notaris RD, et al: Early macronutrient intake and overweight at five years of age. Int J Obes 2000;24:777–781.

28 Dorosty AR, Emmett PM, Cowin S, Reilly JJ: Factors associated with early adiposity rebound. ALSPAC Study Team. Pediatrics 2000;105:1115–1118.

29 Hoppe C, Mølgaard C, Thomsen BL, et al: Protein intake at 9 mo of age is associated with body size but not with body fat in 10-y-old Danish children. Am J Clin Nutr 2004;79:494–501.

30 Agostoni C, Scaglioni S, Ghisleni D, et al: How much protein is safe? Int J Obes 2005;29: S8–S13.

31 Moore LL, Bradlee ML, Gao D, Singer MR: Low dairy intake in early childhood predicts excess body fat gain. Obesity 2006;14:1010–1018.

32 Heaney RP, Davies KM, Barger-Lux MJ: Calcium and weight: clinical studies. J Am Coll Nutr 2002;21:152S–155S.

33 Zemel MB: Role of dietary calcium and dairy products in modulating adiposity. Lipids 2003;38: 139–146.

34 Jacobsen R, Lorenzen JK, Toubro S, et al: Effect of short-term high dietary calcium intake on 24-h energy expenditure, fat oxidation, and fecal fat excretion. Int J Obes Relat Metab Disord 2005;29:292–301.

35 Westerterp-Plantenga MS: The significance of protein in food intake and body weight regulation. Curr Opin Clin Nutr Metab Care 2003;6:635–638.

36 Anderson GH, Moore SE: Dietary proteins in the regulation of food intake and body weight in humans. J Nutr 2004;134:974S–979S.

37 Pupovac J, Anderson GH: Dietary peptides induce satiety via cholecystokinin-A and peripheral opioid receptors in rats. J Nutr 2002;132:2775–2780.

38 Martin RM, McCarthy A, Davey Smith G, et al: Infant nutrition and blood pressure in early adulthood: The Barry Caerphilly Growth study. Am J Clin Nutr 2003;77:1489–1497.

39 Ulbak J, Lauritzen L, Hansen HS, Michaelsen KF: Diet and blood pressure in 2.5-y-old Danish children. Am J Clin Nutr 2004;79:1095–1102.

40 Hoppe C, Mølgaard C, Michaelsen KF: Cow's milk and linear growth in industrialized and developing countries. Annu Rev Nutr 2006;26:131–173.

41 Hoppe C, Udam TR, Lauritzen L, et al: Animal protein intake, serum insulin-like growth factor I, and growth in healthy 2.5-y-old Danish children. Am J Clin Nutr 2004;80:447–452.

42 Hoppe C, Mølgaard C, Vaag A, et al: High intakes of milk, but not meat, increase s-insulin and insulin resistance in 8-year-old boys. Eur J Clin Nutr 2005;59:393–398.

43 Hoppe C, Mølgaard C, Juul A, Michaelsen KF: High intakes of skimmed milk, but not meat, increase serum IGF-I and IGFBP-3 in eight-year-old boys. Eur J Clin Nutr 2004;58:1211–1216.

44 Chellakooty M, Juul A, Boisen KA, et al: A prospective study of serum IGF-I and IGFBP-3 in 942 healthy infants: associations with birth weight, gender, growth velocity and breastfeeding. J Clin Endocrinol Metab 2006;91:820–826.

45 Savino F, Fissore MF, Grassino EC, et al: Ghrelin, leptin and IGF-I levels in breast-fed and formula-fed infants in the first years of life. Acta Paediatr 2005;94:531–537.

46 Socha P, Janas R, Dobrzanska A, et al; EU Childhood Obesity Study Team: Insulin like growth factor regulation of body mass in breastfed and milk formula fed infants. Data from the EU Childhood Obesity Programme. Adv Exp Med Biol 2005;569:159–163.

47 Dewey KG, Peerson JM, Brown KH, et al: Growth of breast-fed infants deviates from current reference data: a pooled analysis of US, Canadian, and European data sets. World Health Organization Working Group on Infant Growth. Pediatrics 1995;96:495–503.

48 Michaelsen KF, Petersen S, Greisen G, Thomsen BL: Weight, length, head circumference, and growth velocity in a longitudinal study of Danish infants. Dan Med Bull 1994;41:577–585.

49 Ben-Shlomo Y, Holly J, McCarthy A, et al: An investigation of fetal, postnatal and childhood growth with insulin-like growth factor I and binding protein 3 in adulthood. Clin Endocrinol (Oxf) 2003;59:366–373.

50 Ong K, Kratzsch J, Kiess W, Dunger D: Circulating IGF-I levels in childhood are related to both current body composition and early postnatal growth rate. J Clin Endocrinol Metab 2002;87:1041–1044.

51 Martin RM, Holly JM, Smith GD, et al: Could associations between breastfeeding and insulin-like growth factors underlie associations of breastfeeding with adult chronic disease? The Avon Longitudinal Study of Parents and Children. Clin Endocrinol (Oxf) 2005;62:728–737.

52 Martin RM, Smith GD, Mangtani P, et al: Association between breast feeding and growth: the Boyd-Orr cohort study. Arch Dis Child Fetal Neonatal Ed 2005;87:F193–F201.

53 Victora CG, Barros F, Lima RC, et al: Anthropometry and body composition of 18 year old men according to duration of breast feeding: birth cohort study from Brazil. BMJ 2003;327:901.

54 Renehan AG, Zwahlen M, Minder C, et al: Insulin-like growth factor (IGF)-I, IGF binding protein-3, and cancer risk: systematic review and meta-regression analysis. Lancet 2004;363:1346–1353.

55 Voskuil DW, Vrieling A, van't Veer LJ, et al: The insulin-like growth factor system in cancer prevention: potential of dietary intervention strategies. Cancer Epidemiol Biomarkers Prev 2005;14:195–203.

56 Juul A, Scheike T, Davidsen M, et al: Low serum insulin-like growth factor I is associated with increased risk of ischemic heart disease: a population-based case-control study. Circulation 2002;106:939–944.

Discussion

Dr. Ziegler: You showed us the fatty acid composition of cow's milk but you did not mention that this fat is very poorly absorbed by normal infants. Butter fat is the fat of cow's milk. If you do a fat-balance study you find that about 60% is absorbed. Compared to fat absorption from breast milk which is 95%, there is a substantial amount of fat loss in the stool of an infant who is fed cow's milk. About introducing cow's milk at 9 months, to which I do not object, I showed you that blood loss disappears toward the end of the first year of life. And most importantly, the dehydration concern diminishes as children acquire the ability to express and communicate thirst, which protects them against dehydration.

Dr. Simell: I have an experimental comment from real life from the STRIP study where children were introduced to the study at the age of 6 months and randomized to an intervention and a control group [1]. In the intervention group the children received regular dietary and lifestyle counseling at half-year intervals from 6 months of age, and they are now between 16 and 17 years of age. We have been looking at obesity development in these children because part of the counseling in the early years was that they be switched to fat-free skimmed milk at the age of 1 year, from formula or breast milk to skimmed milk. We have found no difference in the proportions of obesity and overweight in boys, but in girls there is a very significant difference between the proportions: much fewer obese girls in the intervention group through the years. In the counseling we actually have not concentrated on the amount of fat but on the quality of fat; we have been supporting the higher intake of polyunsaturated and monounsaturated fat as compared to saturated fat. The goal has never really been to focus on the total intake, and surprisingly it has been very effective, actually much better than any other obesity prevention programs we have seen.

Dr. Ribeiro: Regarding your comments that the possible use of these milk sources could be beneficial in countries where stunting is prevalent: we have seen some publications showing that people with stunting are potentially more vulnerable to become obese later in life than the rest of the population. Perhaps this is one of the reasons for the paradox in Brazil now where the proportions of children with malnutrition and obesity are the same. We see in this recommendation just the opposite; we are very concerned about the use of cow's milk or other sources of high energy and high protein in the stunting population.

Dr. Michaelsen: If you are talking about obesity I think it is a question of reducing the fat intake at an early age using fat-reduced milk, and there are some data suggesting that this might have a beneficial effect on the development of obesity later on. So from the available data, it is difficult to say exactly when and how fast the fat content of the milk should be reduced. But if semi-skimmed milk is introduced at an early age and then later skimmed milk, I think the milk will not promote later obesity.

Dr. Ribeiro: But the IGF impact is one of the concerns. The possible recovery from stunting needs to be considered as a potential because of the later compensation growth, but the same effect is also a response here.

Dr. Michaelsen: I think the data that IGF-1 is involved in obesity development is not the response, that was part of the original hypothesis. Obese children will have normal or increased IGF-1 levels, but the increased IGF-1 level is because they eat more. They are also taller up to the age of puberty, then they are not taller, and that is because they get a lot of fuel and that also increases IGF-1 and linear growth. But I don't think it because of the increase in IGF-1.

Dr. Solomons: I think in the dialogue between you and Dr. Ribeiro, your response was that taller people were obese and had more IGF. Meanwhile, Dr. Ribeiro's question was about stunting and the risk of obesity. But I think the difference – or the missing piece of dialogue – is the constraint that makes the stunting in countries like Brazil or Guatemala. In these settings, for reasons other than diet, one may not grow, therefore you are forcing more body mass onto a non-elongated frame. Then you get a kind of obesity that is certainly not IGF-driven, and may not even be IGF-associated. It would be interesting to study.

217

Dr. Michaelsen: So if you give milk you can increase the frame?

Dr. Solomons: No, because the constraint would be running against even giving milk. A lot of stunting is related to the same mechanism why animals don't grow in an infected environment, that there is a constant immuno-stimulation which is essentially catabolic and anti-growth. No matter how much you pour into them they are not going to grow because the mechanisms for forward growth are disrupted by the environment. That is the reality for the countries in the world with more than 20% stunting, it is a massive number of countries in the world.

Dr. Michaelsen: But there are still some intervention studies showing increased growth after animal foods. Then there is the question of what is the effect of meat and what is the effect of milk.

Dr. Solomons: There are more dietary intervention trial studies that are failures with regard to achieving growth than there are successes. Moreover, if one pushes a nutrient-rich diet on children who are already of established short stature, obesity may be the obvious result.

Dr. Shahkhalilli: Can you please comment on what the contribution of fat is in the total energy content of the diet (percent of fat energy) in developed and developing countries? Does the present level of fat in complementary diets need to be modified?

Dr. Michaelsen: In our society we recommend that the family diet should be below 30%, perhaps it should be 25–30%, and breast milk has 52%. So there should be a gradual decline, and there is much debate as to how fast that should go. Some reviews say that in developing countries caution should be taken not to get below 20–25%. In Denmark and in some other countries we have seen that there was a tendency to go from the 52% to very low levels down to 20%. Most families will have a diet with about 30 or 35 or even 40%. So we saw a surprising pattern where at 12 months the children actually had a lower fat energy percentage than the family diet, and I think it is important not to have that. But again at 2 years the energy fat level should be down to 25%–30% in developed countries, and in developing countries where the concern is that it is getting too low and it should be increased to at least 20–25%.

Dr. Biasucci: As a pediatrician, what would you suggest with regard to the time of introduction of cow's milk in the case of infants who do not easily accept meat during the weaning process? Would you still suggest introducing cow's milk at 9 months or would you suggest it later on?

Dr. Michaelsen: If you think about introducing cow's milk at 9 months then you should be sure that there is sufficient iron intake, and this is a problem when they won't eat any meat. You could use infant formula. I am not saying that cow's milk is better from the age of 9 months, I am just saying that I think it is a possibility. I also have a conflict of interest because I am from a country where this is recommended, but we give the mothers a choice to shift to cow's milk at 9 months and then give iron drops or continue with infant formula, and we are not really saying that one is better than the other. In that situation you want to be sure that the iron needs are covered which could be done with infant formula, fortified cereals, or iron drops.

Dr. Haschke: One thing is really missing in the data set and probably the data are not available. If you consider that the breastfed infant should be the reference, at least until 12 months of age and even beyond, we don't have the data on their metabolic outcome, IgF_1 and so on, to really compare what would be the pattern of an infant who is exclusively breastfed until 6 months of age and then a weaning diet is introduced. So if we consider this as the reference, as far as I am aware there are not enough data to really compare with another milk, such as cow's milk, which is substantially different in protein content. Would you agree?

Dr. Michaelsen: I do agree that we know very little about the whole programming concept from 9 to 18 months, so we don't know the long-term consequences. I showed some potentially positive and some negative effects.

Dr. Giovannini: When we speak about whole cow's milk, 9 months is the age at which it is introduced in Denmark whereas the Italian Society of Pediatric Nutrition recommends not using it in the first year of life. But the biggest problem is compliance in Western countries. When mothers taste the formula and also taste cow's milk, they find that cow's milk tastes better because of the saturated fatty acids. For this reason I think we have a big problem regarding education. This is a reality and we should not forget that the mothers taste all the formulas and they think that their children will have the same taste which is a big mistake. Moreover, the problem is also to check later between the early introduction of cow's milk and later nutrition with too much sweets and cakes. I think that the mothers should receive nutritional education before delivery, during pregnancy.

Dr. Michaelsen: It is interesting that the mothers taste the infant formula. That could be the reason why in southern Europe or in some European countries there are some formulas with sugar instead of lactose. I don't know if they are still on the market, but previously there were some formulas with sugar.

Reference

1 Kaitosaari T, Ronnemaa T, Viikari J, et al: Low-saturated fat dietary counseling starting in infancy improves insulin sensitivity in 9-year-old healthy children: The Special Turku Coronary Risk Factor Intervention Project for Children (STRIP) study. Diabetes Care 2006;29:781–785.

Agostoni C, Brunser O (eds): Issues in Complementary Feeding.
Nestlé Nutr Workshop Ser Pediatr Program, vol 60, pp 221–233,
Nestec Ltd., Vevey/S. Karger AG, Basel, © 2007.

Meat as an Early Complementary Food for Infants: Implications for Macro- and Micronutrient Intakes

Nancy F. Krebs

Section of Nutrition, Department of Pediatrics, University of Colorado School of Medicine,
Denver, Colo., USA

Abstract

Optimal complementary feeding is recognized to be critical for prevention of infectious morbidity and mortality and for optimal growth and development. The nutrients which become limiting in human milk after approximately 6 months of exclusive breastfeeding are predictable based on the dynamic composition of human milk and the physiology of infant nutritional requirements. Iron and zinc are two micronutrients for which the concentrations in human milk are relatively independent of maternal intake, and for which the older infant is most dependent on complementary foods to meet requirements. Traditional feeding practices, including reliance on cereals and plant based diets, do not complement these recognized gaps in human milk. Meats or cellular animal proteins are richer sources of these critical minerals as well as other essential nutrients. Yet, cellular animal proteins are often introduced only late in infancy in developed countries, and may be only rarely consumed by young children in developing countries. Plant-based diets result in a predominance of energy from carbohydrates, often including highly refined carbohydrates that are also likely to have a high glycemic index. This pattern of macronutrient intake is contrary to that of the period when the human genome evolved, and may influence the metabolic profile in young children, especially under conditions of nutritional abundance.

Introduction

Optimal complementary feeding is recognized to be critical for meeting the nutritional needs of the older infant and young child who is still breastfed. Indeed, provision of nutritionally adequate complementary foods has been cited as one of the most important measures to prevent infectious morbidity and mortality in children under 5 years of age [1]. Furthermore, the period from birth to 24 months also represents a critical window of brain development, and thus of vulnerability to harm from micronutrient deficiencies that may have permanent effects on neurocognitive development [2]. In contrast to the universal and simple message of exclusive breastfeeding for the first 6 months which has yielded improvements in breastfeeding rates and exclusivity, guidelines and implementation strategies for complementary feeding are inevitably more complex, involving issues related to food availability and economics, cultural customs, preferences and norms, and the developmental readiness of the infant [3]. Thus, while the nutritional needs of the older infant have been extensively considered [4, 5], there is less consensus about the most feasible way(s) to meet energy and nutrient needs. Strategic options, many of which will be discussed in other articles in this series, include food-based approaches, food fortification, biofortification through plant breeding and agricultural practices, micronutrient 'sprinkles' added to local foods, and micronutrient supplements.

Here, the rationale for an approach to complementary feeding that encourages early and regular consumption of meat and flesh (cellular animal protein, CAP) for older infants and toddlers will be discussed, as well as some of the potential barriers to this approach.

Adequacy of Exclusive Breastfeeding

Human milk provides a biologically robust source of nourishment ideally suited for the human infant. The composition is also relatively consistent over a wide range of maternal dietary quality, although there are some exceptions. Regardless of the maternal nutritional status, however, the composition of human milk is dynamic, as are the infant's nutritional requirements. The result of this is that at some point human milk alone will not adequately meet the infant's nutritional needs. Although the exact timing of this point has been an area of some controversy [6], and it is certain to vary among individual infants, the recommendation to introduce complementary foods around 6 months of age recognizes the increasing risk thereafter for development of deficiencies of specific micronutrients for which intake from human milk alone will be marginal. This is not to imply that breastfeeding is not nutritionally important after 6 months, but rather that the combination of high quality complementary foods in addition to continued breastfeeding results in optimal growth, development and immunoprotection.

The concentrations of iron and zinc in human milk are minimally influenced by maternal intake. The relatively low concentration of iron in human milk is adequate for the first several months until the infant's iron endowment at birth is expended. To provide adequate iron for active hematopoiesis and growth after the first 6 months of life, the infant is almost entirely dependent on complementary foods as a dietary source [7, 8]. The situation for zinc is different in that the concentration of zinc in human milk is initially quite high but rapidly declines over the first 5–6 months postpartum; zinc intake by the exclusively breastfed infant follows a similar declining pattern [9, 10]. After this time, as for iron, the majority of the infant's requirement will also need to be provided by complementary foods [7, 8]. Iron deficiency is one of the most prevalent nutritional deficiencies on a global scale [2]. Likewise zinc deficiency, though more difficult to document, is also likely to be very common and to be a major causative factor for susceptibility to infectious morbidity and stunting [1, 11].

Complementary Foods to Meet the Micronutrient Gaps of Exclusive Breastfeeding

Despite knowledge of the nutrient gaps for the older breastfed infant, complementary feeding practices common in both developed and developing countries often do not emphasize foods which fill these gaps. For at least the past century, cereal gruels have been a common early food offered to infants in the US [6, 12]. With the recognition of the relatively high iron requirements of the older infant, iron fortification of infant cereal has provided a major vehicle to meet iron needs [13], thus further promoting the value of cereal as a first food for infants in the US. Fruits and vegetables are typically offered next, despite the fact that these are poor sources of the nutrients most likely to be limiting in older breastfed infants. Specific protein sources are gradually introduced, often not until late in the first year of life. This pattern is not unique to the US. Review of the complementary feeding guidelines described for the six sites participating World Health Organization Multicenter Growth Reference Study also indicates this a similar pattern in other affluent cultures [14].

In developing countries, various types of plant-based gruels or thin soups are common early foods offered to infants. These gruels are made from cereal grains or starchy roots and tubers [3, 4, 8], which not only are low in energy and nutrient content but also contain phytic acid and polyphenols, factors which impair the bioavailability of zinc and iron. Not only are these foods less than ideal, lack of diversity of complementary foods further compromises nutritional adequacy for older infants.

In contrast to the plant-based complementary foods, meats and flesh foods are excellent sources of bioavailable iron and zinc, as well as vitamins B_{12} and B_6, micronutrients which may also be marginal in the diets of older infants and young children. Liver is an excellent source of most micronutrients, and is particularly high in vitamin A, deficiency of which is also very common in developing countries. These animal-source foods also provide high quality protein and typically have a higher caloric density. Thus meats provide a nutrient profile more consistent with and 'complementary' to the nutritional needs of the older breastfed infant. Furthermore, as described by Cordain et al. [15], prior to the agricultural revolution, cereals, especially refined grain flours, were likely to be a relatively small part of the 'hominin diet', presumably including infants' diets. Rather, the human diet was primarily reliant on animal flesh and fruits. Historical review of complementary feeding practices suggests that minced or pre-masticated meats were among early weaning foods prior to the 1800s [12]. Even 50–60 years ago in the US, common practice was to introduce meats, as well as the other major food groups, within the first 2 months of life [12]. Although such early introduction of any complementary foods is now considered undesirable, this illustrates the precedent for acceptance of meats much earlier than is typical in contemporary infant feeding.

Evidence for Benefits of Cellular Animal Protein Intake

A few studies have reported the benefit of meats, or CAPs, on growth and iron status in young children. For example, in a surveillance study of breastfed infants and toddlers in Peru, linear growth was positively associated with intake of animal-product foods (including meats) in those children with low intakes of complementary foods, and in those who had low breastfeeding frequency. Similarly, at low energy intakes, intake of animal source foods was positively associated with linear growth [16]. A cross-sectional survey of 12- to 23-month-old children in Delhi, India, reported higher length-for-age scores associated with parental education and non-vegetarian diets [17]. A nutrition intervention trial targeting improved complementary feeding in Peru, and specifically including a message to offer liver, eggs or fish every day, demonstrated a significant improvement in nutritional intakes and, importantly, a reduction in stunting [18]. In contrast, a similar intervention trial in India, which promoted consumption of higher quality plant-based complementary foods, including legumes and thickened gruels, was not associated with improvements in growth [19].

In developed countries, a handful of studies have examined the potential benefits of meats in the diets of older infants and toddlers. In one prospective observational study, infants were enrolled at 4 months and followed through 24 months of age; dietary intakes were documented by 7-day food diaries. Modest meat intake (<28.3 g/day) was positively associated weight gain in the first year of life, and with psychomotor development at 24 months [20]. An intervention study in Denmark randomized 8-month-old breastfed infants to receive high or low meat diets for 2 months. Despite having a total iron intake from fortified foods similar to the intake of the high meat group, the low meat group had a significantly greater decline in hemoglobin compared to the high meat group [21].

A trial in Denver randomized breastfed infants to either commercial pureed meat (beef) and gravy or iron-fortified rice cereal as the first complementary food [22, 23]. At 7 months, intake of zinc was significantly higher in the meat group, and the amount of zinc absorbed from a test meal was approximately 16-fold greater in the meat group [22]. The mean intake of ~56.6 g meat and gravy/day provided the estimated average requirement of 2.5 mg zinc/day [7]. Infants in the meat group had a significantly greater increase in head circumference from 7 to 12 months; no other significant differences in functional outcomes between the groups were observed. The iron and zinc status at 9 months was suboptimal in over 1/3 of the infants, regardless of the group. Since the feeding intervention ended at 7 months, it is not possible to know whether outcomes, including iron and/or zinc status, would have been improved if the emphasis on meats had been sustained [23].

Macronutrient Intakes with Plant- versus Animal-Based Complementary Feeding Patterns

As the focus on the prevalence of micronutrient deficiencies in older infants and toddlers has emerged over the past decade, somewhat less attention has been directed to the macronutrient distribution of the typical weaning diet [3]. The reliance on cereals, with or without micronutrient fortification, results in a low fat, low energy dense diet. Although continued reliance on human milk will contribute to the quantity and quality of lipid intakes, as the percentage of energy from this source gradually declines, the composition of complementary foods contributes substantially to the macronutrient distribution in the total diet. At a time of development when a high energy dense diet, including high fat intake, is considered to be beneficial, the emphasis on cereals and other plant foods counters this pattern.

In the study described above on breastfed infants in Denver, at 7 months the group assigned to rice cereal as the first weaning food (with ad libitum introduction of fruits and vegetables) consumed more than 80% of the calories from complementary foods as carbohydrate, predominantly refined, and only 8% of calories were from fat. Assuming an average intake of human milk, the overall contribution of fat intake to energy would be only ~35%. Although the study design dictated the introduction of cereal as the first complementary food, it is worth noting that this represents typical feeding patterns for US infants. The intake of calories, iron, and zinc for the cereal group were essentially identical to intakes reported a decade earlier for 7-month-old breastfed infants in Denver [10].

In contrast, the infants assigned to start with meat (also with ad libitum introduction of fruits and vegetables) consumed 50% of energy from complementary foods as carbohydrate and 22% as fat. At 9 months, when the majority of infants were still predominantly breastfed but complementary feeding was entirely ad libitum, carbohydrate continued to dominate, providing 64–75% of energy from complementary foods for the two groups, while energy from fat was <20% for both groups. Data from the Feeding Infants and Toddlers Study of US infants, the majority of whom were formula-fed, showed a similar pattern [24], with the mean percent of total calories from fat of about 35% for 7- to 11-month-olds [24].

The long-term effects of different macronutrient distributions during the critical developmental period of late infancy are unknown. Data from the STRIP Baby Project, in which infants randomized at 7 months to diets low in total fat (~30% of energy), and specifically low in saturated fat, indicated no adverse effects on growth or development after 3 years [25]. On the other hand, an analysis of food balance data in young Latin American children concluded that diets providing <22% of energy from fat, including low animal fat content, were associated with underweight and stunting, and that animal food products were critical to support normal child growth [26].

As noted above, the human genome adapted to an environment, including diet, profoundly different from that of the past 10,000 years when agriculture and animal husbandry were introduced. Not only were cereal grains not routinely consumed prior to this, until only 150–200 years ago the grains that were consumed were unrefined. In the late 1800s, milled grains came to dominate and the germ and bran were routinely removed and discarded [15]. Although the cereals and grains consumed by young children in developing countries in rural areas may be relatively unprocessed, this is likely not the case in urban and peri-urban areas where more refined products are more readily available.

Refined carbohydrates are generally associated with higher glycemic load and have been proposed to cause chronic hyperglycemia and hyperinsulinemia. These metabolic conditions have been proposed to predispose to obesity, type 2 diabetes, cardiovascular disease, and chronic elevation of inflammatory markers [27]. To date, few studies have examined the effects of infant feeding beyond breastfeeding versus formula feeding on obesity and metabolic profiles, but it is possible that the early introduction of a 'westernized diet', with predominance of refined carbohydrates predisposes to risk of later chronic diseases. If a high carbohydrate load is concurrent with micronutrient deficiencies, there may be further exacerbation of adverse metabolic effects. There are many potentially confounding factors, including genetic risk of insulin resistance, birth weight (reflecting intrauterine exposure), early weight gain and subsequent weight status, in addition to the impact of type of feeding. The theoretical issues raised about the relationship of current complementary feeding practices to the later risk of chronic diseases of westernization warrant further consideration and research in view of global concerns about rising rates of childhood obesity and its comorbidities, including insulin resistance.

Acceptability and Safety of Meats as an Early Complementary Food

Although a common perception about the introduction of meats and liver as an early complementary food is that infants will not accept them, our experience does not support this. We found no difference in parents' ratings of infants' acceptance between cereal and meat groups in the Denver study described above [23]. In unpublished observations, we have also found no hesitation to eating pureed cooked liver in 7- and 12-month-old infants in rural Guatemala.

Theoretical concerns may also be raised about the potential for allergic sensitization from different complementary feeding patterns. A recent consensus document cites the major foods posing allergy risks are bovine milk, egg, peanut, tree nuts, fish, and seafood [28]. Wheat especially is associated with both food allergies and celiac disease (gluten enteropathy), and rice is stated to be an important allergen in Asia. The consensus document concludes that well-cooked or freeze-dried meats have low allergenicity [28].

Recognition of the nutritional value of animal source foods, especially meats and flesh foods, for complementary feeding has been noted by several organizations, including the American Academy of Pediatrics, World Health Organization, and the Centers for Disease Control and Prevention [6, 13, 29–30]. Thus, in developed countries, the main barrier to broader adoption of these recommendations seems to be primarily one of education of physicians and care providers who advise breastfeeding mothers on complementary feeding. The lack of a definitive evidence base for optimal feeding for predominantly breastfed infants, however, and the relatively small numbers of these infants also contribute to the lack of consensus in practice.

In developing countries, the issues are quite different, and the availability of meat and flesh foods may be much more limited, due at least in part, to the relative expense of animal source foods. However, this is clearly not the only issue. In many settings, customs rather than availability are the major barrier. Offering the older infant meat is simply not recognized as an appropriate or valuable practice. In some cultures, religious beliefs prohibit the consumption of CAP, although some accept the use of eggs and dairy products. Several initiatives from non-governmental organizations have been undertaken to increase production, accessibility and consumption of animal source foods in efforts to combat coexisting micronutrient deficiencies. These programs have not been universally successful, and emphasize the importance of formative research to characterize and understand a population's perceptions about nutrition, health and infant and child feeding prior to undertaking major interventions. Critically needed are also efficacy studies of meat consumption as part of overall improved complementary feeding practices for older infants and toddlers. At present, the lack of a strong evidence base may foster ambivalence about the benefits of advancing a feeding strategy that has broad sociocultural and economic implications contrary to the status quo.

Conclusion

Optimal complementary feeding is recognized to be critical for optimal growth and development during early childhood. The nutrients which become limiting in human milk after approximately 6 months of exclusive breastfeeding are predictable based on the dynamic composition of human milk and the physiology of infant nutritional requirements. Iron and zinc are two micronutrients for which the concentrations in human milk are relatively independent of maternal intake, and for which the older infant is most dependent on complementary foods to meet requirements. Traditional feeding practices, including reliance on cereals and plant-based diets, do not complement these recognized gaps in human milk. CAP sources are rich in these critical trace minerals as well as other essential nutrients, and limited intervention studies have suggested good acceptance by the infants and beneficial outcomes. The distribution of macronutrients also varies greatly between plant-based diets and those including CAP, which may have implications for metabolic predisposition toward obesity and insulin resistance, both of which are increasingly prevalent in developing countries. Thus, although there is a strong theoretical rationale for the earlier introduction of CAP, there is a great need for both efficacy and effectiveness studies.

References

1   Jones G, Steketee RW, Black RE, et al: How many child deaths can we prevent this year? Lancet 2003;362:65–71.
2   World Bank: Repositioning Nutrition as Central to Development: A Strategy for Large-Scale Action. Washington, World Bank, 2006.
3   Lutter CK, Rivera JA: Nutritional status of infants and young children and characteristics of their diets. J Nutr 2003;133:2941S–2949S.
4   World Health Organization: Complementary Feeding of Young Children in Developing Countries: A Review of Current Scientific Knowledge. Geneva, World Health Organization, 1998.
5   Dewey KG, Brown KH: Update on technical issues concerning complementary feeding of young children in developing countries and implications for intervention programs. Food Nutr Bull 2003;24:5–28.
6   American Academy of Pediatrics Committee on Nutrition: Complementary feeding; in Kleinman RE (ed): Pediatric Nutrition Handbook. Elk Grove Village, American Academy of Pediatrics, 2004, pp 103–115.
7   Food and Nutrition Board, Institute of Medicine: Dietary Reference Intakes for Vitamin A, Vitamin K, Boron, Chromium, Copper, Iodine, Iron, Manganese, Molybdenum, Nickel, Silicon, Vanadium and Zinc. Washington, National Academy Press, 2001.
8   Gibson RS, Ferguson EL, Lehrfeld J: Complementary foods for infant feeding in developing countries: their nutrient adequacy and improvement. Eur J Clin Nutr 1998;52:764–770.
9   Krebs NF, Reidinger CJ, Hartley S, et al: Zinc supplementation during lactation: effects on maternal status and milk zinc concentrations. Am J Clin Nutr 1995;61:1030–1036.

10 Krebs NF, Reidinger CJ, Robertson AD, et al: Growth and intakes of energy and zinc in infants fed human milk. J Pediatr 1994;124:32–39.
11 Brown KH, Peerson JM, Rivera J, et al: Effect of supplemental zinc on the growth and serum zinc concentrations of prepubertal children: a meta-analysis of randomized controlled trials. Am J Clin Nutr 2002;75:1062–1071.
12 Fomon SJ: Nutrition of Normal Infants, ed 3. St. Louis, Mosby-Year Book, 1993.
13 American Academy of Pediatrics, Committee on Nutrition: Iron deficiency; in Kleinman R (ed): Pediatric Nutrition Handbook, ed 5. Elk Grove Village, American Academy of Pediatrics, 2004, pp 299–312.
14 de Onis M, Garza C, Victora CG, et al; The WHO Multicenter Growth Reference Study (MGRS): Rationale, planning, and implementation. Food Nutr Bull 2004;25:S5–S89.
15 Cordain L, Eaton SB, Sebastian A, et al: Origins and evolution of the Western diet: health implications for the 21st century. Am J Clin Nutr 2005;81:341–354.
16 Marquis GS, Habicht JP, Lanata CF, et al: Breast milk or animal-product foods improve linear growth of Peruvian toddlers consuming marginal diets. Am J Clin Nutr 1997;66:1102–1109.
17 Bhandari N, Bahl R, Taneja S, et al: Growth performance of affluent Indian children is similar to that in developed countries. Bull World Health Organ 2002;80:189–195.
18 Penny ME, Creed-Kanashiro HM, Robert RC, et al: Effectiveness of an educational intervention delivered through the health services to improve nutrition in young children: a cluster-randomised controlled trial. Lancet 2005;365:1863–1872.
19 Bhandari N, Bahl R, Nayyar B, et al: Food supplementation with encouragement to feed it to infants from 4 to 12 months of age has a small impact on weight gain. J Nutr 2001;131: 1946–1951.
20 Morgan J, Taylor A, Fewtrell M: Meat consumption is positively associated with psychomotor outcome in children up to 24 months of age. J Pediatr Gastroenterol Nutr 2004;39:493–498.
21 Engelmann MD, Sandstrom B, Michaelsen KF: Meat intake and iron status in late infancy: an intervention study. J Pediatr Gastroenterol Nutr 1998;26:26–33.
22 Jalla S, Westcott J, Steirn M, et al: Zinc absorption and exchangeable zinc pool sizes in breast-fed infants fed meat or cereal as first complementary food. J Pediatr Gastroenterol Nutr 2002;34:35–41.
23 Krebs NF, Westcott JE, Butler N, et al: Meat as a first complementary food for breastfed infants: feasibility and impact on zinc intake and status. J Pediatr Gastroenterol Nutr 2006;42: 207–214.
24 Devaney B, Ziegler P, Pac S, et al: Nutrient intakes of infants and toddlers. J Am Diet Assoc 2004;104:s14–s21.
25 Rask-Nissila L, Jokinen E, Terho P, et al: Neurological development of 5 year old children receiving a low-saturated fat, low-cholesterol diet since infancy: a randomized controlled trial. JAMA 2000;284:993–1000.
26 Uauy R, Mize CE, Castillo-Duran C: Fat intake during childhood: metabolic responses and effects on growth. Am J Clin Nutr 2000;72:1354S–1360S.
27 Ludwig DS: The glycemic index: physiological mechanisms relating to obesity, diabetes, and cardiovascular disease. JAMA 2002;287:2414–2423.
28 Fiocchi A, Assa'ad A, Bahna S: Food allergy and the introduction of solid foods to infants: a consensus document. Adverse Reactions to Foods Committee, American College of Allergy, Asthma and Immunology. Ann Allergy Asthma Immunol 2006;97:10–20.
29 PAHO/WHO: Guiding Principles for Complementary Feeding of the Breastfed Child. Washington, PAHO/WHO, 2003.
30 Centers for Disease Control and Prevention: Recommendations for preventing and controlling iron deficiency in the United States. MMWR Morb Mortal Wkly Rep 1998;47:1–36.

Discussion

Dr. Michaelsen: You compared meat and liver and there was much more zinc and iron in liver. But the meat factor that is enhancing iron absorption, is that mainly in muscle foods? I got the impression that the meat factor, although it is not well identified, is more in muscle food than in liver. So does meat perhaps have a better capacity to enhance iron absorption?

Dr. Krebs: As I said the iron in liver, though it is a very high isn't all heme. So if you were going to predict you would not predict that the absorption would be efficient. Whether it is efficient enough to make use of all that is there has not been done in a head-to-head comparison. The liver of course is richer in several nutrients.

Dr. Kruger: I haven't seen many studies that looked at head circumference and it was a very important result that the zinc status actually predicted head circumference and also the Bayley scores. That to me was one of the really important observations that you made.

Dr. Krebs: I want to be very cautious about this, especially on the Bayley testing, as it is just a trend and the behavior score on that version of the Bayley is still a fairly rudimentary score, but nevertheless it was done blinded and so on. As far as the head circumference is concerned, there has actually been a difference in head circumference according to the amounts of zinc that breastfed infants get depending on what the mother's secretion was. I am beginning to think that this actually may be a real finding. It was a surprise but it was actually the only anthropometric measure that was different. I have become very attuned to measuring that now in any of our intervention trials.

Dr. Solomons: It is really unfortunate that there was only one month of intervention and perhaps there are other populations in which you could increase the amount of time in which the randomized comparison is continued. But in the one month that you had, was there any differential effect on the consumption of breast milk across the two groups? I ask this because these women were presumably still breastfeeding. In the study in Denver you could have chosen a cereal with any amount of fortification with zinc and iron; you could have designed a cereal that was like meat, or a cereal that was like Guatemalan cereals. The real comparison then is in the real world of places where the complementary food, cereal, a grain product, is not a prepared processed infant cereal but is rather something mixed with water. Such a cereal would not have any fortification. So in the real world there would not be the option for the iron- and zinc-fortified cereal side to the equation, so that the contrast between meat and cereal in Pakistan or Guatemala would be much more dramatic than it could be with whatever fortified cereal you used.

Dr. Krebs: You are right, the cereals actually weren't fortified at that time with zinc. So this was a non-fortified cereal and there was very little zinc. There was a lot of electrolytic iron and it is not very well absorbed. Yes, a longer intervention would have been very good. I was actually very nervous about doing the study at the time and I felt it was probably unethical to withhold meat, not really recognizing that many infants go much longer without really having meat introduced. If I did it now I would probably put them on dinners that are low in zinc and iron but actually have enough protein. Regarding the beast milk intake, we didn't do test weighing but they were all exclusively breastfed and none of them used a formula at the 7-month point. By 9 months about 50% were on a formula up to between 110 and 225 g/day. We didn't see any difference between the two groups.

Dr. Mello: What is the amount of the meat necessary?

Dr. Krebs: The average intake was over 2 mg/day of zinc and that was from about 57 g of a commercial product. It would actually only take about 28 g/day of beef and gravy, a pureed product, and so if you are actually just using straight meat, we predict that they actually take less than 57 g.

Dr. Guno: For practical clinical application, it appears from the data that only on the days that liver is fed will the iron and zinc requirements be met. We also say that the babies should be fed a variety of foods on the days that the mother gives a fish or a vegetable source of protein. Is it prudent to say that the mothers should also use other iron-fortified products or give an iron supplement?

Dr. Krebs: That is an interesting question. It is always hard to match reality with the daily requirements, and I don't know if you have to have meat every single day. In many populations if meat were available several times a week, we would be doing much better than we had been. It probably becomes too complicated to recommend a supplement on the days that you don't have meat. By consuming meats you are getting a better iron intake, but it may be difficult to fine tune recommendation of alternating meat with supplementation.

Dr. Brown: One comment about real world situations. The last time I looked at this in Bangladesh using the FAO food balance sheets, the per capita availability of meat was about 4 g/person/day. So even if we are talking about adjusting an ounce of meat, we are far away from being able to meet that requirement in much of the developing world in terms of availability, so there is a big challenge there. I have two questions. In Dr. Ferguson's presentation the other day, it was very interesting to me that with the cereal-based fortified processed complementary foods there has been very little impact on any indicator of physical growth, but in several studies in which mixed diets usually with animal source foods were provided, there has been a growth impact. I am not quite sure what might explain that, you looked at protein and zinc but I also note that there are differences in fat intake. I wonder if you might comment on that. The second question is just for my information. When you looked at the exchangeable zinc for size in relation to zinc intake, did you also look back at the serum zinc concentration?

Dr. Krebs: It was a small subgroup in which we did the isotope that I doubt we would have seen a relationship. The other question was about the fat intake. The calories were so remarkably close, but whether the fat in itself could have had some effect, besides just straight energy, I guess possibly.

Dr. Brown: I raised the question because in the study I presented 2 days ago from Ghana, we saw no differences in the energy intake in the 3 groups that received the different micronutrient supplements, but there was a difference in the weight gain and linear growth in the group that received the 'Nutributter'. We also found a significant increase in the α-linoleic acid concentration in plasma which was directly associated with the differences in growth and explained about 50% of the differences in growth across groups. It is not the ideal study design to address this question, but I was curious if anybody else has experience in that area.

Dr. Krebs: Until we have a really important initiative involving NGOs or ministries of health, it is difficult to say whether there is a true benefit to using animal source foods, meat and flesh. The data are accumulating anyway and that is really why we need controlled trials. So much has been invested in trying to figure out appropriate supplementation and fortification programs, if an equal amount of energy went into how we can deliver meat to the population, that might actually be time well spent. I know it is the norm that there is very little meat available, but it doesn't mean that it has to be that way.

Dr. Agostoni: May I add two comments regarding fat composition. Arachidonic acid is supposed to be a growth promoter, not directly but through eicosanoid synthesis to improve the cell to cell talking. On the other hand, an association of DHA with growth has been observed, even if it is difficult to explain in terms of biologic plausibility. So in both cases we are dealing with fat quality more than quantity. As a further hypothesis on growth promotion with some supplements, we should keep in mind a possible role for branched chain amino acids, even if supplied in minimal amounts, as this could also increase the biologic value of vegetal proteins supplied together.

Dr. Fewtrell: One of the reasons mothers in the UK don't use much meat is they start complementary feed before 6 months and they find it quite difficult to puree foods into a suitable consistency. The alternative is to use jars that actually have very little meat. We don't actually have commercially available single meat products which might actually help. Liver is very unpopular among mothers in the UK, and it is a hard job to persuade them to adopt it. In developing countries where calcium intake may not be good, I wonder whether we should have any concern about giving a lot more meat and increasing calcium excretion in urine, and whether that might potentially have any downsides? It is not something that we particularly thought about before, and I guess in developed countries it is not going to be an issue, but in certain areas of the world I imagine that could be a potential problem.

Dr. Krebs: The protein calcium relationship is very complicated. In our meat study, the actual increase in protein isn't that huge an intake, it wasn't to fortify 4 g/kg/day. I would not worry about that, and in terms of what is holding up growth and what is affecting meal status and so on, it's really iron and zinc, it is not calcium. There is no evidence that in general the bone status of breastfed infants differs in formula-fed infants even though the formula-fed infants absorb a lot more calcium and so on. So to me calcium hasn't been really such a compelling issue in terms of how we think about complementary feeding. It is hard to get it from the plant-based diet and you do need to supplement them, but I don't think it is as critical. I find it hard to believe that the amount of meat these babies were eating would have affected their calcium homeostasis.

Dr. Solomons: There are a lot of fully available studies on electrolytic iron in adults [1]. Electrolytic iron is the source in infant formulas before 6 months and follow-up formulas and cereals, and children in the United States are not iron-deficient. In your study, although the difference was small and the sample size was small, there was more anemia in the meat-fed than in the cereal-fed children. Recent data on anemia rates in a national representative sample show that the United States is so very different from the rest of the world in anemia that it is bizarre to the point where we have overcorrected anemia in young children.

Dr. Krebs: That is a fair comment. It is not that we never see iron deficiency in older breastfed infants who have been on cereals, but in general, absolutely on a population basis, it seems to have done the job. In the US it is very hard to find just breastfeeders and know if it is really doing the job in breastfed infants because there are so few infants in the community who are still predominantly breastfed passed 6 months. So when you look at national data they are reflecting iron-fortified formula.

Dr. Solomons: The in vitro bioavailability of electrolytic iron has been found to be acceptable [2].

Dr. Bulusu: I liked it when you asked if we at all need non-vegetarian food or is there a need for meat. There are two issues here, as Dr. Brown mentioned one is the 4 g of meat in a Bangladesh diet. In India it is not necessarily a socioeconomic issue, it is also a cultural issue. So what would you recommend under those conditions? Secondly Dr. Agostoni mentioned that there are vegetarian bodybuilders. How do you explain that? I come from a Brahmin family. Brahmins are a specific caste that never touches meat, fish or eggs One of my professors at university used to tease me saying that I was a grass-eating lady. Once I had finished my MSC and entered the PhD program, he was still one of my professors. After several such occasions I said, 'For the last two years I have been hearing this from you, sir. We are all nutritionists in this department, can we have a real anthropometric, clinical, biochemical and intellectual study here?' So among 14 research colleagues in the laboratory, and I was the tallest among the girls and scored 81% at my MSC level and had no clinical sign of any deficiency. The only test left was biochemical; my hemoglobin was 13.8, and that too being a vegetarian, the highest, not only among my female colleagues but also among the males. So how can you explain this? To date I have never touched any non-vegetarian food.

Dr. Krebs: There are probably a number of factors here. It is obviously a real dilemma in truly vegetarian communities where it is based on religious practices. I don't want to counter that, but I think we have to recognize, as the WHO has and as you discussed in your presentation, that if you are not going to use animal source foods then you may well need a micronutrient supplement to meet those needs in that vulnerable time period. With regard to the vegetarian bodybuilder, I don't know what that person or that population was fed as young infants, but once you have passed early infancy and toddlerhood your requirements go down, and all of us in this room can do just fine on a vegetarian diet as far as the zinc requirements. So infancy and early childhood are a very vulnerable time, and this is the time in life when it is going to be a challenge to be a vegetarian. But if you are vegetarian then you would be prudent to think about supplementation, again on a population basis as you talked about in your country. The other factor is that there are so many in the world who are not vegetarian for religious purposes, including the US where we simply just don't get this message out; it is just a custom not really a specific religious practice.

Dr. Bulusu: I would just like to add that through the Micronutrient Initiative I promote supplementation and fortification, but I always believe in diversification, a balance diet.

References

1 Zimmermann MB, Winichagoon P, Gowachirapant S, et al: Comparison of the efficacy of wheat-based snacks fortified with ferrous sulfate, electrolytic iron, or hydrogen-reduced elemental iron: randomized, double-blind, controlled trial in Thai women. Am J Clin Nutr 2005;82: 1276–1282.
2 Wortley G, Leusner S, Good C, et al: Iron availability of a fortified processed wheat cereal: a comparison of fourteen iron forms using an in vitro digestion/human colonic adenocarcinoma (CaCo-2) cell model. Br J Nutr 2005;93:65–71.

Agostoni C, Brunser O (eds): Issues in Complementary Feeding.
Nestlé Nutr Workshop Ser Pediatr Program, vol 60, pp 235–250,
Nestec Ltd., Vevey/S. Karger AG, Basel, © 2007.

Functional Fermented Milk Products

O. Brunser, M. Gotteland, S. Cruchet

Institute of Nutrition and Food Technology, University of Chile, Santiago, Chile

Abstract

Fermented foods have been used since prehistoric times. Their number, variety
and geographic origin are considerable, and different substrates and agents including
bacteria, yeasts and moulds have been used in their preparation. In the last few decades
the scientific approach to the study of the participating microorganisms and the
resulting products have provided a better understanding of their biological importance. Among the many health-related properties of fermented foods, effects on blood
pressure have been described after casein hydrolysis by lactic acid bacteria. Peptides
with antimicrobial activity, mainly against Gram-negative bacteria, and derived from
casein have also been identified. This could explain, at least in part, the antidiarrheal
effects of fermented products including those on traveler's diarrhea and against colonization by *Helicobacter pylori*. One of the best known advantages of fermented milk
products is their capacity to improve lactose tolerance in hypolactasic subjects. With
the growing prevalence of allergies and inflammatory bowel diseases, considerable
interest has been focused on the effects of lactic acid bacteria in these conditions;
there is evidence that these agents are associated with improvements in allergy; no
such evidence exists for Crohn's disease or ulcerative colitis. A cholesterol-lowering
capacity has also been described for some microorganisms. Not all the fermenting
microorganisms have probiotic capacities as the latter are strain-specific.

Copyright © 2007 Nestec Ltd., Vevey/S. Karger AG, Basel

Milk and milk-derived products constitute a significant part of the diet of
all ethnic groups at all ages. Because it is difficult to preserve foodstuffs, all
cultures have resorted to fermentation as one of the procedures used to preserve foods for longer periods of time. As these are consumed routinely by
the population, children also consume them as part of their diet from weaning. Fermented products derived from milk have become predominant; some
of these, such as kefir, koumiss and shubat from goat, mare and camel milks,
respectively, contain a wide range of nonpathogenic microorganisms including bacteria, moulds and yeasts which generate complex ecosystems. The

preparation of fermented foodstuffs was initially an empirical process; however interest has increased about the participating microorganisms, the chemical reactions implicated in the fermentation process, the compounds formed and their health benefits. Improvements in systems of food preservation and the massive industrialization of food elaboration during the second part of the last century decreased the consumption of fermented foodstuffs and, consequently of live microorganisms. It is tempting to speculate that this may have resulted in changes in the human resident microbiota and may be related to the increased prevalence of allergies and chronic inflammatory and autoimmune diseases [1].

Milk Fermentation and Metabolite Production

Fermented products derived from milk result from metabolism of lactose by different bacteria. The Codex Alimentarius of 1992 defines yogurt as coagulated milk resulting from fermentation of lactose by *Lactobacillus bulgaricus* and *Streptococcus thermophilus*. Other lactic acid bacteria (LAB), such as other species of *Lactobacillus, Streptococcus* and *Bifidobacterium*, can be added to starter strains to produce fermented milks with specific textural, organoleptic or functional (in the case of probiotic strains) characteristics.

The elaboration of fermented milks results from an intense fermentation process by the LAB, sometimes in association with yeast, acetic bacteria or moulds. A permease transports lactose into the bacterial cell where the disaccharide is hydrolyzed by a β-galactosidase into glucose and galactose; the latter is exported out of the cell while glucose is phosphorylated and converted first to pyruvic acid by an aldolase and then to lactic acid by lactate dehydrogenase [2]. There is a synergistic relation between *S. thermophilus* and *L. delbrueckii* ssp. *bulgaricus* throughout the process: the former uses for its growth the amino acids and peptides produced by *L. bulgaricus* from the milk proteins while the growth of *L. bulgaricus* is stimulated by the carbon dioxide and short chain fatty acids produced by *S. thermophilus* [3]. Twenty to forty percent of the lactose in milk is transformed into lactic acid during yogurt elaboration such that in the final product the lactose concentration is 3.8–4.0 g/dl. The lactic acid concentration in yogurt ranges between 0.7 and 1.2 g/dl and the pH between 3.9 and 4.2. Bacterial lactase improves the intestinal hydrolysis of the residual lactose by hypolactasic individuals. In addition, the orocecal transit of fermented milk products is slower compared with the unfermented milk, allowing a more efficient action of both the bacterial lactase and any residual intestinal lactase. These processes explain why yogurt improves the intestinal digestion of lactose and at the same time the symptomatology in hypolactasic individuals [4].

During milk fermentation some vitamins such as pantothenic acid and vitamin B_{12} decrease while folic acid and niacin increase. Cow's milk proteins represent a complex mixture of which about 80% are caseins with four main fractions

(α_{S1}-, α_{S2}-, β- and κ-caseins) in an approximate proportion of 38:11:38:13. One to two percent of the casein is hydrolyzed by LAB proteases releasing amino acids and peptides which are metabolized by the bacteria or accumulate in the product. Milk triglycerides are not modified during fermentation due to the absence of lipases in LAB. Fermented milks also contain growth factors, hormones and immune-stimulating molecules such as peptidoglycans, polysaccharides and teichoic acid. Some bioactive peptides derived from milk protein hydrolysis modulate the immune system, inhibit pathogen growth, or exert anti-inflammatory activities [5]. Some peptides, such as the casein macropeptide, also stimulate the growth of colonic *Bifidobacterium* populations [6].

Fermentation and Production of Peptides with Hypotensive Properties

Milk protein fermentation by some LAB results in the release of tripeptides with blood pressure-lowering activities. Two of these, Isoleucyl-Prolyl-Proline (Ile-Pro-Pro) and Valyl-Prolyl-Proline (Val-Pro-Pro), isolated from casein digests by *L. helveticus*, lower blood pressure in spontaneously hypertensive rats and in humans with mild hypertension [7]. Although hypertension is considered a disease of mature and old age, the precursor conditions are often present at a young age; furthermore, hypertension secondary to a number of conditions (kidney, endocrine, neurological diseases, etc.) are frequent in childhood and it is important to consider all useful preventive and therapeutic possibilities, including those associated with the effect of LAB upon food constituents [8].

In vivo and in vitro angiotensin-converting enzyme (ACE)-inhibitory activity originating from casein fractions has been detected during milk fermentation by different LAB strains [9]. These peptides are also of low molecular weight but their activities become apparent only after further proteolysis by pepsin and by trypsin. ACE is one of the main molecules that regulate blood pressure through its effects on the synthesis of angiotensin II, a potent vaso-constrictor which, also induces the degradation of bradykinin, a powerful vasodilator. The net result is that ACE inhibition causes the lowering of the blood pressure. In a study carried out with kefir prepared from goat's milk, ACE-inhibitory peptides were detected in 16 sequences of amino acids that showed anti-hypertensive activity. Further hydrolysis of the original peptides with gastric and pancreatic enzymes resulted in new molecules with vasomotor effects [10].

In another study, middle-aged individuals with moderate hypertension received twice daily 150 ml of a milk fermented with *L. helveticus* LBK-16H for 10 weeks with 7.5 mg/100 g of Ile-Pro-Pro and 10 mg/100 g of Val-Pro-Pro. The control group received same product without the added active peptides. During a 4-week run in and in the course of a follow-up period of equal duration, patients and controls received either a product fermented by a different probiotic or the control product. There was a significant decrease in the systolic and diastolic pressures in the groups receiving the milk fermented by the *Lactobacillus* or peptides [7]. Such reductions in blood pressure are of epidemiologic significance from the point of view of public health. Although both Ile-Pro-Pro and Val-Pro-Pro have been reported to be powerful inhibitors of ACE, no changes in its activity were observed in any of these participants, suggesting that another mechanism may be operating.

Antimicrobial Activity in Fermented Foodstuffs

A number of bioactive antimicrobial polypeptides encrypted in milk proteins have been identified; these are released during fermentation and/or digestion in the gastrointestinal tract, where they are released either as propeptides or as mature C- or N-terminal peptides. The antimicrobial peptides from casein are very potent and include caseicidins, isracidins, casocidin-I, kappacin and lactoferricin [11]. They exert lytic activities on bacteria by becoming inserted in the bacterial membrane to form channels which disrupt the microorganisms, allowing the income of water and the outward diffusion of electrolytes and small molecules. These antibacterial peptides have specificity for prokaryotic membranes. Fermentation of casein by *L. acidophilus* DPC6026 produces three peptides that represent fragments of isracidin, two of them with potent activity mostly against Gram-positive but also against Gram-negative bacteria such as *Streptococcus mutans*, *Escherichia coli* O157:H7 and *Enterobacter zakazakii*. The latter has been recognized as an etiological agent for meningitis in neonates, and infant formulae have served as a reservoir. The possibility of incorporating caseicins A or B may protect against *E. zakazakii* and should increase interest in these ingredients for protective purposes [12, 13].

Fermented Foodstuffs in the Prevention and Treatment of Acute Diarrhea

Fermented milks and cheeses have been used since Biblical times for their medicinal properties, particularly in the management of gastrointestinal diseases. The origin of yogurt is unknown and it has been prepared with the milk of buffaloes, cows, donkeys, sheep, camels and goats.

Marriott and Davidson [14] postulated that acidified milks would be easier to digest by children and would prevent diarrhea. This was confirmed by in vitro studies showing that they inhibit the growth of enteropathogens. Early studies supported the idea that the administration of some bacteria exerted positive effects on bacterial diarrhea; it was suggested that this resulted from the modulation of immunity [15].

Effects on Bacterial Diarrhea

Few studies relate the administration of fermented milks to diarrhea associated with enteropathogenic bacteria. A study in the Karelian Republic showed that *L. casei rhamnosus* GG (LGG) did not shorten the duration of diarrhea in infants and children [16]. Studies on the preventive capacity of lactobacilli on diarrhea associated with enterotoxigenic *E. coli* in adults were also negative, even when high doses of LAB were administered at frequent intervals [17]. This was confirmed by other studies showing that the duration of the episodes was not shortened, although stool volumes decreased significantly.

Fermented products not derived from milk have also been evaluated for the management of diarrhea, mostly in Africa and Asia and, again, the number of studies is small. The effectiveness of a fermented maize gruel was compared with the unfermented preparation and with the WHO/UNICEF oral rehydration solution in children. No differences in stool frequency and duration of diarrhea were observed but the fermented product was better accepted [18]. Children who regularly consumed other fermented gruels had a 40% lower frequency of diarrhea during a 9-month follow-up compared to a control group. Some fermented cereals have been shown to exert antibacterial activity in vitro [19]. A study in Ghana evaluated the effect of a fermented millet product in 13-month-old children whose diarrhea had lasted 48 h; 24.4% of them were dehydrated and 90.2% had malaria, and the mean number of episodes of diarrhea in the preceding year was 2.7. Neither the enteropathogens, the LAB in the product nor their possible variations along time were characterized [20]. The product improved neither the cure rate nor the duration of the episodes compared with the heat-inactivated control; furthermore, many patients were receiving antibiotics and anti-malarial drugs concomitantly and it is not known to what extent this affected the results.

In Chile, 82 weaned infants less than 12 months of age received an acidified milk with *L. helveticus* and *S. thermophilus* for 6 months; the control group received a comparable, nonfermented milk. Patients were contacted twice weekly for detection of diarrhea. The acidified product exerted a preventive effect on the incidence of diarrhea, the number of days during which the children were affected and the duration of the episodes. No differences were observed in the enteropathogens detected [21] (table 1).

Effects on Viral Diarrhea

Different species and strains of *Lactobacillus* have been evaluated for their capacity to modify viral diarrhea; LGG has been the most extensively tested, especially in rotavirus infection in children. When administered with a fermented milk, a shorter duration of the disease was observed (table 2) [22]. A recent study in children from day care centers who received *L. reuteri* or *Bifidobacterium lactis* Bb12 revealed lower numbers of episodes of fever of shorter duration when *L. reuteri* was administered [23]. This suggests that there is specificity in these effects, and is in agreement with earlier results

Table 1. Incidence of episodes of acute diarrhea in relation to age in children who received an acidified formula or a control non-acidified formula

Age months	Acidified formula				Control formula		
	children/ month	episodes of diarrhea	incidence		children/ month	episodes of diarrhea	inci-dence
3–5	7				18	3	16.7
6–8	81	8	9.9	$\chi^2 = 7.1235$ $p < 0.005$			
9–11	150	19	12.6	$\chi^2 = 7.6726$ $p < 0.005$	159	41	25.8
12–15	165	12	7.3	$\chi^2 = 15.085$ $p < 0.005$	329	71	21.6
Total	403	39	9.7	$Z = 3.517$ $p < 0.001$	586	137	23.3

From Brunser et al. [21].

Table 2. Effect of *Lactobacillus casei rhamnosus* GG (LGG) on the recovery from acute diarrhea in infants and preschool children (mean ± SD)

Group	Duration of diarrhea, days	
(1) Fermented milk with LGG	1.4 ± 0.8	
		1 vs. 3 and 2 vs. 3:
(2) Freeze-dried LGG	1.4 ± 0.8	$F = 8.70; p < 0.001$
(3) Pasteurized yogurt	2.4 ± 1.1	

The study was carried out on 71 well-nourished children 4–45 months of age; 82% of the cases were associated with rotavirus. The amounts of LGG provided were: 10^{10-11} CFU in 125 g of fermented milk twice daily; freeze-dried LGG 10^{10-11} CFU once daily; pasteurized preparation 125 g twice daily.
Modified from Isolauri et al. [22].

obtained in Finland comparing the effect of LGG, or a combination of *S. thermophilus* and *L. delbruekii* in children with diarrhea. LGG significantly shortened the duration of diarrhea. The number of immunoglobulin- secreting cells stimulated by these bacteria was comparable, but during convalescence LGG was associated with enhanced numbers of IgA specific antibody-secreting cells and higher levels of serum IgA antibodies to rotavirus [24].

In addition to the specific mechanisms activated by LAB as part of the defensive responses against pathogens, other benefits probably relate to the activation of innate immunity, the modulation of the resident colonic microbiota, the stimulation of mucus secretion, and protection of the gastrointestinal barrier function [15, 25].

Table 3. Serum cholesterol changes in individuals randomly allocated to receive a fermented milk (FM) containing *Lactobacillus acidophilus* L1 (L1 FM) of human origin or *Lactobacillus acidophilus* ATCC 43211 (ATCC)

Group	Number	Baseline average	Week 2	Week 2 minus baseline	% change
1st study					
L1 FM	14	6.27 ± 0.19	6.06 ± 0.17	−0.21 ± 0.08	3.2 ± 1.2
ATCC FM	15	6.38 ± 0.23	6.30 ± 0.23	−0.08 ± 0.09	1.2 ± 1.4
2nd study					
L1 FM	21	6.53 ± 0.17	6.27 ± 0.18	−0.26 ± 0.10	3.8 ± 1.7
Placebo	19	6.30 ± 0.14	6.40 ± 0.13	−0.10 ± 0.10	1.9 ± 1.6
Combined					
L1 FM	35	6.42 ± 0.13	6.18 ± 0.13	−0.24 ± 0.07	−3.6 ± 1.2
P vs. baseline			0.0015		
P vs. placebo					0.008
ANOVA					0.03

Placebo = Fermented milk without active bacteria. Values are expressed as mmol/l (means ± SEM).
Modified from Anderson and Gilliland [45].

Fermented Foods and *H. pylori* Colonization

H. pylori is a highly prevalent bacterial agent that colonizes the human gastric mucosa; it is considered as an etiological factor for gastroduodenal ulcers and a risk factor for gastric cancer. In developing countries the colonization begins early in life and affects a high proportion of the pediatric population; most individuals remain asymptomatic. Antibiotic treatments have a high cost and are not 100% effective because of resistance and difficulties with patient compliance due to gastrointestinal intolerance. Furthermore, children are rapidly recolonized after treatment. Products containing LAB or probiotics have been proposed to manage *H. pylori* colonization in at-risk populations. A multicenter, prospective, randomized, double-blind, controlled study was carried out in symptomatic *H. pylori*-positive children to compare 7 days of treatment with antibiotics and omeprazole with the same regime supplemented with a fermented milk containing *L. casei* DN-114 001 for 14 days [26]. The fermented product significantly increased the eradication rate from 57.5 to 84.6% (p = 0.0045). In another study, 65 children received the 7-day standard triple therapy supplemented with 250 ml of a commercial yogurt containing *B. animalis* and *L. casei*, or milk during 3 months. No differences in the rate of eradication were observed between the groups [27]. Cruchet et al. [28] used a commercial product containing either *L. johnsonii* La1 or *L. paracasei* ST11 or the respective heat-inactivated controls in 326 asymptomatic *H. pylori*-positive children during 4 weeks. No eradication was observed but a significant decrease in the values of the ^{13}C-urea breath test (^{13}C-UBT) was detected only in children receiving live La1. The decrease in the UBT values induced by La1 correlated directly with the basal values before treatment [28]. In another study, a yogurt containing *L. gasseri* OLL 2716 (LG21) was administered daily to 12 children colonized with *H. pylori* for 8 weeks. The ^{13}C-UBT and the serum levels of pepsinogen I and II were measured after 4 and 10 weeks; while no differences in ^{13}C-UBT values at 4 and 10 weeks were observed, the pepsinogen I/II ratio at 4 weeks was significantly higher, suggesting a decrease in *H. pylori*-associated gastric mucosal inflammation [29]. These results suggest that fermented milk products and probiotics may be used to maintain low densities of *H. pylori* in colonized subjects.

Such protective effects may be due to the inhibition of *H. pylori* growth through the release by some LAB strains of bacteriocins or of organic acids, and to the decrease in the adhesion of the pathogen to gastric epithelial cells. In addition, probiotics and fermented milk products may stabilize the gastric barrier function, decrease mucosal inflammation, and stimulate healing; the antioxidant and anti-inflammatory properties of LAB may also participate.

Gluten Digestion by Microorganisms in the Management of Celiac Disease

The celiac patients should remain on a strict gluten-free diet for life; however, this is complicated and many abandon this diet. Another problem with the gluten-free diet is that wheat flour and gluten are used to thicken, increase the consistency, palatability and 'mouth' of a considerable number of foodstuffs and culinary preparations. The possibility of using microorganisms to neutralize the pathogenic capacity of gluten and gliadin for celiac patients is currently being explored in many laboratories. The rationale of this is that some LAB, yeasts and molds express proteases which should hydrolyze the deleterious peptide sequences in gluten. The resulting products should be harmless for the patients and acceptable from the culinary point of view [30]. There have been a few preliminary assays in celiac patients but the results have not been clear-cut due to methodological problems.

Fermentation of Carbohydrates: Solving the Problem of Lactose Maldigestion and Intolerance

Congenital deficiency of lactase activity is exceptional. Lactose malabsorption may develop after damage to the intestinal mucosa by pathogens or, more frequently, due to the genetically programmed disappearance of lactase activity in adolescents and adults. Hypolactasic individuals may experience symptoms when the disaccharide load is high enough (lactose intolerance). The symptoms are bloating, flatulence, cramping pain and liquid stools, sometimes expelled explosively. Affected individuals learn instinctively how much lactose and lactose-containing products they can tolerate. The relationship between the amount of lactose and the magnitude of the symptoms is not lineal as there is considerable variation in the responses to the same dose.

Because many LAB have lactase activity and survive their passage through the gastrointestinal tract, their intake improves the symptoms of intolerance and the efficiency of lactose digestion. Their β-galactosidase is released into the intestinal lumen by the bile salts and remains functional. *L. acidophilus* and *L. delbrueckii* ssp *bulgaricus*, the species most frequently used for production of yogurts and fermented milk products, have high levels of lactase activity [7]. Some probiotics have low lactase activity and do not contribute significantly to lactose digestion.

Lactose fermentation by LAB results in the production and absorption of D(−)-lactate; as the human body lacks a D(−)-lactate dehydrogenase, the question arises as to whether this may cause acidosis when feeding yogurt and fermented products to infants. Studies carried out in Santiago on 6-month-old infants demonstrated that this does not occur [31], a finding corroborated elsewhere [32].

Probiotics and Fermented Foods for Control of Inflammatory Bowel Disease

It has been postulated that ulcerative colitis and Crohn's disease are associated with alterations in the resident colonic microbiota and in the responses this elicits from the local and systemic immunity. Considerable interest has been awakened about the effects of probiotics and LAB on their severity, remission and relapse-free interval. A preliminary study in Crohn's disease by Guandalini [33] showed that it was possible to taper corticosteroids. This has been contradicted by subsequent randomized, controlled studies [34]. The question whether LAB or probiotics exert beneficial effects remains so far unanswered.

Fermented Milk and Probiotics in the Management of Allergy

Atopic diseases such as eczema, allergic rhinitis and asthma are chronic allergic disorders whose prevalence has increased considerably during the past 20 years. According to the hygiene hypothesis, there is an inverse association between infections early in life and atopy. The higher frequency of allergies may be related to changes in food consumption patterns, industrial treatments resulting in the disappearance of naturally occurring LAB, alterations in the intestinal microbiota and decreases in intestinal infections. It is estimated that food allergies affect 3.5% of adults and 8–10% of children; the allergens most frequently involved are egg, peanut, milk, fish, nuts, shellfish, wheat, kiwi and mustard.

Various studies have shown a relationship between allergic conditions and the composition of the gut microbiota. The fecal counts of bifidobacteria in allergic infants, particularly those with atopic eczema, are significantly lower than in healthy peers [35]. *Clostridium, Bacteroides* and *Staphylococcus* may also be altered and their numbers may correlate with the IgE serum levels. The colonic population of *Bifidobacterium* of allergic infants shows higher counts of *B. adolescentis* and *B. longum* and lower counts of *B. bifidum*, in contrast to their healthy peers [36]; such a microbiota is associated with the synthesis of TNF-α and IL-12 by macrophage-like cells in vitro [37]. The gut microbiota participates in the establishment of immune oral tolerance by reorienting the Th2 responder phenotype of newborns towards the Th1 cell-mediated immune response and through the secretion of TGF-β and IgA. The microbiota also participates in the regulation of the gut barrier, which blocks the transfer of food antigens and microorganisms across the epithelium, processes which are implicated in the altered immune responses of atopic children.

It has been proposed that fermented food products containing LAB could modulate the homeostasis of the gut microbiota and decrease the risk and symptoms of allergy. Randomized, double-blind, placebo-controlled clinical trials have evaluated whether probiotic intake alleviates atopic eczema in children. LGG, and sometimes *Bifidobacterium* Bb12, decrease SCORAD as well as the fecal α_1-antitrypsin and TNF-α, plasmatic sCD4 and the eosinophil protein X in urine [38]. A decrease in atopic eczema in infants from atopic families was observed when mothers were given LGG prepartum and during lactation (23 vs. 46% in the probiotic and placebo groups, respectively) [39]; TGF-β_2 levels were increased in their milk [40]. The protective effect persisted until 4 years of age [41]. In atopic dermatitis, the daily administration of LGG for 4 weeks decreased SCORAD in those children with high IgE levels [42]. on the contrary, no improvement in SCORAD and inflammatory parameters was observed in infants less than 5 months of age receiving a hydrolyzed, whey-based formula alone or supplemented with LGG or with *L. rhamnosus* for 3 months [43].

Effect of Fermented Foodstuffs on Blood Lipids

The effect of fermented foodstuffs and LAB on lipid metabolism, especially the triglyceride and cholesterol blood levels, has aroused considerable interest. Studies in the Massai of Kenya reported decreases of up to 18% in blood cholesterol, but with the daily intake of large volumes of fermented milk and consequent weight gain. In other studies, fermented milk products have shown cholesterol-lowering effects, especially for total cholesterol and LDL-cholesterol, with some of these even inducing modest increases of HDL-cholesterol in healthy and in moderately hypercholesterolemic adults. Similar effects have also been observed with fermented soy products [44]. These could be due to the incorporation of cholesterol by the bacteria, synthesis of conjugated linoleic acid, deconjugation of bile salts, production of propionic acid which inhibits the expression of hepatic enzymes implicated in the de novo synthesis of lipids [45]. These studies have been conducted in adults, and little is known about the possible responses of children and the long-term repercussions later in life.

In summary, fermented foods have a long history as components of the human diet; the recent application of modern research methodologies is demonstrating that LAB and their products participate in a variety of metabolic processes that are beneficial for health.

References

1 Bach JF: Infections and autoimmune diseases. Autoimmunity 2005;25(suppl):74–80.
2 Marshall V, Cole WM: Threonine aldolase and alcohol dehydrogenase activities in *Lactobacillus bulgaricus* and *Lactobacillus acidophilus* and their contribution to flavour production in fermented milk. J Dairy Res 1983;50:375–379.
3 Torriani S, Vescovo M, Dicks LMT: *Streptococcus thermophilus* and *Lactobacillus delbrueckii* subsp. *bulgaricus*: a review. Ann Microbiol Enzimol 1997;47:29–52.
4 Shermak MA, Saavedra JM, Jackson TL, et al: Effect of yogurt on symptoms and kinetics of hydrogen production in lactose-malabsorbing children. Am J Clin Nutr 1995;62:1003–1006.
5 Menard S, Candalh C, Bambou JC, et al: Lactic acid bacteria secrete metabolites retaining anti-inflammatory properties after intestinal transport. Gut 2004;53:821–828.
6 Etzel MR: Manufacture and use of dairy protein fractions. J Nutr 2004;134:996S–1002S.
7 Seppo L, Korojoki O, Suomalainen T, Korpela R: The effect of a *Lactobacillus helveticus* LBK-16H fermented milk on hypertension – a pilot study in humans. Milk Sci Int 2002;57: 124–127.
8 Jones JE, Jose PA: Hypertension in young children and neonates. Curr Hypertens Rep 2005;7:454–460.
9 Gobbetti M, Ferranti P, Smacchi E, et al: Production of angiotensin-I-converting-enzyme inhibitory peptides in fermented milks started by *Lactobacillus delbrueckii* subsp. *bulgaricus* SS1 and *Lactococcus lactis* subsp. *cremoris* FT4. Appl Environment Microbiol 2000;66: 3898–3904.
10 Quirós A, Hernández-Ledesma B, Ramos M, et al: Angiotensin-converting enzyme inhibitory activity of peptides derived from caprine kefir. J Dairy Sci 2005;88:3480–3487.
11 Malkoski M, Dashper SG, O'Brien-Simpson NM, et al: Kappacin, a novel antibacterial peptide from bovine milk. Antimicrob Agents Chemother 2001;45:2309–2315.
12 Nazarowec-White M, Farber JM: Thermal resistance of *Enterobacter zakazakii* in reconstituted dried infant formula. Lett Appl Microbiol 1997;24:9–13.
13 Hayes M, Ross RP, Fitzgerald GF, et al: Casein-derived antimicrobial peptides generated by *Lactobacillus acidophilus* DPC6026. Appl Environment Microbiol 2006;72:2260–2264.
14 Marriott WMK, Davidson IT: Acidified whole milk as routine infant feed. JAMA 1923;81: 2007–2010.
15 Perdigón G, Nader de Macias ME, Alvarez S, et al: Immunopotentiating activity of lactic bacteria administered by oral route. Favorable effect in infantile diarrheas (in Spanish). Medicina (B. Aires) 1986;46:751–754.
16 Shornikova AV, Isolauri E, Burkanova L, et al: A trial in the Karelian Republic of oral rehydration and *Lactobacillus* GG for treatment of diarrhea. Acta Paediatr 1997;86:460–465.

17 Clements ML, Levine MM, Ristaino PA, et al: Exogenous lactobacilli fed to man – their fate and ability to prevent diarrheal disease. Prog Food Nutr Sci 1983;7:29–37.
18 Yartey J, Nkrumah H, Hori H, et al: Clinical trial of fermented maize-based oral rehydration solution in the management of acute diarrhea in children. Ann Trop Paediatr 1995;15:61–68.
19 Willumsen JF, Darling JC, Kitundu JA, et al: Dietary management of acute diarrhoea in children: effect of fermented and amylase-digested weaning foods on intestinal permeability. J Pediatr Gastroenterol Nutr 1997;24:235–241.
20 Lei T, Friis H, Fleischer Michaelsen K: Spontaneously fermented millet product as a natural probiotic treatment for diarrhoea in young children: an intervention study in Northern Ghana. Int J Food Microbiol 2006;110:246–253.
21 Brunser O, Araya M, Espinoza J, et al: Effect of an acidified milk on diarrhoea and the carrier state in infants of low socio-economic stratum. Acta Paediatr Scand 1989;78:259–264.
22 Isolauri E, Juntunen M, Rautanen T, et al: A human *Lactobacillus* strain (*Lactobacillus casei* sp strain GG) promotes recovery from acute diarrhea in children. Pediatrics 1991;88:90–97.
23 Weizman Z, Asli G, Alsheikh A: Effect of a probiotic infant formula on infections in child care centers: comparison of two probiotic agents. Pediatrics 2005;115:5–9.
24 Majamaa H, Isolauri E, Saxelin M, Vesikari T: Lactic acid bacteria in the treatment of acute rotavirus gastroenteritis. J Pediatr Gastroenterol Nutr 1995;20:333–338.
25 Dai D, Walker WA: Protective nutrients and bacterial colonization in the immature gut. Adv Pediatr 1999;46:353–382.
26 Sykora J, Valeckova K, Amlerova J, et al: Effects of a specially designed fermented milk product containing probiotic *Lactobacillus casei* DN-114 001 and the eradication of *H. pylori* in children: a prospective randomized double-blind study. J Clin Gastroenterol 2005;39: 692–698.
27 Goldman CG, Barrado DA, Balcarce N, et al: Effect of a probiotic food as an adjuvant to triple therapy for eradication of *Helicobacter pylori* infection in children. Nutrition 2006;22: 984–988.
28 Cruchet S, Obregón MC, Salazar G, et al: Effect of the ingestion of a dietary product containing *Lactobacillus johnsonii* La1 on *Helicobacter pylori* colonization in children. Nutrition 2003;19:716–721.
29 Shimizu T, Haruna H, Hisada K, Yamashiro Y: Effects of *Lactobacillus gasseri* OLL 2716 (LG21) on *Helicobacter pylori* infection in children. J Antimicrob Chemother 2002;50: 617–618.
30 De Angelis M, Rizzello CG, Fasano A, et al: VSL#3 probiotic preparation has the capacity to hydrolyze gliadin polypeptides responsible for celiac sprue. Biochim Biophys Acta 2006;1762: 80–93.
31 Brunser O, Haschke-Becher M, Gotteland M, et al: Urinary excretion of D(−)-lactic acid after intake of a milk formula that contains pre- or probiotics (abstract 27). Proc Latin Am Soc Pediatr Res, Ushuaia, Argentina, 2000.
32 Connolly E, Abrahamsson Th, Björkstén B: Safety of D(−)-lactic acid producing bacteria in the human infant. J Pediatr Gastroenterol Nutr 2005;41:489–492.
33 Guandalini S: Use of *Lactobacillus* GG in paediatric Crohn's disease. Dig Liver Dis 2002;34 (suppl 2):S63–S65.
34 Bousvaros A, Guandalini S, Baldassano RN, et al: A randomized, double blind trial of *Lactobacillus* GG versus placebo in addition to standard therapy in children with Crohn's disease. Inflamm Bowel Dis 2005;11:833–839.
35 Sepp E, Julge K, Mikelsaar M, Bjorksten B: Intestinal microbiota and immunoglobulin E responses in 5-year-old Estonian children. Clin Exp Allergy 2005;35:1141–1146.
36 He F, Ouwehand AC, Isolauri E, et al: Comparison of mucosal adhesion and species identification of bifidobacteria isolated from healthy and allergic infants. FEMS Immunol Med Microbiol 2001;30:43–47.
37 He F, Morita H, Ouwehand AC, et al: Stimulation of the secretion of pro-inflammatory cytokines by *Bifidobacterium* strains. Microbiol Immunol 2002;46:781–785.
38 Isolauri E, Arvola T, Sutas Y, et al: Probiotics in the management of atopic eczema. Clin Exp Allergy 2000;30:1604–1610.
39 Kalliomaki M, Salminen S, Arvilommi H, et al: Probiotics in primary prevention of atopic disease: a randomized placebo-controlled trial. Lancet 2001;357:1076–1079.

40 Rautava S, Kalliomaki M, Isolauri E: Probiotics during pregnancy and breast-feeding might confer immunomodulatory protection against atopic disease in the infant. J Allergy Clin Immunol 2002;109:119–121.

41 Kalliomaki M, Salminen S, Poussa T, et al: Probiotics and prevention of atopic disease: 4-year follow-up of a randomized placebo-controlled trial. Lancet 2003;361:1869–1871.

42 Viljanen M, Kuitunen M, Haahtela T, et al: Probiotic effects on faecal inflammatory markers and on faecal IgA in food allergic atopic eczema/dermatitis syndrome infants. Pediatr Allergy Immunol 2005;16:65–71.

43 Brouwer ML, Wolt-Plompen SA, Dubois AE, et al: No effects of probiotics on atopic dermatitis in infancy: a randomized placebo-controlled trial. Clin Exp Allergy 2006;36:899–906.

44 Anderson JW, Gilliland SE: Effect of fermented milk (yogurt) containing *Lactobacillus acidophilus* L1 on serum cholesterol in hypercholesterolemic humans. J Am Coll Nutr 1999;18: 43–50.

45 Heber D, Yip I, Ashley JM, et al: Cholesterol-lowering effects of a proprietary Chinese red-yeast-rice dietary supplement. Am J Clin Nutr 1999;69:231–266.

Discussion

Dr. Ribeiro: I just want to return to a comment that was made during the discussion about probiotics in diarrhea. With all respect to the data of Isolauri and Guandalini, our experience definitely does not confirm what has been stressed. But the point is when we really look for severe dehydrating diarrhea, in the methodological design we all include really dehydrated patients with less than 3 days of diarrhea, meaning that we have a very uniform group with an average of 3–6 ml/kg/h of stool output, and we use strong variables to control the study. At least in our common vulnerable population, we don't see the effect of LGG or several other probiotics. We are still not convinced that probiotics could be useful in the treatment, not the prevention, of acute diarrhea in settings like here in Brazil or countries where the conditions are similar.

Dr. Brunser: That is a good point. If you are dealing mostly with diarrhea of bacterial origin probably the effect of probiotics will not be as evident. However, there are studies showing that the addition of probiotics to oral rehydration solutions results in better outcomes. With regard to viral diarrhea we have little personal experience but the situation in Finland is different, of course, from the situation here in Brazil. I would like to make a comment on the Finnish studies; they used a special formula which is whey predominant and with partially hydrolyzed protein to which LGG are added. I wonder what effect this substrate has because in general people just add a probiotic to regular milk or a regular formula.

Dr. Barclay: I would just like to come back to the very interesting results you showed on the effect of certain peptides on blood pressure. The Dietary Approach to Stop Hypertension (DASH) [1] studies in the United States in hypertensive adults showed that increased dairy product intake and also fruit and vegetable intakes resulted in a remarkable lowering of blood pressure. One hypothesis from the DASH studies is that it could be the ratio of dietary calcium, magnesium and potassium versus sodium that could be having an effect on blood pressure. I am just wondering whether there are any data in children on this; whether dietary intake in this period could have an effect on blood pressure in adult life?

Dr. Brunser: Not as far as I know, but pediatric nephrologists regularly check blood pressure in the children. There are studies in the Afro-American population which show that about 25% of the children, when they are 12–15 years old, are mildly hypertensive. The intake of milk is also associated with lower systolic blood pressure levels in adults.

247

Dr. Silveira: I would like your opinion on the relation between the process of fermentation and celiac disease.

Dr. Brunser: There are a few studies on the effect of gluten fermentation by different combinations of bacteria to destroy or reduce the epitopes that damage the mucosa in celiac disease. The general idea is that through fermentation you decrease the complexity of the gluten, and you probably decrease the number and concentration of intact epitopes; I wonder if it can be reduced to zero because that is what is needed. There are no studies that have tested these results in celiac patients. I also think that it is an ethical problem. One study was done in Italy in which they incubated ex vivo biopsies of intestinal mucosa with hydrolysates of gluten, and the authors stated that there was no increase in the infiltration of the lamina propria or outflows of cytokines from the biopsies. The Italian study produced pasta with this fermented gluten, and it tastes good and it could be positive for the patients; however, in celiac disease there should probably be no gluten in the diet whatsoever.

Dr. Uy: I have two questions. In your opinion is there any deleterious effect from an excess intake of probiotics? As the probiotics, the bacteria, are not made equally, they have different effects. Can all the identified bacteria be incorporated in a capsule and then one capsule taken per day?

Dr. Brunser: As more and more probiotics in yogurt products are being consumed in the Western world, there have been increases in the reports of individuals having bacteremia due to some kind of *Lactobacillus*, a few of these apparently originated from the food that was ingested. But there are cases of people who ingest enormous amounts of yogurt and nothing has happened: individuals with AIDS eat yogurt and they are advised to eat yogurt for its effects in stabilizing the resident microbiota of the gastrointestinal tract, and there are apparently no deleterious effects in these patients. So the conclusion is that yes, they are safe, if anything can be absolutely safe in this world. As for the combinations, that is an interesting field because you may combine different capacities, for example for the stimulation of the immune system and to obtain better results, but it requires very careful clinical evaluation.

Dr. Fisberg: In many countries and many societies there is a common habit of introducing yogurts and fermented dairy products very early. In the last years pediatric societies are trying to postpone the introduction of these products until probably 1 year of age. What is your opinion on this?

Dr. Brunser: If you eat yogurt you provide a load of $D(-)$-lactic acid and lactic acid in general. With Dr. Haschke-Becher we showed that the amount of $D(-)$-lactate excreted in 12-hour collections of urine is not excessive. Recently Connolly et al. [2] measured the blood concentration of $D(-)$-lactic acid in children eating yogurt and again levels were normal. Giving or not giving fermented products depends on many things, many of which escape us pediatricians. In Chile, mothers give yogurt without asking their pediatrician. On the other hand if you take into account the potential positive effects, it is difficult to say no. Then again, when children don't like milk, yogurt becomes a good source of proteins and minerals. So there is no straight answer to that.

Dr. Solomons: The overlap is that the starter cultures for yogurts are lactic acid bacteria and that fermented milk products, yogurt and acidified milks, are fed as complementary food. It would be nice to have a review of that experience. But what confuses me is that we tend to conflate discussion of the simple fermented products with probiotics – which don't ferment. I have always had a problem with the co-discussion of fermented milk products and lactic acid bacteria, that we are interested in being probiotics, and the fact that sometimes we combine the two, one is a vehicle and the other is a probiotic.

Dr. Brunser: Fermented milks and yogurt are produced by specific starters. You may add probiotics to those fermented products and yogurt. Some probiotics are able to ferment lactose, but most are not. So you have a baseline product which is the fermented milk and you add a strain of bacteria, or whatever, that has specific functional capacities, and this is the whole problem: to distinguish what is produced by the basic product and what by the probiotics. We are beginning to understand that these bacteria are more complex and more plastic in their capacities to adapt to the environment and to acquire new genes by mechanisms such as conjugation and to synthesize all kinds of molecules. Let's not forget that, for example, antibiotics originated initially from the activity of bacteria, and that desferoxamine, used to combat iron poisoning, is the product of a bacterium. We have used bacteria for many years, sometimes in empirical ways. We are beginning to understand bacteria as very complex organisms whose synthetic capabilities we are harnessing for our purposes.

Dr. Solomons: I would assert that the benefits historically ascribed to fermented yogurts and fermented and acidified milks have nothing to do with what is currently the molecular biology of probiotics. If they did, it would be very casual and coincidental – not systemic. On the other hand, the fermented byproducts have a potential danger for the consumption of fermented milks that has never really been raised, and that is the bacterial metabolism in lactose. The simple sugar, galactose which persists in the system along with lactic acid, can represent a danger. As 'free' galactose in the circulation, this sugar damages the lens of the eye. Normally, an epimerase enzyme in the liver immediately converts absorbed galactose to glucose. But the enzyme is inhibited by alcohol in very low concentrations. So that by having alcohol and a fermented beverage at the same time, one can get very high levels of galactose in the blood which accumulate in the lens of the eye, as in a galactosemic child. There are all sorts of drinks which are combined milk or fermented milk and alcohol (White Russian, Sombrero, etc.). By drinking several of those in an evening, you can get blind drunk because over time it will lead to an accumulation of galactose. Thus a combination of two kinds of fermentation has the potential for adverse consequences.

Dr. Brunser: Your point is very interesting. When you introduce galactose in the small intestine, it will be absorbed very efficiently by Sglut1. Now there are fermented products that naturally contain alcohol, for example kumiss and kefir contain alcohol. I haven't seen any reports on individuals from areas where they consume kumiss or kefir exhibiting signs of excessive alcohol intake. I don't think the amount of ethanol is that big.

Dr. Agostoni: I go back to my own experience regarding Dr. Solomons' fundamental question. This has been largely debated over the last 3 years within the Committee on Nutrition of ESPGHAN. Just to make clear there are 3 different types of products: formula with probiotics; formula with prebiotics, and fermented formulas without live bacteria. These are 3 totally different conceptual products, and there are trials investigating their effects. In my opinion, the black hole of the literature is represented by the role of yogurt, a simple fermented milk product in the first part of the complementary feeding period.

Dr. Brunser: I think in the use of fermented milk and yogurts and similar products in infants and children, there is the problem of empirism. If we want to transform empirism into scientifically proven truth, carefully planned clinical observations will have to be made over time. Humankind has carried out empirical observations for centuries in very large numbers of individuals to validate some ideas, and in this way a large body of knowledge about foodstuffs and their properties has been acquired. I am sure people have been giving all kinds of fermented milks and other products to their children for hundreds or thousands of years and they probably never observed any effects that they considered deleterious. What we want now is to have a statistical analysis for every variable to assure that it is scientifically valid.

Dr. Fisberg: Certainly one of the empirical situations that we have is based on allergy, especially because pediatricians appear to give these products based on allergy. The data that we have show that there are no allergies with these kinds of products.

Dr. Michaelsen: It is just a comment on fermented cereal products. When we talk about complementary feeding in developing countries, fermented cereal products might or might not have probiotic effects. Apart from that, there are some very interesting benefits: they have very good food safety; a low pH and with a low pH minerals are better absorbed; there is also a decrease in phytate content and thereby a better absorption, and because of the decrease in phytate and fiber there is better energy density. So there are a lot of good reasons to try to promote fermented cereal foods, especially in developing countries.

References

1 Appel LJ, Moore TJ, Obarzanek E, et al: A clinical trial of the effects of dietary patterns on blood pressure. DASH Collaborative Research Group. N Engl J Med 1997;336:1117–1124.
2 Connolly E, Abrahamsson T, Bjorksten B: Safety of D(−)-lactic acid producing bacteria in the human infant. J Pediatr Gastroenterol Nutr 2005;41:489–492.

Agostoni C, Brunser O (eds): Issues in Complementary Feeding.
Nestlé Nutr Workshop Ser Pediatr Program, vol 60, pp 251–258,
Nestec Ltd., Vevey/S. Karger AG, Basel, © 2007.

Concluding Remarks

The focus of this workshop was 'Issues in Complementary Feeding', and the meeting opened with the generally agreed assertion that complementary feeding should be started around 6 months of life. However there are a number of important exceptions, for instance in the prevention or amelioration of the symptoms of celiac disease, as emphasized further on. There is a growing body of evidence supporting the rationale for anticipating the administration of gluten-containing food. It is also important to keep in mind that this advice about awaiting the administration of a complementary food must be issued on an individualized basis, because it depends on very personalized circumstances.

A second relevant point is that complementary feeding should not interfere with breastfeeding. It is known from previous observations that adding fats (especially oils) as a source of energy for breastfed infants during complementary feeding displaces the same amount of energy intake from human milk. In consequence, emphasis should be placed on solid foods that are true complements and not supplements, and that, if used as supplements, they should not replace the central role of human milk in infant nutrition. With respect to quality from a microbiological standpoint, complementary feeding should be appropriate. Concerning its nutritional characteristics, complementary feeding should provide adequate amounts of energy with satisfactory density so as to fulfill the requirements of growing infants.

There is an emerging body of evidence about the susceptibility of infants to the effects of early nutritional influences and insults – generally encompassed in the programming hypothesis. There are considerable experimental data but, unfortunately, they are rather limited in the case of humans. Present knowledge indicates that rapid growth during a critical window of sensitivity may program metabolic processes and pathways in ways that may be detrimental to later health, and this programming may even influence the appearance of some types of endocrine disorders and malignancies in mature or old age. However, those who have to manage the nutrition of low birth weight infants must be aware of the fact that their first duty is to supply adequate amounts of nutrients to enhance their possibilities of survival. Theoretical considerations about the possible consequences of early life programming should not represent a hindrance that could limit nutrient intake aiming at fast growth. It is known that during the first weeks and months of life, particularly for those infants born after 23–24 to 30 weeks of gestation, the risks of mortality are high, energy and protein requirements are high, and growth and neurodevelopment are tightly associated. Therefore, considerations about increased risks of later obesity, diabetes mellitus and hypertension should be considered as secondary to the need to assure the survival and development of these infants.

The role of breastfeeding and its protective effects compared to formula feeding at later ages were emphasized in this workshop. The advantages of breast milk are important in different areas and this was underlined during the discussions. There is accumulating and convincing evidence that breast-feeding during the first months of life is associated later in life with a lower risk of obesity, lower levels of arterial blood pressure and blood cholesterol. This latter aspect is important considering that breastfed babies have higher blood cholesterol levels, probably as a result of the high cholesterol levels in breast milk. In all probability this represents an example of programming in which the lipid metabolism of infants becomes conditioned early in life to handle the large amounts of cholesterol supplied initially by their maternal milk diet. The better cognitive development of young infants has recently been associated with the level of maternal intellectual capacity, but it is not known whether this is the result of the particular composition of the milk of mothers from a better socioeconomic strata, or due to the fact that mothers with higher education levels are better adapted to satisfy their infants' requirements, including not only nutrition but also psychomotor stimulation. As discussed later in this workshop, breastfeeding is also negatively associated with the risk of autoimmune disorders such as type 1 diabetes and immune diseases including Crohn's disease and even celiac disease. During the discussions it was stressed that epidemiological studies on the long-term effects of breastfeeding should be interpreted carefully, paying special attention to sample sizes, and considering that, in general, larger populations are better suited to adjustments for major confounders. The value of human milk was also emphasized not only on a quantitative basis but also from a qualitative standpoint, particularly for the feeding of special groups of infants such as preterm babies and those with inborn errors of metabolism. From an evolutionary perspective, these abnormal genes may be surviving in the human population due to the tempering effects breastfeeding and human milk may have on the consequences of their metabolic derangements.

Besides successful breastfeeding, the availability of safe weaning foods represents a key point for successful weaning programs, particularly in developing countries where the various partners have to be taken into consideration and the traditions of the population respected while trying to improve the quality of complementary feeding. Particularly in rural settings, it may be advantageous to improve the quality of traditional complementary foodstuffs through a holistic approach that includes educating women, particularly mothers, and the creation of effective networks incorporating all participants in the healthcare system, contacting families at their homes, and establishing systems for the control of food quality, preservation, and safety, and taking into account the economical constraints of poor families. Networks such as the one outlined could represent a key to improve the quality of complementary feeding in developing and transition countries. As long as a baby is breastfed, in all probability he/she will never become underfed, but after 6 months appropriate complementary feeding that does not displace human milk should be initiated, otherwise the risk of malnutrition increases considerably. It is worth underlining that commercial complementary foods in those countries may carry potential contaminants if production quality control systems are deficient. Fortunately it is now possible to rely on efficient quality control in the production chain, in which specialized professionals anticipate emerging problems by means of constant sampling and testing and early warning systems along all steps of the food preparation process from 'Mother Earth' to the final product and its final consumer. Finally, efficient coordination systems should be established between national and international regulatory bodies, food processing industries and consumer groups, taking into consideration the rapid development of a new 'industrial food production science' whose purpose is to improve the quality of the products offered to the population.

In addition to dangerous bacterial contaminants from the surrounding milieu, the human body, especially the colon, harbors 'good' bacteria. The way in which the body acquires this complex bacterial population is intriguing because there is accumulating evidence that this is not a process that occurs at random. The gut of newborns, which is initially sterile, is ready for colonization because its epithelial lining presents receptors for certain bacterial species and strains that gain access to the lumen. The potential risks associated with altered colonization processes start during delivery: the vaginal route is associated with a different colonization (normal?) pattern compared with that resulting from birth by cesarean section. The elucidation of the short- and long-term consequences of both birth mechanisms vis à vis the establishment of the resident microbiota is important because of the increasing rates of cesarean sections, and the potential risk of delayed colonization with the bacteria that are considered beneficial. Breastfed infants also receive bacteria through maternal milk. The origin of bacteria is still a matter of debate but they probably reside in the galactophores. Considered as a whole, the mechanism of delivery and the first feedings interact to create in the infant gut the ecological system and the microbiota that will remain with him for the rest of his life. Within this context, molecular biology currently represents a revolution for microbiology as it makes possible the identification of hitherto unknown bacterial species and strains through the analysis of their genes. This is generating more information on the complexity of these systems than was ever available, especially about the enormous number and variety of the microflora and the fact that beneficial, neutral and plainly potentially dangerous bacteria coexist sharing space and receptors, with the former normally controlling the latter. Beneficial bacteria (*Bifidobacteria*, *Lactobacilli*, and probably *Ruminococci*) generally displace the unfavorable bacteroides and clostridia from the human gut during breastfeeding. In the coming years many more species and strains are going to be identified and this will provide more information about the influence of this huge microbiota on health and disease, including obesity, tumorigenesis, etc.

Clearly, food safety has to be associated with satisfactory nutrient quality and availability and this combination represents the real challenge of complementary feeding in the developing world. Food fortification is an effective way of achieving this goal and could be an acceptable way to implement the changes required by disadvantaged population groups. There are many ways in which food fortification can be provided: incorporated directly into local staples or processed foods, or added by parents or caregivers as sprinkles or spreads. One of the basic aspects of any supplementation program is that the target population should accept the supplements being provided. This is achieved by providing information about its effects, by respecting the beliefs and taboos of the population, and by consulting the opinion leaders before the process of fortification is started. One of the important aspects that should be taken into consideration is that the population should not feel that they are the recipients of 'food for the poor'. In this respect there is experience from many parts of the world about resounding successes and failures when these aspects have not been taken into consideration. This holistic approach, taking all aspects of a sound fortification program into consideration, is required for the optimization of resources and to improve knowledge about the healthcare and nutrition of the population. Every fortification program should be evaluated at defined intervals, or when special circumstances arise, to quantify the cost-benefit ratios and to evaluate the opinions of its beneficiaries. Within this context, it is interesting to keep in mind that a wide variety of foodstuffs, including cereals, are possible targets for supplementary programs.

In relation to cereal fortification programs in developing countries, it was emphasized that fortification/supplementation activities must have reasonable costs and attain levels and coverage that are truly effective if the nutritional problems they are focused on are to be solved. Cereals are useful vehicles for fortification/supplementation programs as it is possible to use them as vehicles for functional components such as prebiotics, probiotics, nucleotides and combinations of vitamins and micronutrients that enhance their nutritional value. A number of easily detected and quantifiable parameters must be applied for the periodic evaluation of the results. It is also important to understand and take into account the magnitude of the difficulties that may be encountered in expanding from the pilot level to massive distribution programs. Stability, palatability and adequate vehicles are also factors that must be taken into consideration. Furthermore, it is important to keep in mind that if the infants who receive the supplement/fortification are being breastfed, the results of the program may not be as obvious and this may explain why some studies show no apparent effects.

For maximal effect, micronutrients and functional components have to be provided together with adequate levels of dietary protein and energy. The efficiency of the supplements may be decreased by microbiological contamination of the environment (including food and drinking water) that may impair, sometimes to a considerable extent, the efficiency of nutrient absorption and utilization, including that of the supplements/fortifiers. Other points to be considered include the possibility of interactions and synergies between nutrients and the need not only for short-term but also for long-term assessments to appreciate the quality of the results attained. In planning the dosages of supplements to be administered it is important to keep in mind that these have to take into account the possibility that genetic polymorphisms may be the cause of unexpected results, including a lack of response or untoward reactions.

Providing complementary feeding to children with pathologies must address their particular requirements. The complementary food category most commonly introduced early in life is cereals; this occurs later in breast-fed than in formula-fed infants. There is little evidence supporting the choice of the age at which this should be done or the types of cereals that should be used for this purpose. It is now agreed that introducing solid foods before the 4th month of life is detrimental to the infant and there continues to be some discussion as to the age at which solid foods, including those containing gluten, should be introduced. Introducing cereals after 7 months of age results in an increased risk for the appearance of islet cell immunity and insulin-dependent diabetes mellitus compared with introduction at 4–6 months. If the cereals are introduced while the infant is being breastfed, the risk of 'celiac disease autoimmunity' decreases. A protective role for breast-feeding in celiac disease has been ascertained by studies in Scandinavia and the United States. According to these studies, gluten introduction should occur between 4 and 6 months of age for infants at risk of this disease, and while they are still on breast milk. This may lessen the severity of their symptoms or delay the age when the disease will become clinically manifest. Gluten should be provided initially in small amounts as large amounts probably increase the severity of the symptoms. As celiac disease has a strong genetic component, it is advisable to perform measurements of antibodies, anti-tissue transglutaminase and anti-endomysium in those infants in whose families there are antecedents of this disease. The possibility of using oats in the diet of celiac patients is now accepted, although an occasional case may present adverse effects.

In relation to the repercussions of allergic disease on the nutritional status of infants and the role of complementary feeding, it was agreed that in many cases poor growth may result from extreme dietary restrictions and, as a result, this may be considered an iatrogenic effect. This stresses the need for proper evaluation of the relationship between allergic symptoms and the consumption of complementary foods. On the other hand, it is important to keep in mind that the mainstay of the dietary management of food allergy is avoidance of the offending antigens in the diet. Another point that was emphasized is the possibility that infants may be allergic to more than one antigen and that the inflammatory reaction caused by such a situation amplifies the negative nutritional effects of food allergy and restricts the possibilities of achieving adequate nutrition. Unfortunately, elimination diets that exclude potential allergens do not prevent the appearance of allergy to other foods or of other manifestations of allergies and for this reason novel approaches are necessary, such as protocols that aim at inducing tolerance to proven allergens or to potential allergens. It is also important to understand that the diet normally provides components that may play a role in the modulation of allergy, such as polyunsaturated fatty acids, antioxidants and micronutrients that in allergic infants may stimulate the development and normal responses of their immune system. An active approach should include the administration of probiotics that modulate the innate immune system and the immunoregulatory pathways. Developments in this field may reach a point in which it will become possible to demonstrate that positive prevention through the use of dietary components, including special strains of probiotic microorganisms, may have advantages over passive elimination diets.

In many parts of the world, in low-income societies, infants become malnourished very early in life, even if they are still being breastfed, because the complementary foods available for them after 6 months of age may not satisfy their requirements for some nutrients, particularly energy. Among the causes that explain the appearance of malnutrition in these infants are hereditary and congenital abnormalities, underlying chronic infections, lack of adequate foods, low birth size and, finally, adaptive poor growth as a result of intrauterine growth restrictions. Each of these etiologies requires specific forms of intervention and, in addition, the management of each infant should be as individualized as possible, keeping in mind that growth too slow or too fast is undesirable, and that the late repercussions of nutritional rehabilitation that is too accelerated, such as obesity and type 2 diabetes mellitus, should be prevented as much as possible. It is important to keep in mind that the foremost consideration in treating malnutrition is the survival of the infant. In the extreme situations that many infants face in the less developed world, it is important to make them gain weight rapidly to decrease the risks associated with malnutrition: high mortality rates from increased susceptibility to infection, and the possibility of intellectual impairment.

The participants concluded that unmodified cow's milk (UCM) cannot be considered as a complementary food and, furthermore, that it may exert negative effects which manifest themselves on iron nutrition and renal function. The effects of UCM on iron nutrition stem from its low iron content, and from the fact that if not subjected to thermal treatment, it induces blood loss through the feces in about 40% of infants. The cause of this blood loss remains unknown and it decreases with age and disappears by 1 year of age.

The magnitude of the fecal blood loss is such that it may contribute importantly to iron deficiency anemia at a stage when iron stores are low. Iron absorption is also decreased by UCM due to its high casein and calcium contents that inhibit the intestinal transport of the iron provided by other foods. UCM also generates a high solute load for the immature kidneys of infants, derived from its high protein and electrolyte content. This load has to be excreted and requires additional water which, if not provided, and especially in the presence of warm weather and/or acute diarrhea and vomiting, may result in hypernatremic dehydration which carries a high risk of brain damage and death in infants. As for the reasons that children are fed UCM, these are mostly traditional, as milk in all its forms (full-fat, half-skimmed and skimmed) is considered a source of high quality nutrients. Feeding skimmed milk to young infants has the additional inconveniences of its low energy content, its even higher renal solute loads, and higher concentration of lactose. Another cause of concern is that high renal solute loads are considered as one of the factors that condition the appearance of hypertension later in life. It is now recommended in most countries that UCM should not be introduced before 9 months of age and preferably after 12 months of age.

In addition to the concerns about iron nutrition, preoccupation also exists about the fat composition of UCM, with its high percentages of saturated fatty acids, rather low and variable amounts of linoleic (LA) and linolenic (ALA) acids, although the LA/ALA ratio is favorable. These characteristics make the fat of UCM very different from that of human milk and from modern formulae. There is little evidence that the fat in UCM may have undesirable effects on fat metabolism in adult life, including adiposity. The intake of UCM should not exceed 500 ml/day, with the remaining nutrients provided by a varied diet.

The intake of high amounts of protein in cow's milk has been linked to the genesis of obesity through the stimulation of IGF-1 secretion, which increases cell multiplication and accelerates bone maturation. Although this aspect has been discussed at length, this matter has not been entirely settled and, furthermore, it has been shown that individuals who regularly drink milk are on average taller than non-consumers and may have lower systolic blood pressure.

The value of meat in the nutrition of infants is based on the high quality of its proteins, its content of iron, zinc, and other important trace elements which complement those of cereals and other plant-based foods. The viscera also represent useful sources of nutrients, although in the case of the liver, its fat and cholesterol content is high. Cellular animal protein sources are also good sources of energy, taking their fat content into account. When the feed provided to animals contains polyunsaturated fatty acids, these are incorporated into the meat, the eggs, the milk and the viscera. The high protein content of foods of animal origin may have implications for metabolic conditions resulting in a propensity to obesity later in life. The need for studies that will evaluate both the efficacy and the effectiveness of foods of animal origin in complementary feeding is clearly apparent.

Concluding Remarks

Fermentation is a useful tool for the preservation of a variety of foodstuffs. Fermented foods have been used for millennia to feed children since the first months of life. This type of food is useful in the management of lactose intolerance, highly prevalent in many areas of the world and which limits milk consumption by adults. Until recently the lactic acid bacteria (LAB) were chosen on an empirical basis, but they are now being investigated for a number of beneficial properties. In addition to the management of lactose intolerance, these include the treatment and prevention of infantile and traveler's diarrhea, the production of bioactive peptides with antibiotic, and blood pressure- and cholesterol-lowering effects. Fermented foods have been shown to play a role in the prevention or the amelioration of allergy. Fermented foods, such as the milk of different mammalian species, cereals, vegetables, fruits, and honey, are still consumed in many parts of the world, although the microbiota responsible for the fermentation processes remain unknown. LAB are not synonymous with probiotics, as there are LAB which are not probiotics, and probiotics that are neither LAB nor bacteria. The study of fermenting microorganisms and their effects is a rapidly expanding field that is benefiting from the application of techniques borrowed from molecular biology, classical microbiology, gastrointestinal physiology, immunology, nutrition and metabolism, and clinical studies. In all probability, this expansion of knowledge will result in a better understanding of the interrelations between human beings, their nutrition, their resident microbiota, and the environment.

C. Agostoni, O. Brunser

Subject Index

Subject Index